CRC Press
Taylor & Francis Group
6000 Broken Sound Parkway NW, Suite 300
Boca Raton, FL 33487-2742

ISBN-13: 978-0-805-89612-1 (pbk)

DOI: 10.4324/9780203764800

Visit the Taylor & Francis Web site at
http://www.taylorandfrancis.com

Williams Syndrome: 15 Years of Psychological Research

Carolyn B. Mervis
University of Louisville

Williams syndrome is a rare genetic disorder caused by a microdeletion of about 20 genes on chromosome 7q11.23. The importance of this syndrome for theories and models of cognition became apparent about 15 years ago, when Bellugi, Sabo, and Vaid (1988) argued that Williams syndrome was a paradigm case of the independence of language from cognition. In particular, it was argued that individuals with Williams syndrome have "intact" language despite severe mental retardation. More recent findings indicate a more complex relation between language and characteristics associated with this syndrome. The articles in this special issue form 3 overlapping clusters: articles concerned with language development relative to cognitive development, articles concerned with other aspects of cognition, and articles concerned with interpersonal relations and personality. Together, these articles provide strong evidence of the importance of the study of neurodevelopmental genetic disorders for enhancing understanding of the complex manner in which initial genetic differences impact both behavior and processing strategies from infancy through adulthood. Our hope is that this issue will motivate further studies, informed by the genetic–developmental approach, on both Williams syndrome and other neurodevelopmental genetic disorders.

Williams syndrome is a rare developmental disorder associated with mild to moderate mental retardation or (less frequently) learning disabilities. Fifteen years ago, the cause of Williams syndrome was unknown; it had not yet been determined even that the syndrome had a genetic basis. Diagnosis was extremely difficult; many geneticists had never knowingly seen a case of Williams syndrome. Nevertheless, a single chapter published in 1988 (Bellugi, Sabo, & Vaid, 1988), along with conference presentations and reports of conference presentations of this study and its sequels, eventually motivated an increasingly large group of behavioral researchers to devote considerable resources to studying individuals who have Williams syndrome. The

Requests for reprints should be sent to Carolyn B. Mervis, Department of Psychological and Brain Sciences, University of Louisville, Louisville, KY 40292. E-mail: cbmervis@louisville.edu

initial findings of Bellugi et al. (1988) attracted the attention of the National Institutes of Health as well, leading to a conference in 1991 and a Request for Applications by the National Institute for Neurological Disorders and Stroke (NINDS) for proposals on Williams syndrome soon thereafter. Why all this attention to such a rare and difficult-to-diagnose syndrome? What was the message of the 1988 paper and related conference presentations and reports of conference presentations?

The message was this: Williams syndrome represents a clear dissociation between intact language abilities and severe cognitive deficits. Put another way, Williams syndrome provides a strong demonstration of the independence of language (or a language module) from cognition (or a cognitive module). Thus, Williams syndrome became a rallying ground for researchers whose theoretical perspective was consistent with a modular organization of intelligence. At the same time, researchers who took the opposite perspective—that specific aspects of language and cognition were closely linked—were highly motivated to investigate the syndrome that was claimed to provide conclusive evidence that this approach was incorrect. Thus, with this message, Bellugi et al. (1988) catapulted Williams syndrome into the consciousness of researchers interested in the relation (or lack thereof) between language and cognition. It fair to say that without Bellugi's research, none of the primary authors of the articles in this issue would have started a research program on Williams syndrome.

I first was exposed to Bellugi's Williams syndrome research during an invited address on language acquisition by Elizabeth Bates to the International Society for Infancy Studies in 1990 (Bates, 1990). Bates (1990) included a report of Bellugi's initial position that individuals with Williams syndrome had intact language abilities in the face of "profound" mental retardation, thus providing impressive evidence for the independence of language from cognition. The specific finding that Bates cited in support of this position was that adolescents with Williams syndrome produce and comprehend complex grammatical constructions such as reversible passives, conditionals, and tag sentences, yet are unable to conserve quantity or number. Previously, an argument had been made by Piagetian researchers (e.g., Beilin, 1975) that understanding of reversible passives required concrete operational ability, in particular reversible thought as exemplified by success on conservation tasks (Bellugi et al., 1988).[1] The Williams syndrome data clearly contradicted that position.

[1]Ironically, even before Bellugi first made this argument, Maratsos, Kuczaj, Fox, and Chalkey (1979) had shown that typically developing children were able to comprehend and produce reversible passives well in advance of attaining the Piagetian construct of reversibility as exemplified by conservation, thus indicating that there is no link between acquisition of reversible passives and conservation even for typically developing children. More recently, Brooks and Tomasello (1999) found that almost half of the young 3-year-olds in their study were able to produce passive constructions using novel verbs following one or two brief training sessions, providing further evidence that typically developing English-speaking children acquire passives well before they are able to conserve. Studies of the acquisition of non-Indo-European languages in which passive constructions are common have shown that 2-year-olds spontaneously produce reversible passive constructions (Allen & Crago, 1996). For a summary of research on acquisition of passives by young preschoolers, see Guasti (2002).

Bellugi's relatively focused comparison of the ability to comprehend and produce reversible passives despite an inability to conserve was soon forgotten (or never known) by most researchers. Her more general claim, however, that language was intact despite severe mental retardation became the rallying point for researchers and theorists who took a modularity approach. The comparisons cited became those between "intact" language in contrast to severe mental retardation, and between severely disordered drawings composed of isolated and typically unidentifiable parts strewn randomly around the page in contrast to rich linguistic descriptions of the characteristics of the creature or object that had been drawn, using complex grammar and unusual vocabulary. For example, Pinker (1991) argued that Williams syndrome "is one of several kinds of dissociation in which language is preserved despite severe cognitive impairments" (p. 534). Jackendoff (1994) noted that although people with Williams syndrome almost always have mental retardation, "Their language, though, is if anything more fluent and advanced than that of their age-mates" (p. 117). These positions have found their way into textbooks as well. For example, in *Advanced Psychology for Teachers*, Sharpes (1999) presented a "case study" of a teenager who has Williams syndrome as follows:

> [This individual] has a facility with language few possess and can easily recognize faces. So why does this same teenage boy score only 49 on a standard IQ test; struggle with arithmetic; and read, write, and draw poorly? Because he has Williams Syndrome… (p. 210)

In the 15 years since the publication of Bellugi's initial report, multiple studies across the United States, Europe, and Asia have confirmed her finding that the language abilities of people with Williams syndrome are more advanced than their visuospatial constructive abilities such as drawing or pattern construction/block design (e.g., Jarrold, Baddeley, & Hewes, 1998; Mervis et al., 2000; Mervis, Morris, Bertrand, & Robinson, 1999; Pezzini, Vicari, Volterra, Milani, & Ossella, 1999; Udwin & Yule, 1991). Furthermore, more recent research has confirmed Bellugi's finding that the syntactic abilities of individuals with Williams syndrome are more advanced than those of individuals with Down syndrome matched for chronological age (CA) and IQ (Mervis, Robinson, Thomas, Becerra, & Klein-Tasman, in press) and shown that this pattern extends to comparisons with younger children with specific language impairment matched for mean length of utterance (Rice, 1999). However, comparisons to individuals with Down syndrome or specific language impairment are not really relevant to claims of "intact" language abilities; these groups are known to have specific difficulties with regard to expressive language, especially syntax. Evaluation of the claim of "intact" language abilities requires comparisons to typically developing children of the same CA. Even before Bellugi's first study was published, two research groups had published reports indicating that language acquisition in Williams syndrome was not nearly as advanced as would be expected for CA (Kataria, Goldstein, & Kushnick, 1984; Meyerson & Frank, 1987). Thus, language was clearly not intact. The less extreme position of a dramatic dissociation of language abilities from other cognitive abilities also has not fared well. Udwin and Yule (1990) and Gosch, Städing, and Pankau (1994) found that the syntactic abilities of children with Williams syndrome were at the same level as those of children with other developmental disabilities matched for CA and IQ. Similarly, Volterra, Capirci, Pezzini, Sabbadini, and Vicari (1996) found that syntactic abilities of children with Williams syndrome were at the same level as those of younger typically developing children matched for mental age (MA). Furthermore, in languages with more complex morphology, the morphological abilities of individuals with Williams syndrome have been found to be significantly less advanced than those of MA-matched typically developing children (for French, see Karmiloff-Smith et al., 1997; for Italian, see Volterra et al., 1996).

As these findings have emerged, studies of individuals with Williams syndrome have become more sophisticated. Whereas adult-onset right hemisphere (parietal) brain damage had been taken initially as an appropriate model for Williams syndrome (e.g., Bellugi, Wang, & Jernigan, 1994), much of the recent research has started from the premise that Williams syndrome is a developmental disorder and thus the most appropriate models are developmental ones (e.g., Bertrand, Mervis, & Eisenberg, 1997). For example, the parts-scattered-around-the-page drawings produced by many children and adolescents with Williams syndrome initially were compared to those produced by persons with adult-onset right hemisphere damage. In contrast, Bertrand et al. (1997) demonstrated that these types of drawings in fact are part of the normal developmental sequence of learning to draw; such drawings are produced by many young typically developing preschoolers. Global claims for linguistic superiority have largely been replaced by research programs addressing the question of whether the process of language acquisition is similar for children with Williams syndrome and typically developing children, and what these similarities and differences tell us about Williams syndrome in particular and pathways to (processes of) language acquisition more generally (e.g., Mervis & Bertrand, 1997). Similarly, global claims for extreme weakness in visuospatial construction abilities are being replaced by research programs addressing questions parallel to those now being addressed for language (e.g., Bertrand et al., 1997; Hoffman, Landau, & Pagani, in press).

The articles in this special issue form three overlapping clusters: articles concerned with language development, articles concerned with other aspects of cognition, and articles concerned with interpersonal relations and personality. The articles in the language cluster focus on three different languages—English, Italian, and Hebrew—and on language acquisition by individuals at several different points on the CA continuum: preschoolers, school-age children, and adolescents. A recurring theme among several of these articles is the importance of auditory short-term memory for language acquisition by individuals with Williams syndrome.

In the first article, Robinson, Mervis, and Robinson (this issue) consider the relation among receptive grammatical ability, receptive vocabulary ability, and three measures of auditory short-term memory ability for English-speaking children with Williams syndrome and typically developing children matched for receptive grammar ability. Relations between memory ability and grammatical ability differed for the two groups: Whereas forward digit span (a measure of auditory rote memory), backward digit span (a measure of working memory), and nonword repetition (a measure of phonological memory) were all significantly related to grammatical ability for children with Williams syndrome, none of the memory variables was significantly related to grammatical ability for the typically developing contrast group. The relation between backward digit span and grammatical ability was significantly stronger for the children with Williams syndrome than the typically developing children. These findings, along with others, lead Robinson et al. to consider the possibility that children with Williams syndrome are more dependent than typically developing children on working memory and phonological memory to acquire language in general and grammar in particular.

Volterra, Caselli, Capirci, Tonucci, and Vicari (this issue) consider the language abilities of younger Italian-speaking children with Williams syndrome relative to children with Down syndrome matched for CA and expressive vocabulary size and younger typically developing children matched for expressive vocabulary size. They assessed expressive vocabulary using a parental report measure (the Italian version of the MacArthur Communicative Development Inventories; Fenson et al., 1993). The children with Williams syndrome had similar grammatical abilities to the typically developing children whether measured by parental report or a sentence repetition task. The grammatical abilities of the children with Williams syndrome were significantly greater than those of the children with Down syndrome when measured by sentence repetition. Furthermore, grammatical ability was strongly correlated with sentence repetition ability across all three groups, suggesting an important role for verbal memory in early grammatical ability regardless of developmental etiology.

Levy and Hermon (this issue), in a study of Hebrew-speaking adolescents with Williams syndrome in comparison to two groups of typically developing children—one matched to the bottom of the MA range for the Williams syndrome participants and one matched to the top of the MA range—revisit the question of the morphological abilities of individuals with Williams syndrome. The authors argue that the best measure of the "intactness" of morphosyntactic ability in Williams syndrome involves morphemes that are strictly formal (i.e., that do not introduce meaning modulations). Hebrew, a language with very rich morphology, offers an excellent opportunity for this type of study. Based on their findings, Levy and Hermon conclude that performance on even strictly formal aspects of morphology is at or below MA level, confirming that grammatical ability of individuals with Williams syndrome is not selectively preserved.

The ability to comprehend nonliteral language lies at the intersection of language and theory of mind. This aspect of language is crucial for successful social interaction, especially with peers. Sullivan, Winner, and Tager-Flusberg (this issue), in their study of the ability to differentiate lies from ironic jokes, present one of the first examinations of the nonliteral language comprehension abilities of individuals with Williams syndrome. They find that despite the strong interest in social interaction and the relatively good literal language skills evidenced by individuals with Williams syndrome, none of the adolescent participants with Williams syndrome was able to tell the difference between lies and ironic jokes. For the most part, both the lies and the ironic jokes were treated as lies. Furthermore, fewer than half of the participants with Williams syndrome were able to solve second-order theory of mind problems. The participants with Williams syndrome were significantly more likely to justify their interpretation of the joke statements based on a literal interpretation (rather than based on the mental states of the story characters) than were the two contrast groups (CA-, IQ-, and vocabulary-matched individuals with Prader–Willi syndrome or nonspecific mental retardation). Consistent with a developmental approach, the performance of the Williams syndrome participants was similar to that of much younger typically developing children and contrasted with those of adults with adult-onset right hemisphere brain damage.

Landau and Zukowski's article (this issue) bridges research on language acquisition and visuospatial cognition in an examination of the verbal descriptions of videotaped motion events by children with Williams syndrome, MA-matched typically developing children, and adults of normal intelligence. Results showed that the children with Williams syndrome had substantial control over the key linguistic components of motion events, indicating that the visuospatial problems associated with Williams syndrome have relatively little impact on spatial language. The authors raise the possibility that visuospatial short-term memory difficulties may play an important role in the one component of spatial language that was somewhat difficult for children with Williams syndrome, linguistic encoding of the path of motion.

Atkinson et al. (this issue) consider visuospatial cognition and executive function abilities of children with Williams syndrome. In a systematic series of studies, these authors demonstrate that performance is better on visuospatial tasks tapping the ventral stream than those tapping the dorsal stream. However, performance even on the dorsal stream tasks was consistent with a developmental model. On executive function tasks, performance was better on a verbal task than on tasks requiring spatially directed responses, which tap frontal–parietal processing. Atkinson et al. also stress the large individual differences found among children with Williams syndrome: In contrast to the great difficulty that many children with Williams syndrome evidenced on the dorsal tasks, some children with Williams syndrome performed at CA levels even on these tasks.

Farran and Jarrold (this issue) provide a review of prior studies of the visuospatial abilities of individuals with Williams syndrome. They begin with a much-needed discussion of methodological issues. Based on their review, they conclude that contrary to expectations based on a right-hemisphere brain damage model, individuals with Williams syndrome are able to process visuospatial information at both the local and the global levels. However, they argue, performance on constructional tasks is likely to reflect a local processing bias because individuals with Williams syndrome have difficulty using global information in these situations. (Note that a "local processing bias" on visuospatial construction tasks is actually part of the normal developmental sequence, as evidenced by Bertrand et al.'s [1997] drawing findings discussed earlier and the production of broken configurations by young children on block design tasks [Kramer, Kaplan, Share, & Huckeba, 1999].)

Don, Schellenberg, Reber, DiGirolamo, and Wang (this issue) provide the first examination of implicit learning abilities of individuals with Williams syndrome. Implicit learning has been hypothesized to play an important role in the acquisition of language, social, and motor skills and to be relatively independent of CA and IQ (e.g., Reber, 1992). Don et al. (this issue) compared the performance of a group of children and adults with Williams syndrome to a CA-matched group of typically developing individuals on two implicit learning measures: an artificial grammar task and a rotor-pursuit task. As expected, performance was not related to CA. However, contrary to hypothesis, the Williams syndrome group performed substantially and significantly below the contrast group on both implicit learning measures. Once performance on either a nonverbal reasoning measure or a verbal working memory measure was partialled out, the difference in performance among the groups was eliminated, suggesting that performance was broadly consistent with MA. The authors argue, based on effect sizes, that although implicit learning clearly is affected by IQ, the impact of IQ on implicit learning may be less than the impact on vocabulary or verbal working memory.

In the final article concerned with language and other cognitive abilities, Karmiloff-Smith, Brown, Grice, and Paterson (this issue) provide a strong argument that Williams syndrome should not be used to support claims of innately specified independent modules. They review studies showing that not only are language and face processing not "intact" in Williams syndrome, the relatively good abilities that individuals with Williams syndrome have in these areas are at least in part based on different processing strategies than those used by individuals in the general population. Furthermore, they argue, the use of different strategies should not be surprising, given the qualitative differences between the brains of individuals who have Williams syndrome and individuals who are developing typically.

The final section of this special issue is concerned with interpersonal relations and personality. Early case studies of individuals with Williams syndrome almost always included comments on the individuals' personality characteristics, typically mentioning a combination of extreme sociability (including lack of stranger anxiety) and anxiety. However, until now there have been few empirical studies on these topics. In the first article in this section, Mervis and her colleagues (this issue) consider the attentional patterns of infants and toddlers with Williams syndrome during triadic interactions. Findings from the studies reported in this article indicate that not only do very young children with Williams syndrome spend more time looking at other people than do either typically developing children or children with other genetic syndromes, the quality of the gazes of the participants with Williams syndrome when looking at strangers is highly unusual, typically described as "it seems as if her eyes are boring into her partner." The authors argue that these attention patterns presage the temperament and personality characteristics shown by older children with Williams syndrome, in particular the extreme interest in and orientation toward other people. Furthermore, these looking patterns are argued likely to be the result of the hemizygous deletion of one or more genes in the Williams syndrome region, leading to alterations in the typical cascades and gene–gene and gene–environment transactions involved in shaping the developing brain.

Klein-Tasman and Mervis (this issue) address the question of whether there is a consistent quantifiable personality profile for individuals with Williams syndrome. Their study focused on 8-, 9-, and 10-year-olds and compared children with Williams syndrome to CA- and IQ-matched children with other developmental disabilities. Personality profiles with very high sensitivity and high specificity were identified for both of the personality/temperament measures used. These profiles, which were focused on eagerness to interact with others, empathy, sensitivity, and tension, also had high face validity. The measures chosen allow for extension to both older and younger age groups, so that the age course of personality development in Williams syndrome may be determined. The importance of a quantifiable personality profile for genotype/phenotype research on personality characteristics in Williams syndrome is discussed, and at the same time the importance of gene–gene and gene–environment transactions in personality development is stressed.

Dykens (this issue) considers the question of whether Williams syndrome is associated with increased levels of anxiety and fears. Her first two studies compared parental and child reports of fears of a large group of individuals with Williams syndrome across a broad age range (6–48 years) to reports regarding a comparison group of individuals with other forms of developmental disabilities. The Williams syndrome group was found to be significantly more fearful than the comparison group for a wide variety of types of fears, based both on parental and self-report. In a third study, Dykens used a clinical interview measure to determine the extent to which individuals with Williams syndrome met clinical criteria for phobia or other anxiety disorders. More than one third of the participants received a clinical diagnosis of Specific Phobia, and about 18% were diagnosed with Overanxious Disorder (Generalized Anxiety Disorder). These rates are much higher than those for either the general population or other forms of mental retardation. Dykens argues that these highly elevated rates of phobia and overanxiety are likely associated with genetic aspects of Williams syndrome in interaction with life experience and with other aspects of the Williams syndrome personality such as increased social sensitivity.

In summary, the articles in this special issue take a very different approach from that of Bellugi's ground-breaking research (e.g., Bellugi et al., 1988; Bellugi et al., 1994). No longer is Williams syndrome considered to be the paradigm example of an intact language module in the face of a severely impaired cognitive module (Levy & Hermon, this issue). No longer is the adult right-hemisphere brain damage model considered the most appropriate one for Williams syndrome (Farran & Jarrold, this issue; Sullivan et al., this issue). Instead, many of the studies reported in this volume take a genetic–developmental[2] approach. In this approach, the fact that Williams syndrome (a hemizygous microdeletion encompassing at least 17 genes [Osborne et al., 2001]) is present from the time of conception is taken as evidence that the brain may well develop in different ways than in typical development. As a result, even when individuals with Williams syndrome are matched to typically developing individuals for level of performance, these similar levels of performance may be attained through differential emphasis on particular processes (e.g., increased importance of auditory memory for acquisition of grammar [Robinson et al., this issue], increased use of verbal

---

[2]I refer to this approach as "genetic–developmental" to differentiate it from the "developmental" approach initially proposed by Zigler (1969) for individuals with mental retardation due to cultural–familial factors. This approach was developed to contrast with the "difference" approach, according to which individuals with mental retardation differed fundamentally from individuals with average intelligence in specific and fundamental ways beyond simply intellectual slowness (e.g., behavioral rigidity, short-term memory deficits, verbal mediation deficits, attentional deficits). According to the developmental approach, individuals with mental retardation acquire new abilities within a domain in the same sequence as children who are developing typically (similar sequence hypothesis) and do not show particular areas of strength or weakness relative to MA-matched children of average intelligence (similar structure hypothesis). Cicchetti and Pogge-Hesse (1982) argued that the similar-sequence hypothesis is applicable to individuals with mental retardation due to organic (including genetic) causes as well. The similar structure hypothesis, however, does not generally apply to individuals with mental retardation due to organic causes. (See Hodapp, Burack, and Zigler [1998] and Mervis [2001] for brief histories of psychological/educational approaches to mental retardation.) The question of whether children with a particular genetic syndrome might use or emphasize different processes from children who are developing typically to achieve similar levels of ability in a particular domain has not been addressed within the developmental approach. The similar sequence hypothesis is compatible with both the developmental approach and the genetic–developmental approach.

mediation in visuospatial and frontal reasoning tasks [Atkinson et al., this issue], and different event-related potential waveforms and increased reliance on featural processing for face processing [Karmiloff-Smith et al., this issue]). The genetic–developmental approach is explicitly taken by each of the articles addressing interpersonal relations and personality. In these articles, the importance of gene–gene and gene–environment transactions and cascades for the unusual looking patterns shown by infants and toddlers with Williams syndrome in triadic interactions (Mervis et al., this issue), the emerging personality constellation of extreme interest in other people, overfriendliness, and high levels of empathy accompanied by social anxiety (Klein-Tasman & Mervis, this issue), and the unusually large proportion of individuals with Williams syndrome who meet clinical diagnostic criteria for specific phobia or generalized anxiety disorder (Dykens, this issue) are stressed.

The articles in this volume provide strong evidence of the importance of the study of individuals with neurodevelopmental genetic disorders for enhancing our understanding of the complex manner in which initial genetic differences impact on both behavior (performance) and processing strategies from infancy through adulthood. Much work remains to be done, not only from a psychological or a biological perspective, but most importantly from an integrated psychological–biological perspective. Our hope is that the articles in this issue will motivate future studies informed by the genetic–developmental approach both to Williams syndrome and to other neurodevelopmental genetic disorders.

ACKNOWLEDGMENTS

Preparation of this manuscript was supported by Grant No. HD29957 from the National Institute of Child Health and Human Development and by Grant No. NS35102 from the NINDS.

REFERENCES

Allen, S. E., & Crago, M. B. (1996). Early passive acquisition in Inuktitut. *Journal of Child Language, 23,* 129–155.

Atkinson, J., Braddick, O., Anker, S., Curran, W., Andrew, R., Wattam-Ball, J., et al. (2003/this issue). Neurobiological models of visuospatial cognition in children with Williams syndrome: Measures of dorsal-stream and frontal function. *Developmental Neuropsychology, 23,* 141–174.

Bates, E. (1990, April). *Early language development: How things come together and how they come apart.* Paper presented at the International Conference on Infant Studies, Montreal, Quebec.

Beilin, H. (1975). *Studies in the cognitive basis of language development.* New York: Academic.

Bellugi, U., Sabo, H., & Vaid, J. (1988). Dissociation between language and cognitive functions in Williams syndrome. In D. Bishop & K. Mogford (Eds.), *Language development in exceptional circumstances* (pp. 177–189). London: Churchill-Livingstone.

Bellugi, U., Wang, P. P., & Jernigan, T. L. (1994). Williams syndrome: An unusual neuropsychological profile. In S. Broman & J. Grafman (Eds.), *Atypical cognitive deficits in developmental disorders: Implications for brain function* (pp. 23–56). Hillsdale, NJ: Lawrence Erlbaum Associates, Inc.

Bertrand, J., Mervis, C. B., & Eisenberg, J. D. (1997). Drawing by children with Williams syndrome: A developmental perspective. *Developmental Neuropsychology, 13,* 41–67.

Brooks, P. J., & Tomasello, M. (1999). Young children learn to produce passives with nonce verbs. *Developmental Psychology, 35,* 29–44.

Cicchetti, D., & Pogge-Hesse, P. (1982). Possible contributions of the study of organically retarded persons to developmental theory. In E. Zigler & D. Balla (Eds.), *Mental retardation: The developmental–difference controversy* (pp. 277–318). Hillsdale, NJ: Lawrence Erlbaum Associates, Inc.

Don, A. J., Schellenberg, E. G., Reber, A. S., DiGirolamo, K. M., & Wang, P. P. (2003/this issue). Implicit learning in children and adults with Williams syndrome. *Developmental Neuropsychology, 23,* 203–227.

Dykens, E. M. (2003/this issue). Anxiety, fears, and phobias in persons with Williams syndrome. *Developmental Neuropsychology, 23,* 293–318.

Farran, E. K., & Jarrold, C. (2003/this issue). Visuospatial cognition in Williams syndrome: Reviewing and accounting for the strengths and weaknesses in performance. *Developmental Neuropsychology, 23,* 175–202.

Fenson, L., Dale, P. S., Reznick, J. S., Thal, D., Bates, E., Hartung, J. P., et al. (1993). *MacArthur communicative development inventories: User's guide and technical manual.* San Diego, CA: Singular.

Gosch, A., Städing, G., & Pankau, R. (1994). Linguistic abilities in children with Williams–Beuren syndrome. *American Journal of Medical Genetics, 52,* 291–296.

Guasti, M. T. (2002). *Language acquisition: The growth of grammar.* Cambridge, MA: MIT Press.

Hodapp, R. M., Burack, J. A., & Zigler, E. (1998). Developmental approaches to mental retardation: A short introduction. In J. A. Burack, R. M. Hodapp, & E. Zigler (Eds.), *Handbook of mental retardation and development* (pp. 3–19). Cambridge, England: Cambridge University Press.

Hoffman, J., Landau, B., & Pagani, B. (in press). Spatial breakdown in spatial construction: Evidence from eye fixations in children with Williams syndrome. *Cognitive Psychology.*

Jackendoff, R. (1994). *Patterns in the mind.* New York: Basic Books.

Jarrold, C., Baddeley, A. D., & Hewes, A. K. (1998). Verbal and non-verbal abilities in the Williams syndrome phenotype: Evidence for diverging developmental trajectories. *Journal of Child Psychology and Psychiatry, 39,* 511–523.

Karmiloff-Smith, A., Grant, J., Berthoud, I., Davies, M., Howlin, P., & Udwin, O. (1997). Language and Williams syndrome: How intact is "intact." *Child Development, 68,* 274–290.

Karmiloff-Smith, A., Brown, J. H., Grice, S., & Paterson, S. (2003/this issue). Dethroning the myth: Cognitive dissociations and innate modularity in Williams syndrome. *Developmental Neuropsychology, 23,* 229–244.

Kataria, S., Goldstein, D. J., & Kushnick, T. (1984). Developmental delays in Williams ("elfin facies") syndrome. *Applied Research in Mental Retardation, 5,* 419–423.

Klein-Tasman, B. P., & Mervis, C. B. (2003/this issue). Distinctive pesonality characteristics of 8-, 9-, and 10-year olds with Williams syndrome. *Developmental Neuropsychology, 23,* 271–292.

Kramer, J. H., Kaplan, E., Share, L., & Huckeba, W. (1999). Configural errors on the WISC–III block design. *Journal of the International Neuropsychological Society, 5,* 518–524.

Landau, B., & Zukowski, A. (2003/this issue). Objects, motions, and paths: Spatial language in children with Williams syndrome. *Developmental Neuropsychology, 23,* 107–139.

Levy, Y., & Hermon, S. (2003/this issue). Morphological abilities of Hebrew-speaking adolescents with Williams syndrome. *Developmental Neuropsychology, 23,* 61–85.

Maratsos, M., Kuczaj, S. A., Fox, D. E., & Chalkey, M. A. (1979). Some empirical studies in the acquisition of transformational relations: Passives, negatives, and the past tense. In W. A. Collins (Ed.), *Children's language and communication.* Hillsdale, NJ: Lawrence Erlbaum Associates, Inc.

Mervis, C. B. (2001). Mental retardation, cognitive aspects. In N. J. Smelser & P. B. Baltes (Eds. in Chief), W. Kintsch (Ed.), *International encyclopedia of the social and behavioral sciences, Vol. 21. Cognitive psychology and cognitive science* (pp. 9700–9704). Oxford: Pergamon.

Mervis, C. B., & Bertrand, J. (1997). Developmental relations between cognition and language: Evidence from Williams syndrome. In L. B. Adamson & M. A. Romski (Eds.), *Communication and language acquisition: Discoveries from atypical development* (pp. 75–106). New York: Brookes.

Mervis, C. B., Morris, C. A., Bertrand, J., & Robinson, B. F. (1999). Williams syndrome: Findings from an integrated program of research. In H. Tager-Flusberg (Ed.), *Neurodevelopmental disorders* (pp. 65–110). Cambridge, MA: MIT Press.

Mervis, C. B., Morris, C. A., Klein-Tasman, B. P., Bertrand, J., Kwitny, S., Appelbaum, L.G., et al. (2003/this issue). Attentional characteristics of infants and toddlers with Williams syndrome during triadic interactions. *Developmental Neuropsychology, 23,* 245–270.

Mervis, C. B., Robinson, B. F., Bertrand, J., Morris, C. A., Klein-Tasman, B. P., & Armstrong, S. C. (2000). The Williams syndrome cognitive profile. *Brain and Cognition, 44,* 604–628.

Mervis, C. B., Robinson, B. F., Thomas, M. L., Becerra, A. M., & Klein-Tasman, B. P. (in press). Language abilities of people who have Williams syndrome. In L. Abbeduto (Ed.), *International review of research in mental retardation,* Vol. 27. Orlando, FL: Academic.

Meyerson, M. D., & Frank, R. A. (1987). Language, speech and hearing in Williams syndrome: Intervention approaches and research needs. *Developmental Medicine and Child Neurology, 29,* 258–262.

Osborne, L. R., Li, M., Pober, B., Chitayat, D., Bodurtha, J., Mandel, A., et al. (2001). A 1.5 million-base pair inversion polymorphism in families with Williams–Beuren syndrome. *Nature Genetics, 29,* 321–325.

Pezzini, G., Vicari, S., Volterra, V., Milani, L., & Ossella, M. T. (1999). Children with Williams syndrome: Is there a single neuropsychological profile? *Developmental Neuropsychology, 15,* 141–155.

Pinker, S. (1991). Rules of language. *Science, 253,* 530–535.

Reber, A. S. (1992). The cognitive unconscious: An evolutionary perspective. *Cognition and Consciousness, 1,* 93–113.

Rice, M. L. (1999). Specific grammatical limitations in children with specific language impairment. In H. Tager-Flusberg (Ed.), *Neurodevelopmental disorders* (pp. 331–359). Cambridge, MA: MIT Press.

Robinson, B. F., Mervis, C. B., & Robinson, B. W. (2003/this issue). The roles of verbal short-term memory and working memory in the acquisition of grammar by children with Williams syndrome. *Developmental Neuropsychology, 23,* 13–31.

Sharpes, D. K. (1999). *Advanced psychology for teachers*. New York: McGraw-Hill.

Sullivan, K., Winner, E., & Tager-Flusberg, H. (2003/this issue). Can adolescents with Williams syndrome tell the difference between lies and jokes? *Developmental Neuropsychology, 23,* 87–105.

Udwin, O., & Yule W. (1990). Expressive language of children with Williams syndrome. *American Journal of Medical Genetics Supplement, 6,* 108–114.

Udwin, O., & Yule, W. (1991). A cognitive and behavioural phenotype in Williams syndrome. *Journal of Clinical and Experimental Neuropsychology, 13,* 232–244.

Volterra, V., Capirci, O., Pezzini, G., Sabbadini, L., & Vicari, S. (1996). Linguistic abilities in Italian children with Williams syndrome. *Cortex, 32,* 663–677.

Volterra, V., Caselli, M. C., Capirci, O., Tonucci, F., & Vicari, S. (2003/this issue). Early linguistic abilities of Italian children with Williams syndrome. *Developmental Neuropsychology, 23,* 33–59.

Zigler, E. (1969). Developmental vs. difference theories of mental retardation and the problem of motivation. *American Journal of Mental Deficiency, 73,* 536–556.

The Roles of Verbal Short-Term Memory and Working Memory in the Acquisition of Grammar by Children With Williams Syndrome

Byron F. Robinson
Georgia State University

Carolyn B. Mervis
University of Louisville

Bronwyn W. Robinson
Georgia State University

The roles of verbal short-term and working memory were examined in a sample of children with Williams syndrome (mean chronological age 10 years, 2 months) and a sample of grammar-matched children who are developing normally. Forward digit span, nonword repetition, and backward span were all found to be correlated with receptive grammatical ability in the sample of children with Williams syndrome, but not in the sample of children who are developing normally. The relation between working memory, as measured by backward digit span, and grammatical ability was found to be significantly stronger in children with Williams syndrome than in the control group. This finding highlights the possibility that children with Williams syndrome may rely on their working memory to a greater extent than children who are developing normally to learn grammar. Hierarchical regression analyses indicated receptive vocabulary may mediate the relations among forward digit span, backward digit span, and grammatical ability for the children with Williams syndrome. Phonological short-term memory, however, contributed independently to grammatical ability even after receptive vocabulary was taken into account.

Requests for reprints should be sent to Byron F. Robinson, Department of Psychology, Georgia State University, Atlanta, GA 30303. E-mail: bfrobinson@gsu.edu

Individuals with Williams syndrome typically have mild to moderate mental retardation with a particular weakness in visuospatial constructive abilities (Frangiskakis et al. 1996; Mervis, Morris, Bertrand, & Robinson, 1999; Mervis, Robinson, et al., 2000). Language skills, on the other hand, are reported to be relatively good, with some researchers describing them as intact or spared (Bellugi, Marks, Bihrle, & Sabo, 1988; Bellugi, Wang, & Jernigan, 1994). Performance on auditory short-term memory tasks is usually better than expected relative to general level of cognitive ability (Bennett, LaVeck, & Sells, 1978; Mervis & Klein-Tasman, 2000; Udwin & Yule, 1991). Given the good language skills and generally poor performance in nonverbal functioning, some investigators consider the cognitive profile of Williams syndrome to be evidence that language can be dissociated from other cognitive abilities (Bellugi et al., 1988; Bellugi et al., 1994; Clahsen & Almazan, 1998). The argument put forward by these researchers rests on the assumption that individuals with Williams syndrome would have difficulty acquiring their relatively good language skills using inadequate cognitive abilities (Rossen, Klima, Bellugi, Bihrle, & Jones, 1996).

An opposing position questions the language independence view on the grounds that there are significant correlations between language and nonlanguage abilities, despite mean differences between the two domains of cognition (Mervis, 1999; Mervis, Morris, et al., 1999). One correlation in particular, that between working memory and language measures, fits well with research that has found similar relations in children who are developing normally (e.g., Gathercole & Baddeley, 1993; Just & Carpenter, 1992). Therefore, one explanation of the relatively good language abilities of individuals with Williams syndrome is that these abilities may be the result of their auditory short-term and working memory skills. Perhaps these memory skills provide individuals with Williams syndrome an alternate route to more advanced language that relies less on abstract reasoning to extract the rules of language from input and more on working memory. This study is designed to explore this possibility. The remainder of the introduction is devoted to describing the language abilities of individuals with Williams syndrome, their memory abilities, and the possible relation between the two skills.

LANGUAGE ABILITIES OF INDIVIDUALS WITH WILLIAMS SYNDROME

Initial reports portrayed the language skills of individuals with Williams syndrome as normal or intact (Bellugi et al., 1988; Bellugi et al., 1994). In particular, unlike other individuals with mental retardation, their language is described as fluent and expressive (Udwin & Yule, 1990) and consisting of coherent narrative structure (Bellugi et al., 1994). Research indicates that individuals with Williams syndrome have vocabulary skills that are at or above expected levels, given their cognitive deficits (Bellugi et al., 1994; Mervis, 1999). For instance, Mervis, Morris, et al. (1999) found that 48% of a sample of 85 children and adolescents with Williams syndrome scored in the normal range (≥ 70) on the Peabody Picture Vocabulary Test–Revised (PPVT–R), a test of receptive vocabulary. Children with Williams syndrome are also described as being in the normal range on tests of grammatical comprehension (Bellugi, Bihrle, Jernigan, Trauner, & Doherty, 1990). Their utterances are described as grammatically well formed and include grammatically complex constructions such as passives, conditionals, and embedded relative clauses (Bellugi et al., 1994). Clahsen and Alamazan (1998) similarly found that children with Williams syndrome are capable of applying systematic rules of morphology and could comprehend sentences that required the analysis of referential dependences between anaphoric elements.

Despite the evidence supporting the view that language in children with Williams syndrome is preserved, more recent research outlines an uneven profile of language and contradicts the position that the language of individuals with Williams syndrome is completely normal. Scores on the Test for the Reception of Grammar (TROG) typically fall below the level expected for chronological age (CA; Karmiloff-Smith et al., 1997). Mervis, Morris, et al. (1999) found a wide range of grammatical ability in a sample of 77 individuals. Scores on the TROG in this large sample ranged from the 1st to the 73rd percentile, with 56% scoring in the normal range (standard score ≥ 70). However, even those individuals who scored in the normal range on the TROG usually had difficulty processing relative clauses and embedded, left-branching sentences. The authors concluded that, although grammar is a relative strength for individuals with Williams syndrome, their processing of complex syntax is impaired.

In addition to depressed TROG scores, there are reports of abnormalities in grammatical ability. For instance, Volterra, Capirci, Pezzini, Sabbadini, and Vicari (1996) found that, despite an overall level of grammatical ability in the range expected given their mental age (MA), Italian children with Williams syndrome display morphological substitution errors not found during typical development. Similarly, French-speaking children with Williams syndrome are able to display an understanding of gender agreement when pairing an article and a noun, but have problems learning gender agreement across sentence elements such as pronouns and adjectives (Karmiloff-Smith et al., 1997). Gender agreement is typically a very early appearing grammatical skill that normally developing children learning French master with little effort. There also is evidence of deviant preposition use, including incorrect substitutions and omissions of prepositions, by children with Williams syndrome (Rubba & Klima, 1991).

In sum, recent research indicates that the grammatical abilities of individuals with Williams syndrome are delayed, with some aspects not following the typical patterns of development. Thus, it is likely the case that the language of individuals with Williams syndrome is not the result of a completely intact and independent language module. Other factors must be found to explain the grammatical abilities of individuals with this syndrome.

RELATIONS BETWEEN MEMORY AND LANGUAGE ABILITIES

One reason individuals with Williams syndrome originally may have been characterized as possessing intact language skills may be due less to their ability to process and produce advanced grammar and more to some basic grammatical skills coupled with enhanced phonological skills and verbal working memory. Individuals with Williams syndrome are reported to use an excessive amount of unanalyzed stereotypical phrases and sentences (Gosch, Städing, & Pankau, 1994; Udwin & Yule, 1990). It is therefore possible that some of the reported complex language ability of individuals with Williams syndrome is due to the rote memorization of phrases rather than the productive application of grammatical rules. Researchers have suggested that phonological working memory may be a factor that masks underlying deficits in grammatical ability (Klein & Mervis, 1999; Thal, Bates, & Bellugi, 1989).

There is substantial evidence that auditory working memory is a particular strength of individuals with Williams syndrome. Children with Williams syndrome perform significantly better than mental-age matches with Down syndrome on most verbal memory tasks (Klein & Mervis, 1999; Wang & Bellugi, 1994). Mervis, Morris, et al. (1999) found that 73% of a sample of 104 individuals with Williams syndrome scored in the normal range on the digit-span subtest of the Differential Ability Scales (Elliot, 1990). Similarly, in a study investigating the memory abilities of Italian children with Williams syndrome (Vicari, Brizzolara, Carlesimo, Pezzini, & Volterra, 1996), the digit spans of the participants with Williams syndrome were equal to those of MA-matched normally developing controls. Vicari et al. (1996) also performed an analysis of serial position effects in a list recall task. This analysis revealed that the children with Williams syndrome exhibited similar performance to the controls for words at the end of the list, but not the beginning and the middle of the list. The authors concluded that short-term memory is intact, but long-term memory may be a difficulty for these children.

The nonword repetition task, a measure of phonological short-term memory, is considered to be a verbal memory task that is not confounded by familiarity with the items to be recalled (Gathercole & Baddeley, 1989). Children with Williams syndrome have been found to be proficient at repeating nonwords, performing at about their MA level, but below the level expected for their CA (Grant, Karmiloff-Smith, Berthoud, & Christophe, 1996). Moreover, Grant et al. (1996) found that children with Williams syndrome who are learning English perform better on a nonword repetition task based on English phonotactics than on a test based on French phonotactics. This indicates that children with Williams syndrome are not simply skilled at sound imitation, but are able to build phonological representations of their first language.

Individuals with Williams syndrome also perform well on verbal working memory tasks that require the manipulation of items stored in short-term memory. For instance, the backward-digit-span task requires the participant to remember a string of digits, but before repeating the digits the participant must reverse their order. The ability to manipulate verbal items in memory has been associated with the acquisition of complex syntax (Kemper, Kynette, Rash, & O'Brien, 1989). Individuals with Williams syndrome typically perform well on backward-digit-span tasks. In a sample of 86 individuals, 89% scored within the normal range (Mervis, Morris, et al., 1999).

THIS STUDY

In children who are developing normally, verbal working memory is associated with the acquisition of vocabulary (Gathercole & Baddeley, 1989, 1993). Similarly, investigators reported that verbal memory is associated with the comprehension of syntax in elderly adults (Kemper et al., 1989; Norman, Kemper, & Kynette 1992). Bishop, North, and Donlan (1996) suggested that poor performance on a nonword repetition task is a phenotypic marker of language impairment. Despite nonverbal cognitive abilities in the normal range, children with specific language impairment demonstrated reduced performance on phonological working memory tasks relative to language matched children who are developing normally (Dollaghan & Campbell, 1998; Gathercole & Baddeley, 1990; Montgomery, 1996a). Children with Williams syndrome represent an interesting contrast in that they typically have very good verbal short-term and working memory skills, but poor nonverbal cognition and abstract reasoning. Given this profile, further investigation into the role of verbal working memory in the acquisition of language by individuals with Williams syndrome is warranted. Specifically, the goal of the research reported here is to determine whether children with Williams syndrome evidence a stronger relation between working memory and grammatical ability than children who are developing normally. If this is the case, then the language abilities of individuals with Williams syndrome can be explained in part with basic cognitive processing skills.

METHOD

Participants

Children with Williams syndrome were identified based on referrals from geneticists and cardiologists in Georgia, Alabama, North Carolina, Kentucky, and Nevada and through the National Williams Syndrome Association. The diagnosis of Williams syndrome was based on fluorescent *in situ* hybridization tests; all children had a microdeletion of chromosome 7q11.23. The children who are developing normally were identified through private schools, day-care programs,

YMCA after-school programs, and Boys and Girls Clubs in Georgia and Kentucky. The Williams syndrome group consisted of 39 children (21 girls, 18 boys) who ranged in CA from 4.5 to 16.7 years ($M = 10.24$; $SD = 3.70$). The normally developing group consisted of 32 children (17 girls, 15 boys). These children were selected to match the children with Williams syndrome on receptive grammatical skills and were therefore younger, with CAs between 4.08 and 10.26 years ($M = 6.01$; $SD = 1.56$). Additional descriptive statistics are provided in Table 1.

Materials and Procedure

All testing took place in the Byron Robinson and Carolyn Mervis's laboratories, in a quiet room at the participants' schools or homes, or at family conferences of the national or regional Williams syndrome associations. Standardized tests were administered according to procedures outlined in their respective manuals. Descriptions of standardized tests and descriptions and administration procedures for unstandardized tests are presented in the following.

Test for the Reception of Grammar. The TROG (Bishop, 1989) is a measure of grammatical comprehension. The participant is shown four pictures and is asked to choose the one that matches the word, phrase, or sentence produced by the experimenter. It is composed of 20 blocks of four items with each block testing a different grammatical construct. Raw scores on the TROG correspond to the number of blocks in which the participant correctly answered all four items within a block.

TABLE 1
Descriptive Statistics for the Williams Syndrome and Normally Developing Groups

	Williams Syndrome Group				*Normally Developing Group*				
Measure	*M*	*SD*	*Min*	*Max*	*M*	*SD*	*Min*	*Max*	p^a
CA (years)	10.24	3.70	4.51	16.68	6.01	1.56	4.08	10.26	<.001
K–BIT IQ	67.97	14.36	41	96	100.38	11.12	81	120	<.001
K–BIT Matrices raw score	15.87	4.11	8	23	16.66	5.42	7	28	.490
TROG SS	72.21	11.04	<55	96	92.19	11.79	72	111	<.001
TROG raw score	9.92	3.47	3	17	10.31	4.21	1	18	.670
PPVT–R SS	71.26	16.83	31	98	94.59	15.08	68	133	<.001
PPVT–R raw score	76.59	24.04	45	125	63.19	20.12	30	127	.014
Forward digit span	4.00	0.79	3	5	4.16	1.19	2	8	.160
Nonword repetition	16.05	8.26	1	40	14.91	9.03	0	41	.579
Backward digit span	1.33	1.30	0	3	1.69	1.55	0	5	.300

Note. CA = chronological age; K–BIT = Kaufman Brief Intelligence Test; TROG = Test for the Reception of Grammar; PPVT–R = Peabody Picture Vocabulary Test–Revised.
[a] *p*-values are associated with independent sample *t* tests of group differences.

Peabody Picture Vocabulary Test–Revised. The PPVT–R (Dunn & Dunn, 1981) is a commonly used measure of receptive vocabulary. The child selects one picture out of four that matches a word spoken by the experimenter. The test includes words for objects, actions, descriptors, and abstractions.

One-item-per-second forward digit span (SpanF). This is the traditional measure of verbal short-term memory. The participant is asked to repeat strings of digits, which are spoken by the experimenter at a rate of one digit per second. Digit strings are presented in blocks of two strings of the same length and increase in length until the participant incorrectly repeats both strings within a block. Span is scored as the longest string length at which the participant correctly repeated at least one of the two strings within a block.

One-item-per-second backward digit span (SpanB). This measure is designed to assess the participant's ability to manipulate items that are stored in short-term memory. It is identical to SpanF with the exception that participant is asked to reverse the order of the digit string as presented by the experimenter. Because of this additional aspect of processing, backward digit span is thought to play an important role in the comprehension and production of complex syntax (e.g., Kemper et al., 1989; Mervis, Morris, et al., 1999).

Nonword Repetition Task. In the Nonword Repetition Task (NWRT), participants are asked to repeat nonwords that conform to English phonotactics. Nonword repetition is generally preferred to actual word repetition as a measure of verbal short-term memory because it controls for the participants' familiarity with the presented words. Montgomery (1996a) developed the list of 48 nonwords and the presentation procedure for the nonword task used in this study. This particular task has been found to be related to grammatical ability in children with specific language impairment (Montgomery, 1996a, 1996b).

Kaufman Brief Intelligence Test. The Kaufman Brief Intelligence Test (K–BIT; Kaufman & Kaufman, 1990) is a standardized test of intelligence and combines vocabulary and nonverbal intelligence (matrices) subtests to yield an IQ index of general cognitive ability.

RESULTS

Matching and Group Differences

Descriptive statistics for children with Williams syndrome and children who are normally developing and the p values associated with t tests of group differences are presented in Table 1. The children with Williams syndrome were significantly older than the children who are normally developing as assessed by a t test corrected for unequal variances, $t(53.10) = 6.41, p < .001$. As would be expected, the two groups also differed on IQ scores as measured by the K–BIT, $t(69) = 10.45$, $p < .001$. The normally developing group was designed to match the Williams syndrome group on comprehension grammar (the TROG). A t test for independent groups indicated that the two groups were well matched on number of blocks correct, $t(69) = 0.43$, $p = .67$. Given the younger CA and higher IQ of the normally developing group, this leads to the normally developing group earning significantly higher standard scores on the TROG, $t(69) = 7.82$, $p < .001$. The two groups differed significantly on PPVT–R raw scores, $t(69)$, 2.51, $p < .05$, with the Williams syndrome group evidencing slightly higher scores. PPVT–R standard scores, however, demonstrated that for CA level, the children with Williams syndrome were performing significantly worse than the normally developing group, $t(69) = 6.10$, $p < .001$. Interestingly, although not planned, the two groups did not differ on any of the memory measures.

Partial Correlations Between the Memory Measures and Grammatical Abilities

As can be seen in Table 2, the partial correlations, controlling for CA, between the memory measures and number of blocks passed on the TROG (i.e., raw scores) for the Williams syndrome group range from .33 to .52 and are all significant at the $p = .05$ level. On the other hand, none of the partial correlations between the memory measures and the TROG approached significance for the normally developing

TABLE 2
Correlations Controlling for Chronological Age

	SpanF	*NWRT*	*SpanB*	*PPVT–R*
Williams syndrome group				
NWRT	.26			
SpanB	.55***	.16		
PPVT–R	.27	.15	.58***	
TROG	.33*	.48**	.52***	.74***
Normally developing group				
NWRT	.11			
SpanB	.23	.38*		
PPVT–R	–.12	.15	.32	
TROG	.17	.07	.27	.66***

Note. NWRT = Nonword Repetition Task; SpanB = One per-second backward digit span; PPVT–R = Peabody Picture Vocabulary Test–Revised; TROG = Test for the reception of grammar.
*$p < .05$. **$p < .01$. ***$p < .001$.

group. Comprehension vocabulary (PPVT–R raw scores) and TROG scores are significantly correlated in both groups.

All of the correlations between the memory measures and the TROG are larger in the Williams syndrome group. Given the relatively small sample sizes, significance tests of the group differences in the correlations based on asymptotic theory would be suspect. For this reason permutation tests of group differences in the strength of relation between the memory measures and the TROG were performed. The permutation test used was an adapted version of Bakeman and Robinson's (1997) test for slope differences. Group differences in the regression coefficients of each memory measure were tested separately using a model including the TROG raw scores as a dependent variable and CA and the memory measure as independent variables. The test was based on 100,000 permutations of group membership for each set of scores. The procedure yielded exact p values indicating the significance of the difference between the Williams syndrome group and the normally developing group in the strength of the relation between the memory measure and grammatical ability. The permutation tests revealed that, after controlling for CA, the difference between the two groups in the strength of relation between forward-digit-span and TROG raw score was not significant ($p = .14$). However, the relation between backward-digit-span and TROG raw score was significantly greater for the Williams syndrome group than the normally developing group ($p = .02$). The Williams syndrome group also demonstrated a stronger relation between NWRT scores and TROG raw score, but only at the $p = .09$ level.

Exploratory Hierarchical Regressions

In an effort to explore the relations between the memory measures and grammatical ability further, a series of hierarchically nested regressions was performed separately for each group. The hierarchical regression results for a model containing CA, forward span, nonword repetition, and backward span as independent variables is presented in Table 3. For the normally developing group, the memory measures as a set accounted for only 5% additional variance in TROG raw scores beyond CA. For the Williams syndrome group, however, the memory variables taken together accounted for .26 of the variance in TROG raw scores beyond CA. When SpanF is entered before NWRT and SpanB, it accounts for a significant amount of variance beyond CA. However, tests of individual regression coefficients in a simultaneous regression including CA and all of the memory measures indicated that nonword repetition and backward digit span are significant unique predictors of TROG raw scores ($t = 3.105, p < .01$; and $t = 3.14, p < .01$, respectively), but that forward span does not contribute significantly to predicting TROG raw scores.

TABLE 3
Hierarchical Regressions

Variable Entered	*Model* R^2	ΔR^2	Δp
Williams syndrome group			
CA	.414	.414	.000
Forward digit span	.476	.062	.046
Nonword repetition	.573	.097	.008
Backward digit span	.669	.096	.003
Normally developing group			
CA	.426	.426	.000
Forward digit span	.444	.017	.351
Nonword repetition	.445	.002	.776
Backward digit span	.476	.031	.218

Note. CA = chronological age.

Exploratory Hierarchical Regressions Including PPVT–R

Two additional hierarchical regressions were performed to examine the possibility that the relations between the memory measures and grammatical ability are primarily the result of vocabulary ability. In these models, PPVT–R raw scores were entered after CA and before the memory measures. The results of these regressions are presented in Table 4. The PPVT–R raw scores explain a significant amount of variance in the TROG raw scores of the normally developing group, but, as expected given the pattern of correlations, none of the memory measures contributed significantly to the model. For the Williams syndrome group, entering PPVT–R raw scores before the memory measures resulted in nonsignificant increases in R^2 from SpanF and SpanB. Interestingly, however, even after accounting for CA, PPVT–R raw scores, and SpanF, the NWRT accounted for a significant amount of variance in TROG raw scores. Results from a simultaneous regression confirmed these findings, with only the PPVT–R and NWRT regression coefficients attaining significance ($t = 5.12, p < .001$; and $t = 3.60, p < .001$, respectively).

DISCUSSION

The general pattern of cognitive abilities of this sample of children with Williams syndrome is consistent with other reports in the literature (e.g., Mervis, Morris, et al., 1999). As expected, children with Williams syndrome evidenced delayed development. The mean IQ of the Williams syndrome group was in the range of mild mental retardation. There was, however, a wide range of functioning: 21% of the sample scored in the range of moderate mental retardation (40–54), 41% of the sample scored in the mild mental retardation range (55–70), and 38% scored in the low-normal to normal range (> 70). Language scores of the Williams syndrome group

TABLE 4
Hierarchical Regressions Including PPVT–R Raw Score as an Independent Variable

Variable Entered	*Model* R^2	ΔR^2	Δp
Williams syndrome group			
CA	.414	.414	.000
PPVT–R raw score	.731	.317	.000
Forward digit span	.741	.011	.235
Nonword repetition	.813	.071	.001
Backward digit span	.816	.003	.466
Normally developing group			
CA	.426	.426	.000
PPVT–R raw score	.676	.250	.000
Forward digit span	.712	.036	.070
Nonword repetition	.714	.002	.665
Backward digit span	.714	.000	.946

Note. PPVT–R = Peabody Picture Vocabulary Test–Revised; CA = chronological age.

were slightly higher than general IQ levels. With respect to receptive vocabulary (PPVT–R), 56% of the children scored in the normal range. On the measure of receptive grammar (TROG), 46% of the children scored in the normal range.

Despite the relatively good language scores of the children with Williams syndrome, receptive grammar was delayed. The mean CA-equivalent score on the TROG for the Williams syndrome group was 5 years, 6 months. This figure is well below the group's mean CA of 10 years, 3 months. Moreover, the mean CA of the children in the grammar-matched normally developing control group was significantly younger than the mean CA of the children with Williams syndrome. These findings are consistent with research indicating delay in grammatical abilities (Karmiloff-Smith et al., 1997; Vicari et al., 1996), and are inconsistent with the viewpoint that grammar is spared or intact (Bellugi et al., 1988; Bellugi et al., 1994).

Raw scores of the children with Williams syndrome on the PPVT–R were significantly higher than those of the grammar-matched control group. Therefore, as found in previous studies (e.g., Volterra et al., 1996), the children with Williams syndrome displayed receptive vocabulary slightly in advance of grammatical ability. Interestingly, however, there was no difference between the two groups on K–BIT Matrices raw scores. Typically, children with Williams syndrome are found to have nonverbal skills that are significantly delayed relative to language skills. However, the K–BIT Matrices subtest does not include a measure of visuospatial constructive cognition (e.g., block design), which is the most severe nonverbal deficit displayed by most individuals with Williams syndrome (Mervis, Morris, et al., 1999; Mervis, Robinson, & Pani, 1999). Therefore, children with Williams syndrome would be expected to score higher on measures of nonverbal ability, such as K–BIT Matrices, that do not include a visuospatial constructive component.

Relations Between Memory Measures and Grammatical Ability

After controlling for CA, all of the verbal memory measures were significantly correlated with grammatical comprehension in the Williams syndrome group. Taken together, the memory variables accounted for 26% of the variance in TROG raw scores. However, forward digit span alone did not uniquely contribute to variance in the scores once CA, nonword repetition, and backward digit span were taken into account. Nonword repetition, on the other hand, did account for additional unique variance even after CA and the other memory measures were controlled. Although nonword repetition and forward digit span could both be considered tasks requiring short-term memory for verbal items, the nonword repetition task requires participants to repeat unfamiliar strings that are spoken without pauses between syllables and contain stress patterns similar to real English words. The digit-span task, on the other hand, presents potentially familiar words, sounds with pauses between the syllables (with the exception of the two syllables in seven), and little or no stress on individual syllables. Therefore, nonword repetition may be indexing phonological skills, such as the ability to parse strings of phonemes and the efficiency of phonological encoding, in addition to simple storage of sequences of phonological items. It is possible that the nonword-repetition task relies, in part, on a child's ability to relate unknown words to abstract phonological reference frames containing information that would be helpful in processing phonological input (Gathercole, Willis, Emslie, & Baddeley, 1991). According to this hypothesis, nonwords that could be related to abstract wordlike structures (i.e., those containing sublexical structures such as "ment" and "ish") present in English words would be more easily remembered by those possessing enhanced phonological ability.

Some research has found evidence of enhanced phonological skills in children with Williams syndrome (Volterra et al., 1996). Grant et al. (1997) suggested that this facility with phonological processing of nonword items is related to the receptive vocabulary size of children with Williams syndrome. Our study extends this relation to receptive grammatical ability. As with children with specific language impairment (Bishop et al., 1996; Montgomery, 1996b), the ability of children with Williams syndrome to repeat nonwords appears to be related to performance on grammatical measures. The acquisition of grammar is due, in part, to the ability to process grammatical function words and bound morphemes. These units are difficult to perceive in connected speech because they tend to be short, unstressed, and deformed in their phonetic structure (Bates & Goodman, 1997). It is therefore reasonable to assume that an enhanced ability to parse phonetic units from the speech stream and efficiently encode and store them would be a requirement of acquiring grammatical structures.

The strong relation between memory and receptive grammar does not necessarily imply that the grammatical ability of children with Williams syndrome is simply the result of rote memorization of unanalyzed phrases. Few, if any, of the TROG items could be answered by simply recognizing previously heard sentences. Thus, even if explicit grammatical rules are not mastered by children with Williams syndrome, some basic pattern extraction of grammatical rules must be taking place for the children to answer the TROG items correctly.

Backward digit span accounted for the largest proportion of variance in TROG raw scores for both groups, but the correlation was significant only for the Williams syndrome group. The exploratory regressions revealed that, for the children with Williams syndrome, backward digit span accounted for a significant proportion of the variance in TROG raw scores after controlling for CA, forward digit span, and nonword repetition. The significant and unique contribution of backward digit span indicates that additional processing capacity required to manipulate (i.e., reverse) items stored in short-term memory is important in the acquisition of grammar.

There are two compatible hypotheses that could explicate the relation between working memory as measured by backward digit span and grammatical ability. One explanation is primarily linguistic and the other involves more general processing abilities. The linguistic explanation suggests that facility with the storage of phonological items allows a word or phrase to be held in memory longer, thereby increasing the likelihood that the language item will be maintained in long-term memory (Gathercole & Baddeley, 1989, 1993). Moreover, the facility to manipulate the items in memory would be required to process sentence elements that are presented sequentially into a coherent representation (Daneman & Carpenter, 1980). In addition to the processing of linguistic elements, however, the acquisition of grammatical structures requires the ability to associate the meaning of the phrase from the context (i.e., the results of perceptual/cognitive/social processing of the scene associated with an utterance) and integrate that meaning with the stored linguistic form. This process is not purely a function of phonological memory (i.e., encoding and storage), but would fall in the domain of the central executive according to Baddeley and Hitch's (1974) working memory model. More recent research suggests that the defining feature of working memory and the central executive, as opposed to simple short-term memory, is the ability to switch attention between the items in storage and the processing component of the task (Engle, Tuholski, Laughlin, & Conway, 1999). Learning grammar requires not only the encoding and storage of the linguistic items (the aforementioned linguistic hypothesis), but also the processing of extralinguistic cues to meaning available from other systems. The ability to integrate the stored linguistic representation of an utterance with the extralinguistic cues necessary for the interpretation of the utterance may require attention-switching capacities as much as the more traditional abilities associated with working memory. Further investigation of the attentional capacities of individuals with Williams syndrome may help clarify the role of these abilities in the language learning context.

Group Differences in the Relations Between Working Memory and Grammatical Ability

The finding that backward digit span shared a stronger relation with grammatical ability in the Williams syndrome group than in the normally developing group suggests that the children with Williams syndrome may be learning language in a manner different from normally developing children. Learning a grammar requires the online integration of multiple cues to the meaning of a specific grammatical form in an utterance. These cues may be visual perceptual, pragmatic, cognitive, or linguistic. The efficient processing of these nonlinguistic cues facilitates the attachment of meaning to the phonological representation of an utterance that is held in short-term memory. For a typically developing child, these cues can be processed easily and integrated seamlessly with the phonological representation of the utterance to be comprehended. For a child with mental retardation, additional time and cognitive resources are necessary to process the nonlinguistic cues. Therefore, the ability to maintain the phonological representation in working memory longer and then integrate it with the nonlinguistic cues may be more central to a child with mental retardation than a normally developing child.

One unexpected finding is that the normally developing children did not show any significant correlations between the memory measures and the scores on the test of receptive grammar. This is likely due to the relatively simple grammatical structures probed by the TROG. The amount of working memory required to acquire basic grammatical structures may be minimal for normally developing children. Instead, abstract reasoning skills and the ability to apply language learning strategies may play a larger role in the typical path through language development. The contrast between the normally developing and the Williams syndrome groups with respect to the role of working memory does highlight the possibility that children with Williams syndrome rely on working memory to offset deficits in the application of language learning strategies. Mervis and Bertrand (1997) found that young children with Williams syndrome do not display some of the typical developmental relations between cognition and language found for normally developing children. For instance, children who are developing normally usually acquire the ability to fast-map words (i.e., rapid single-trial learning of new words) at about the same time they experience a rapid acceleration in their rate of word learning (the vocabulary spurt). Mervis and Bertrand (1994) suggested that the ability to fast-map new words is based on the novel name–nameless category (N3C) principle. Children who display this word-learning strategy realize that, when a novel (unknown) word is heard in the presence of an object for which they do not have a label, the unknown word must refer to the category of objects that contains the nameless object. Normally developing children (Mervis & Bertrand, 1994), children with Down syndrome (Mervis & Bertrand, 1995), and children with mental retardation who use visual-graphic symbols to speak (Romski, Sevcik, Robinson, Mervis, & Bertrand, 1996) all display a temporal relation between the vocabulary spurt and the emergence of the ability to use the N3C principle in an experimental situation. Children with Williams syndrome, however, typically experience a vocabulary spurt well before they show evidence of the ability to use the N3C principle. Therefore, in the case of learning words, children with Williams syndrome initially rely on verbal memory skills to a greater extent than the application of more sophisticated strategies. It is possible that a similar process occurs with the acquisition of grammar. Normally developing children may rely on more advanced conceptual abilities to learn grammar, which place fewer demands on working memory, whereas children with Williams syndrome, who are not able to apply some of these strategies, place a higher demand on working memory to acquire the same grammatical rules.

Relation Between Lexical and Grammatical Acquisition

Previous research with children who are developing normally found a relation between productive vocabulary size and early grammatical ability (Bates, Thal, Finlay, & Clancy, 2003). A strong nonlinear relation between productive vocabulary size and number of constructions in a child's grammatical inventory is evident in normally developing children, late talkers (Bates & Goodman, 1997), and children with Williams syndrome (Mervis, Rausch, & Robinson, 2000). Relations between vocabulary size and specific grammatical constructions have been found between verbs and acquisition of past-tense morphology (Marchman & Bates, 1994) and between nouns and acquisition of the plural –s morpheme (Robinson & Mervis, 1998). The results of the second exploratory regressions in our study demonstrate a link between receptive vocabulary and receptive grammar, as evidenced by the relation between PPVT–R and TROG scores, in children who are developing normally and children with Williams syndrome. Moreover, after vocabulary skills are taken into account, backward digit span is no longer a significant predictor of grammatical ability. Therefore, it is possible that the ability to manipulate items in memory enhances vocabulary acquisition and the acquisition of basic grammatical constructs in a similar manner. Phonological memory as measured by the nonword repetition task, on the other hand, contributes a unique skill to grammar acquisition, even after receptive vocabulary is controlled. Therefore, as discussed previously, phonological skills necessary for isolating grammatical morphemes from the speech stream may facilitate grammatical development. The sample sizes of this study do not allow a more in-depth investigation of the interrelations among grammar, vocabulary, and working memory. Further research will shed light on the theoretically important relations among these skills.

SUMMARY

This study provides evidence that children with Williams syndrome share a stronger relation between working memory and grammatical ability than do normally developing children. Importantly, the ability to manipulate items in memory, rather than simple rote short-term storage of verbal items, appears to be a key component in the acquisition of grammar. The importance of working memory to the grammatical development of children with Williams syndrome highlights a basic difference between how children with Williams syndrome and children who are developing normally acquire language. It is an open question as to whether this difference is a matter of extremes or whether children with Williams syndrome acquire language using significantly different mechanisms from those used by children who are developing normally. Further research is required to determine whether children with Williams syndrome utilize similar language learning strategies to those used by typically developing children, but apply them less consistently and therefore need to rely more heavily on working memory, or whether children with Williams syndrome use altogether different strategies to acquire basic grammatical constructs.

ACKNOWLEDGMENTS

This research was supported by National Institute of Child Health and Human Development Grant No. HD29957, National Institute of Neurological Disorders and Stroke Grant No. NS35102, and the Research Enhancement Program of Georgia State University. We thank the children and their parents for their enthusiastic participation in this research. Deborah Deckner, Janell Kalina, Echo Meyer, Beth Lehue, Andrea Burkhead, Florence Chang, Mary Beth Whittle, Amy Haney, and Carey Kennedy assisted with data collection, reduction, and analysis.

REFERENCES

Baddeley, A. D., & Hitch, G. (1974). Working memory. In G. A. Bower (Ed.), *The psychology of learning and motivation* (Vol. 8, pp. 47–89). New York: Academic.

Bakeman, R., & Robinson, B. F. (1997). When *N*s do not justify the means: Small samples and scientific conclusions. In L. B. Adamson & M. A. Romski (Eds.), *Communication and language acquisition: Discoveries from atypical development* (pp. 49–72). Baltimore: Brookes.

Bates, E., & Goodman, J. (1997). On the inseparability of grammar and the lexicon: Evidence from acquisition, aphasia, and real-time processing. *Language and Cognitive Processes, 12,* 507–586.

Bates, E., Thal, D., Finlay, B. L., & Clancy, B. (2003). Early language development and its neural correlates. In F. Boller & J. Grafman (Series Eds.) & S. J. Segalowitz & I. Rapin (Vol. Eds.), *Handbook of neuropsychology, Vol. 8, Child neurology* (2nd ed., pp. 525–592). Amsterdam: Elsevier.

Bellugi, U., Bihrle, A., Jernigan, T., Trauner, D., & Doherty S. (1990). Neuropsychological and neuroanatomical profile of Williams syndrome. *American Journal of Medical Genetics, 6,* 115–125.

Bellugi, U., Marks, S., Bihrle, A., & Sabo, H. (1988). Dissociation between language and cognitive functions in Williams syndrome. In D. Bishop & K. Mogford (Eds.), *Language development in exceptional circumstances* (pp. 177–189). London: Churchill Livingstone.

Bellugi, U., Wang, P., & Jernigan, T. L. (1994). Williams syndrome: An unusual neuropsychological profile. In S. H. Broman & J. Grafman (Eds.), *Atypical cognitive deficits in developmental disorders: Implications for brain function* (pp. 23–56). Hillsdale, NJ: Lawrence Erlbaum Associates, Inc.

Bennett, F. C., LaVeck, B., & Sells, C. J. (1978). The Williams elfin facies syndrome: The psychological profile as an aid in syndrome identification. *Pediatrics, 61,* 303–306.

Bishop, D. V. M. (1989). *Test for the reception of grammar* (2nd ed.). Manchester, England: Chapel.

Bishop, D. V. M., North, T., & Donlan, C. (1996). Nonword repetition as a behavioral marker for inherited language impairment: Evidence from a twin study. *Journal of Child Psychology and Psychiatry, 37,* 391–403.

Clahsen, H., & Almazan, M. (1998). Syntax and morphology in Williams syndrome. *Cognition, 68,* 167–198.

Daneman, M., & Carpenter, P. A. (1980). Individual differences in working memory and reading. *Journal of Verbal Learning and Verbal Behavior, 19,* 450–466.

Dollaghan, C., & Campbell, T. F. (1998). Nonword repetition and child language impairment. *Journal of Speech, Language, and Hearing Research, 41,* 1136–1146.

Dunn, L. M., & Dunn, L. M. (1981). *Peabody Picture Vocabulary Test–Revised.* Circle Pines, MN: American Guidance Services.

Elliott, C. D. (1990). *Differential Ability Scales.* San Diego, CA: Harcourt Brace.

Engle, R. W., Tuholski, S. W., Laughlin, J. E., & Conway, A. R. A. (1999). Working memory, short-term memory, and general fluid intelligence: A latent-variable approach. *Journal of Experimental Psychology: General, 128,* 309–331.

Frangiskakis, J. M., Ewart, A. K., Morris, C. A., Mervis, C. B., Bertrand, J., Robinson, B. F. et al. (1996). LIM-kinase1 hemizygosity implicated in impaired visuospatial constructive cognition. *Cell, 86,* 59–69.

Gathercole, S. E., & Baddeley, A. D. (1989). Evaluation of the role of phonological STM in the development of vocabulary in children: A longitudinal study. *Journal of Memory and Language, 28,* 200–213.

Gathercole, S. E., & Baddeley, A. D. (1990). The role of phonological memory in vocabulary acquisition: A study of young children learning new names. *British Journal of Psychology, 81,* 439–454.

Gathercole, S. E., & Baddeley, A. D. (1993). *Working memory and language.* Hillsdale, NJ: Lawrence Erlbaum Associates, Inc.

Gathercole, S. E., Willis, C., Emslie, H., & Baddeley, A. D. (1991). The influences of number of syllables and wordlikeness on children's repetition of nonwords. *Applied Psycholinguistics, 12,* 349–367.

Gosch, A., Städing, G., & Pankau, R. (1994). Linguistic abilities in children with Williams–Beuren syndrome. *American Journal of Medical Genetics, 52,* 291–296.

Grant, J., Karmiloff-Smith, A., Berthoud, I., & Christophe, A. (1996). Is the language of people with Williams syndrome mere mimicry? Phonological short-term memory in a foreign language. *Cahiers de Psychologie Cognitive, 15,* 615–628.

Grant, J., Karmiloff-Smith, A., Gathercole, S. A., Paterson, S., Howlin, P., Davies, M., et al. (1997). Phonological short-term memory and its relationship to language in Williams syndrome. *Cognitive Neuropsychiatry, 2,* 81–99.

Just, M. A., & Carpenter, P. A. (1992). A capacity theory of comprehension: Individual differences in working memory. *Psychological Bulletin, 99,* 122–149.

Karmiloff-Smith, A., Grant, J., Berthoud, I., Davies, M., Howlin, P., & Udwin, O. (1997). Language and Williams syndrome: How intact is "intact"? *Child Development, 68,* 274–290.

Kaufman, A. S., & Kaufman, N. L. (1990). *Kaufman Brief Intelligence Test.* Pines, MN: American Guidance Services.

Kemper, S., Kynette, D., Rash, S., & O'Brien, K. (1989). Life span changes to adults' language: Effects of memory and genre. *Applied Psycholinguistics, 10,* 49–66.

Klein, B. P., & Mervis, C. B. (1999). Contrasting patterns of cognitive abilities of 9- and 10-year-olds with Williams syndrome or Down syndrome. *Developmental Neuropsychology, 16,* 177–196.

Marchman, V. A., & Bates, E. (1994). Continuity in lexical and morphological development: A test of the critical mass hypothesis. *Journal of Child Language, 21,* 399–366.

Mervis, C. B. (1999). The Williams syndrome cognitive profile: Strengths, weaknesses, and interrelations among auditory short-term memory, language, and visuospatial constructive cognition. In E. Winograd, R. Fivush, & W. Hirst (Eds.), *Ecological approaches to cognition: Essays in honor of Ulric Neisser* (pp. 193–227). Mahwah, NJ: Lawrence Erlbaum Associates, Inc.

Mervis, C. B., & Bertrand, J. (1994). Acquisition of the novel name–nameless category (N3C) principle. *Child Development, 65,* 1646–1662.

Mervis, C. B., & Bertrand, J. (1995). Acquisition of the novel name–nameless category (N3C) principle by children with Down syndrome. *American Journal on Mental Retardation, 100,* 231–243.

Mervis, C. B., & Bertrand, J. (1997). Developmental relations between cognition and language. In L. B. Adamson & M. A. Romski (Eds.), *Communication and language acquisition: Discoveries from atypical development* (pp. 75–106). Baltimore: Brookes.

Mervis, C. B., & Klein-Tasman, B. P. (2000). Williams syndrome: Cognition, personality, and adaptive behavior. *Mental Retardation and Developmental Disabilities Research Reviews, 6,* 148–158.

Mervis, C. B., Morris, C. A., Bertrand, J., & Robinson, B. F. (1999). Williams syndrome: Findings from an integrated program of research. In H. Tager-Flusberg (Ed.), *Neurodevelopmental disorders* (pp. 65–110). Cambridge, MA: MIT Press.

Mervis, C. B., Rausch, J. M., & Robinson, B. F. (2000, July). *Patterns of early grammatical development of children with Williams syndrome.* Poster presented at the International Professional Meeting of the Williams Syndrome Association, Dearborn, MI.

Mervis, C. B., Robinson, B. F., Bertrand, J., Morris, C. A., Klein-Tasman, B. P., & Armstrong, S. C. (2000). The Williams syndrome cognitive profile. *Brain and Cognition, 44,* 604–628.

Mervis, C. B., Robinson, B. F., & Pani, J. R. (1999). Visuospatial construction. *American Journal of Human Genetics, 65,* 1222–1229.

Montgomery, J. A. (1996a). Examination of phonological working memory in specifically language-impaired children. *Applied Psycholinguistics, 16,* 355–378.

Montgomery, J. A. (1996b). Sentence comprehension in children with specific language impairment: The role of phonological working memory. *Journal of Speech and Hearing Research, 38,* 187–199.

Norman, S., Kemper, S., & Kynette, D. (1992). Adult reading comprehension: Effects of syntactic complexity and working memory. *Journal of Gerontology, 47,* 258–265.

Robinson, B. F., & Mervis, C. B. (1998). Disentangling early language development: Modeling lexical and grammatical acquisition using an extension of case-study methodology. *Developmental Psychology, 34,* 363–375.

Romski, M. A., Sevcik, R. A., Robinson, B. F., Mervis, C. B., & Bertrand, J. (1996). Mapping the meanings of novel visual symbols by youth with moderate or severe mental retardation. *American Journal on Mental Retardation, 100,* 391–402.

Rossen, M., Klima, E. S., Bellugi, U., Bihrle, A., & Jones, W. (1996). Interaction between language and cognition: Evidence from Williams syndrome. In J. H. Beitchman, N. J. Cohen, M. M. Kostantareas, & R. Tannock (Eds.), *Language, learning, and behavior disorders: Developmental, biological, and clinical perspectives* (pp. 367–392). Cambridge, England: Cambridge University Press.

Rubba, J., & Klima, E. S. (1991). Preposition use in a speaker with Williams syndrome: Some cognitive grammar proposals. *Newsletter of the Center for Research in Language, University of California, San Diego, CA, 5,* 3–12.

Thal, D., Bates, E., & Bellugi, U. (1989). Language and cognition in two children with Williams syndrome. *Journal of Speech and Hearing Research, 32,* 489–500.
Udwin, O., & Yule W. (1990). Expressive language of children with Williams syndrome. *American Journal of Medical Genetics Supplement, 6,* 108–114.
Udwin, O., & Yule, W. (1991). A cognitive and behavioral phenotype in Williams syndrome. *Journal of Clinical and Experimental Neuropsychology, 13,* 232–244.
Vicari, S., Brizzolara, D., Carlesimo, G. A., Pezzini, G., & Volterra, V. (1996). Memory abilities in children with Williams syndrome. *Cortex, 32,* 503–514.
Volterra, V., Capirci, O., Pezzini, G., Sabbadini, L., & Vicari, S. (1996). Linguistic abilities in Italian children with Williams syndrome. *Cortex, 32,* 503–514.
Wang, P. P., & Bellugi, U. (1994). Evidence from two genetic syndromes for a dissociation between verbal and visual–spatial short-term memory. *Journal of Experimental and Clinical Neuropsychology, 16,* 317–322.

Early Linguistic Abilities of Italian Children With Williams Syndrome

Virginia Volterra, M. Cristina Caselli, and Olga Capirci
Institute of Cognitive Sciences and Technology
National Research Council (CNR)
Rome, Italy

Francesca Tonucci and Stefano Vicari
Children's Hospital Bambino Gesù
Rome, Italy

Previous studies of linguistic and memory abilities in Italian-speaking children with Williams syndrome (WS) and Down syndrome (DS) are briefly reviewed. New data on linguistic performance of 6 Italian children with WS between 3 and 6 years of age are presented and compared with data on linguistic performance of 6 children with DS selected from a larger sample and matched for chronological age and vocabulary size and of 6 typically developing (TD) younger children matched for mental age and vocabulary size. The language measures also included a parent report of early phrase structure, a naming test, and a sentence repetition task. Analyses revealed that the 3 groups of children were at the same productive vocabulary level, but showed different patterns in sentence production and repetition. Children with WS produced more complete sentences, similar to TD children at the same vocabulary size, whereas children with DS produced more telegraphic and incomplete sentences. The difference between children with DS and those with WS was more marked on the repetition task, suggesting that phonological short-term memory may play a greater role when sentence production is measured through repetition. In addition, qualitative analysis of errors produced in the repetition test revealed interesting differences among the 3 groups. These results from younger children confirm and extend previous findings with older children and adolescents with WS. They further suggest that the apparently spared linguistic abilities of children with WS could emerge as an artifact of comparisons made to

Requests for reprints should be sent to Virginia Volterra, Istituto di Scienze e Tecnologie delle Cognizione via Nomentana, 56, 00161 Rome, Italy. E-mail: volterra@ip.rm.cnr.it

children with DS, whose sentence production competence is more compromised relative to other verbal and nonverbal abilities.

The study of language acquisition in special populations can offer particular insight into the relation between language and cognition. Early studies carried out by Bellugi, Bihrle, Neville, Jernigan, and Doherty (1992) underscored that "Williams syndrome presents a rare decoupling of language from other cognitive capacities...: linguistic functioning is selectively preserved in the face of severe general cognitive deficits" (p. 228). The particular cognitive and linguistic profile of children and adolescents with Williams syndrome (WS) has inspired some new thinking about the independence of language and cognition (e.g., Pinker, 1994, 1999; for a discussion see also Maratsos & Matheny, 1994).

The hypothesized dissociation between language and nonverbal cognition seems to emerge most clearly when performance by children with WS is compared to performance by children with Down syndrome (DS) on the same verbal and nonverbal tasks. The behavioral phenotypes of these two genetically determined syndromes appear to mirror each other.

Children with WS:

> ...have an unusual command of language: their comprehension is usually far more limited than their expressive language, which tends to be grammatically correct, complex and fluent at a superficial level, but verbose and pseudo-mature. Most individuals have a well-developed and precocious vocabulary, with excessive and frequently inappropriate use of clichés and stereotyped phrases. The children tend to be very chatty, and auditory memory, mimicry skills and social use of language are particularly well developed. (Udwin & Dennis, 1995, pp. 202–203)

In contrast, children with DS have

> specific difficulties with speech and language ... For most teenagers some aspects of expressive language are around a 3-year level. While vocabulary may progress quite well, the syntactic element of language is severely retarded (Fowler, 1990). Short sentence length and key word speech are characteristic. Speech production difficulties complicate the picture ... Many adults with the syndrome have mild/moderate hearing impairment. (Udwin & Dennis, 1995, pp. 106–107)

Comparative studies of adolescents with WS and adolescents with DS showed that the WS group was significantly more competent in terms of lexical abilities and semantic fluency, morphological abilities, and narrative abilities (Bellugi, Bihrle, Jernigan, Trauner, & Doherty, 1990; Bellugi et al., 1992; Reilly, Klima & Bellugi, 1991; Wang & Bellugi, 1993).

More recent studies, however, report partially different results. A study by Klein and Mervis (1999) showed that receptive lexical abilities are equivalent for 9- and 10-year-old children when the two syndrome groups were closely matched for chronological age (CA) and mental age (MA). Another study involving large numbers of children with WS and DS in the early stages of language development (Singer Harris, Bellugi, Bates, Jones, & Rossen, 1997) found that both syndrome groups were delayed in the onset of language. Expressive vocabulary acquisition was equivalent for the WS and DS groups. However, children with WS displayed a significant advantage over children with DS in the early stages of grammar. Finally, a study by Mervis and Robinson (2000) on very young groups of children with DS and WS, carefully matched for CA, confirmed that both syndromes evidence a language delay. However, in contrast to some of the results reported by Singer Harris et al. (1997), an expressive advantage for children with WS relative to children with DS was apparent even at age 2 years, 2 months (2:2).

Over the last 10 years various studies of Italian-speaking children and adolescents with WS and DS have been conducted by our laboratory with particular attention to linguistic and memory abilities. In this article we briefly review these studies. Then we report the first results of a major program for investigating and comparing early stages of language development of children with WS and children with DS. Our main goal is to investigate whether children with comparable levels of general cognitive impairment, but genetically distinct syndromes, are equivalently delayed in language acquisition, and if and how their linguistic profiles differ early in development.

PREVIOUS STUDIES OF ITALIAN CHILDREN WITH WS AND DS

In a first study (Volterra, Capirci, Pezzini, Sabbadini, & Vicari, 1996) we investigated linguistic abilities of Italian children with WS to answer specifically two relevant questions: (a) Are children with WS ahead of, behind, or equivalent to typically developing (TD) children of the same MA on language measures? (b) Do children with WS display unique patterns of grammatical morphology in a richly inflected language like Italian?

Lexical and morphosyntactic abilities of 17 individuals with WS between 4:10 and 15:3 were explored. The mean MA was 5:2 (range 3:8–6:8), reflecting a mean IQ of 56 (range 38–90). On all of the relevant language measures, lexical and grammatical, children with WS were compared to samples of TD children whose CA corresponded to the MA range of the WS group.

Results of the comparison showed that the two groups did not differ on the Peabody test for lexical comprehension, the Category Test for Semantic Fluency, or the mean length of utterance calculated from the story descriptions. However, individuals with WS did obtain significantly poorer scores than TD controls on the Test for the Reception of Grammar, the Boston Naming Test, and the Sentence

Repetition Test. In contrast, the participants with WS performed significantly better than TD controls on the Phonological Fluency test. However as the authors pointed out, children with WS "have had several years of experience with letter and alphabet games in school, while younger MA matched controls have had very little experience with letters" (Volterra et al., 1996, p. 673).

Our answer to the first question was that the language produced by participants with WS in this age range was for the most part not ahead of their MA, and that our data offered very little evidence for a dissociation between language and cognition. As to our second question, the language produced by our participants with WS was unusual from several points of view. By investigating language development in children with WS exposed to Italian we were able to see some patterns that would be difficult to detect in English. In particular, individuals with WS produced some grammatical errors that were qualitatively different from anything that has usually been reported for TD children acquiring Italian, including errors of gender agreement and verb conjugation.

We also conducted a detailed longitudinal study of the first stages of cognitive and linguistic development of an Italian girl with WS followed through weekly observations from 18 months to 58 months of age and systematically tested every 2 months (Capirci, Sabbadini, & Volterra, 1996). The results of the study confirmed a delayed and partially atypical profile of language development in children with WS. Following an initial delay which appeared less marked than is usually reported for children with WS, Elisa's rate and sequence of development seemed to be similar to those observed for TD children. However, in contrast to TD children, she displayed an uneven pattern of within-domain dissociations. Elisa exhibited fluent vocabulary and proficient use of syntax, at least in some contexts, but failed with simple grammatical agreement: She made several kinds of grammatical errors (gender agreement between article and noun and in pronominalization) that are rarely made by TD children at the same syntactic level.

More recently, we have explored the question of variability in performance among individuals with WS. Comparing Italian children and adolescents with WS to a group of younger TD children on the same visuospatial and linguistic tasks, we found results suggesting that individuals with WS do not exhibit a single cognitive profile. Instead, considerable variability across individuals was found. In the four individual cases we examined in detail, each child showed a different pattern of sparing and impairment on the linguistic and visual–spatial tasks. However, all four cases showed a particular difficulty in visuomotor construction in a block construction test (Pezzini, Vicari, Volterra, Milani, & Ossella, 1999).

In another study reporting a case of dizygotic twins, 1 boy with WS and 1 TD girl, our goal was to verify whether the child with WS displayed a cognitive profile unique to the syndrome (Volterra, Longobardi, Pezzini, Vicari, & Antenore, 1999). The special case gave us a unique opportunity to compare in more detail the neuropsychological profile of a child with WS with that of a TD control matched for CA and family background. At age 10:9, compared to his sister, the boy with WS displayed developmental delay in many nonverbal and verbal abilities. He achieved a level of performance similar to his sister only in facial recognition, phonological word fluency, and memory for phonologically similar words. However, despite the overall delayed performance of the boy with WS, both twins displayed a cognitive profile characterized by strength in lexical comprehension and relative weakness in visuomotor abilities.

Studies conducted by our laboratory have demonstrated that children with WS present, in the presence of well-preserved phonological processes, slightly impaired lexical–semantic and morphosyntactic abilities. A complex pattern of spared and impaired functions in both the linguistic and the visuospatial domains is the emerging picture of mental architecture in children with WS, replacing the previous interpretation of a simple dichotomy between language and visuospatial abilities (see also Karmiloff-Smith, 1985; Karmiloff-Smith et al., 1997; Mervis, Morris, Bertrand & Robinson, 1999).

Dissociations within the linguistic domain for individuals with WS, including greater efficiency of phonological than lexical–semantic encoding processes, are also supported by recent studies conducted by our group focusing on both short-term and long-term memory (Vicari, Brizzolara, Carlesimo, Pezzini, & Volterra, 1996; Vicari, Carlesimo, Brizzolara, & Pezzini, 1996). These studies demonstrated that memory abilities of children with WS appear to be characterized by a dissociation between normal short-term and deficient long-term verbal learning.

Specifically, Vicari, Brizzolara, et al. (1996), studying the position effect in a free recall of words task, demonstrated that the WS group recalled significantly more words from the terminal part (recency effect) than from the early part of the list (primacy effect). It is well known that recall of terminal items in a list-learning task is mostly based on the phonological encoding of stimuli (Basso, Spinnler, Vallar, & Zanobio, 1982; Shallice & Warrington, 1970). Furthermore, comparing the performance of children with WS to that of TD children in a word span task, it was found that the WS group revealed normal phonological similarity and length effects, but a reduced frequency effect (Vicari, Carlesimo, et al., 1996). These findings demonstrate a dissociation between normal phonological encoding and a reduced contribution of lexical–semantic encoding mechanisms to word span in children with WS.

Children with DS, with rare exceptions (Rondal, 1995; Vallar & Papagno, 1993), usually exhibit impairments in language acquisition. Indeed, as we have already seen, problems in morphology and syntax are frequently reported (Chapman, 1995; Fowler, 1990, 1995; Miller, 1992). Moreover, Fowler (1995) pointed out that the linguistic difficulties of persons with DS may be a consequence of "more basic difficulties at the phonological level, both in perceiving speech and in encoding incoming acoustic information into a representational format that can be accurately, and readily, retrieved to serve memory, production, and comprehension" (p. 127).

In recent years we have focused our attention on early communicative and linguistic development in Italian children with DS. Two studies investigated the relation between gestures and words in the early stages (Caselli, Longobardi, & Pisaneschi, 1997; Caselli et al., 1998), revealing a more extensive use of communicative gestures by children with DS compared to TD children at the same stage of communicative–linguistic development. This advantage in the gestural modality can be interpreted as an indirect sign of difficulty in the development of spoken language.

Another study (Vicari, Caselli, & Tonucci, 2000) explored the acquisition of language in children with DS, focusing on the potential dissociation between MA and specific aspects of language. Particular attention was given to the emergence of morphosyntactic abilities compared to the lexicon. Fifteen children with DS (from 4–7 years) and 15 TD children matched on MA participated in the study. For children with DS, results showed lower performance in language abilities compared to TD children. No dissociation was evident between lexical and cognitive abilities in either group, but specific morphosyntactic difficulties emerged both in comprehension and production for the DS group.

Fabbretti, Pizzuto, Vicari, and Volterra (1997) compared linguistic production in a story description task for older children and adolescents with DS (from 6–15 years) relative to TD controls matched on mean length of utterance. The results revealed strong individual differences in the sample of individuals with DS. Data analysis focused on a subset of lexical, morphological, and syntactic aspects of language use. The results showed that the children and adolescents with DS and their TD matches used a similar lexical repertoire. However, the two groups differed with respect to omission of free morphemes (more common in the DS group) and some aspects of syntactic and pragmatic abilities.

Children with DS, consistently with their linguistic difficulties, have been shown to have defective phonological short-term as well as long-term memory (Carlesimo, Marotta, & Vicari, 1997; Vicari, Carlesimo, & Caltagirone, 1995). In particular, Vicari et al. (1995) investigated verbal and spatial short-term memory abilities in persons with DS and with intellectual disability of different etiologies and documented a deficit of verbal and spatial backward spans in persons with DS, confirming a phonological memory deficit.

Most of our studies have been conducted separately on WS or DS populations. For example, children with WS were compared to TD children whose CA corresponded to the MA of the WS group and their linguistic performance was never directly compared to that of children with DS on the same tasks. Given the remarkable individual differences observed in the WS group in this study, we concentrate here on a qualitative analysis of early linguistic production of a small sample of young children with WS, comparing their performance with that of children with DS matched for CA and vocabulary size. The performance of both groups is compared to that of younger TD children matched for vocabulary size.

We pay particular attention to the selection of participants in each group because this is the first study in which we directly compared linguistic performance on different tasks across the three groups, that is, children with WS, children with DS, and TD controls.

METHOD

Participants

All the children with WS or with DS included in this study were tested at the Children's Hospital (Bambino Gesù) of Santa Marinella. The sample consisted of 6 children with WS, matched on the basis of CA, MA, and productive vocabulary size to 6 children with DS and 6 TD children matched on the basis of MA and vocabulary size. We first identified the children with WS and then tested children with DS until we found 6 who matched the 6 children with WS.

In all three groups, MA was assessed by the Brunet–Lezine Scale (1967) or the Leiter International Performance Scale (LIPS; Leiter, 1980).[1] Vocabulary repertoire was assessed with the Italian version of the MacArthur Communicative Development Inventory (CDI; Fenson et al., 1993). For present purposes, total words checked on the vocabulary list of the Words and Phrases Form (670 words) was taken.

The sample was further selected on the basis of the following criteria: a positive fluorescent *in situ* hybridization test for elastin deletion for children with WS and a free trisomy 21 documented by karyotyping for children with DS, the absence of any neurosensory deficits such as serious auditory or visual impairment, and absence of epilepsy and psychopathological disorders. The three groups of children were given the same tests. For evaluation purposes the children with WS and those with DS were examined in the hospital on two occasions across an approximately 2-week period. TD toddlers were examined individually at school. All the observations were videotaped and subsequently transcribed and analyzed after obtaining informed consent from the families. The CA in months and the expressive vocabulary

---

[1]The Brunet–Lezine Scale is used for assessing development of children from 1 to 36 months of age. Tests are distributed in four domains: postural control and motor ability; language; eye–hand coordination or adaptation to objects; and social and personal relationships. The LIPS is a culture-fair, nonverbal intelligence test of general mental ability that can be used from 2 to 18 years of age. Subtest items are categorized according to skills considered essential for problem solution, in eight categories. The subscales used in the first 3 years of life include matching (e.g., matching colors, block design, picture completion) and quantitative discrimination (e.g., number discrimination, counts four). It is likely that MAs based on the Brunet–Lezine and Leiter measures are not equivalent because the two tests partially differ in the domains that they assess. For this reason we will refer to the vocabulary size as a more reliable matching measure for the rest of the article.

size for all children are reported in Table 1 (including means and standard deviations for each group). As can be seen in Table 1, CA (mean and range) is very similar for the WS and DS children. As expected, the TD children are about 2 years younger than the other two groups, but the MA for each group is equivalent: mean 29 months for the WS group, 29 months for the DS group, and 30 months for the TD group (ranges 24–33, 25–36, and 25–37 respectively). An analysis of variance (ANOVA) demonstrated no statistical differences in MA in the three groups, $F(2, 15) = 0.02$. CA was significantly different, $F(2, 15) = 33.69$, $p < .0001$. Planned comparisons revealed significant differences between the TD and DS groups, $F(1, 15) = 59.3$, $p < .0001$, and between the TD and WS groups, $F(1, 15) = 39.8$, $p < .0001$, but no difference between the WS and DS groups, $F(1, 15) = 1.9$. The means and standard deviations for expressive vocabulary size were very similar in the three groups of children and correspond to the mean number of words reported for the Italian normative sample on the Primo Vocabolario del Bambino (PVB) for 30-month-old toddlers ($M = 446$, $SD = 168$; Caselli & Casadio, 1995). An ANOVA performed with group as the independent variable and number of words produced as the dependent variable showed no significant differences among the three groups, $F(2, 15) = 0.5$, *ns*, indicating that the three groups were well matched for productive vocabulary size.

Instruments

The First Child Vocabulary (PVB). The PVB (Caselli & Casadio, 1995) is the Italian version of the CDI (Fenson et al., 1993). The Words and Phrases Form of the PVB was used for this study, appropriate for the MA of the children (the

TABLE 1
Participants

	Williams Syndrome Group		*Down Syndrome Group*		*Typically Developing Group*	
Participant Number	*CA*	*Vocabulary Size*	*CA*	*Vocabulary Size*	*CA*	*Vocabulary Size*
1	44	306	64	298	31	331
2	58	345	48	385	29	395
3	41	349	61	430	31	478
4	62	369	58	433	30	530
5	56	578	64	500	31	565
6	55	630	51	521	28	603
M	53	430	58	428	30	484
SD	8.3	137.7	6.8	80.8	1.3	104.1

Note. CA = chronological age.

Words and Phrases Form is recommended and normed for TD children 18–30 months of age). The PVB consists of a section on vocabulary production and a section on grammar production. This section includes 37 pairs of phrases, with each phrase presented in two versions: the first is an incomplete phrase (telegraphic style), without any function words or lacking a predicate or necessary argument (e.g., "Medicine no!"); the second is a morphosyntactically complete version of the same phrase (e.g., "I don't want any medicine"). Parents were asked to fill out the questionnaire and were told the aim was to collect detailed information about their child's language development. Specifically, they were asked to mark with a cross on the vocabulary checklist those words that their child produces in spontaneous conversation. In the grammar scale, for each pair of phrases parents were asked to choose the one closest to the kinds of expressions spontaneously used by their child. All parents willingly participated in the data collection, showing interest in the instrument, which, as they often said, made them observe their child more carefully and become more aware of his or her real abilities.

On the grammar scale, three mutually exclusive scores were computed for each child: total number of pairs in which the more complete option was checked, total number of pairs in which the telegraphic option was checked, and total number items left unanswered.

First Language Test (Test del Primo Linguaggio [TPL]). This is an Italian standardized test for evaluating the first stages of language development (Axia, 1995). In this study we used the subscale for lexical production of nouns. This subscale consists of 20 pictures (plus 2 training pictures) depicting very common items from different lexical categories: vehicles, animals, people, and everyday objects. The child is requested to name each picture presented. We considered the total number of correct productions, the total number of nonresponses, and the total number of lexical substitutions taking into account the lexical categories of substituted words.

Sentence Repetition Test (Test di Ripetizione Frasi [TRF]). This is a word and sentence repetition test designed to assess Italian children's ability to imitate verbal stimuli, with an emphasis on both morphological and syntactic aspects of repetition (Devescovi, Caselli, Ossella, & Alviggi, 1992). All the words used in the test are appropriate for children in this MA age range, based on item analyses reported in Caselli and Casadio (1995). The test is accompanied by a set of 51 cards plus 3 training cards. Each card depicts the meaning of each noun and the overall meaning of each utterance. The repetition test was presented to each child individually as a game, introduced as follows: "Now let's play a game together: I will say something and you say the same thing." If the child did not respond at the first presentation of the stimulus phrase, it was repeated a second time, leaving the figure in view. For present purposes, three scores were derived from the repetition results, corresponding as closely as possible to the three mutually exclusive scores derived for the grammar scale of the PVB; a fourth score concerned correctness and accuracy of repetitions:

1. Total number of complete repetitions, where *complete* was defined as a repetition that reproduced (in some fashion) all the content words and function words in the target sentence. Children were not penalized on this measure if they altered or substituted words in their repetitions. Hence this is a measure of completeness, but not necessarily a measure of accuracy (e.g., the target sentence "Maria mette la bambola a letto" [Maria puts the doll in the bed] was repeated by the child as "Maria mette la bimba a letto" [Maria puts the child in the bed]).
2. Total number of incomplete repetitions, where *incomplete* was defined as a repetition that omits one or more content or function words in the target sentence (e.g., the target sentence "Il bimbo mangia la cioccolata" [The child eats the chocolate] was repeated by the child as "Bimbo mangia" [Child eats]).
3. Nonresponses, defined as failures to reproduce any part of the target (including silence or irrelevant comments).
4. Total number of phrases repeated correctly out of the total number of phrases repeated, where *correct* was defined as exact reproductions of all elements of the target sentence (e.g., the target sentence "Maria mette la bambola a letto" [Maria puts the doll in the bed] repeated by the child as "Maria mette la bimba a letto" [Maria puts the child in the bed] was considered not correct).

All omissions or alterations of content or function words were calculated. Further analyses of specific error types within these sentence repetitions (omission, lexical substitution, error of bound morphology, addition of new elements, word order inversion) were conducted.

RESULTS

Grammatical Complexity (PVB Section)

Table 2 reports the number of phrases (both telegraphic and morphosyntactically complete) checked by parents for each child of our sample, in addition to the means and standard deviations for each group of children. Considering the number of complete phrases relative to the telegraphic ones, we note that each TD child produced many more complete than telegraphic sentences; 4 of the 6 children with WS showed a similar trend, whereas all but 1 child with DS produced more telegraphic than complete sentences.

TABLE 2
PVB: Grammatical Complexity

Participant	*Williams Syndrome Group*			*Down Syndrome Group*			*Typically Developing Group*		
Number	*Complete*	*Telegraphic*	*No Response*	*Complete*	*Telegraphic*	*No Response*	*Complete*	*Telegraphic*	*No Response*
1	4	7	26	10	24	3	37	0	0
2	12	2	23	4	19	14	12	5	20
3	13	4	20	4	30	3	31	3	3
4	5	22	10	4	29	4	31	0	6
5	37	0	0	12	18	7	37	0	0
6	37	0	0	35	1	1	36	1	0
M	18.0	5.83	13.17	11.5	20.17	5.33	30.67	1.5	4.83
SD	15.1	8.4	11.6	12	10.6	4.7	9.6	2.1	7.8

Note. PVB = IL Primo Vocabulario del Bambino (The First Child Vocabulary).

To evaluate these trends statistically, we began by conducting three separate between-subject analyses of variance across the three groups, one for each of the three (mutually exclusive) measures of sentence complexity/completeness. In the category of nonresponses (sentence pairs left unchecked), there was no significant effect of group, $F(2, 17) = 1.82$, *ns*. Hence we focused the rest of our attention on the two more interesting categories of complete/complex versus incomplete/telegraphic phrases.

The analysis of number of complete options checked by parents did yield a significant group difference, $F(2, 17) = 3.67, p < .05$. To explore this effect further, a post-hoc analysis (Tukey HSD test) was conducted comparing each pair of groups. The difference between the WS and DS groups did not reach significance ($p = .65$), nor was there a significant difference between the children with WS and the TD children ($p = .2$). However, the contrast between the DS group and the TD controls did reach significance ($p < .05$), reflecting substantially fewer complete phrases checked by the parents of children with DS.

The analysis of number of incomplete or telegraphic options checked by parents also yielded a significant group difference, $F(2, 17) = 9.20, p < .002$. Post-hoc analysis (Tukey HSD test) of each pair of groups indicated that children with DS were reported to produce significantly more incomplete phrases than both children with WS ($p < .02$) and TD controls ($p < .003$). In contrast, there was no difference between the WS and TD groups in number of incomplete or telegraphic options checked ($p = .62$).

Results of these separate analyses for each variable suggest that the three groups differ in the relation between telegraphic and complete utterances. To confirm this impression, we constructed a new measure: the number of incomplete or telegraphic options checked, divided by the sum of complete and incomplete selections (ignoring nonresponses). As we shall see, this new proportional measure also proves useful in the sentence repetition analyses presented later, including comparisons between the two tasks. A visual representation of this relation for each of the three groups is presented in Figure 1.

This figure shows that the highest proportion of telegraphic/complete speech was observed in children with DS ($M = .653$, $SD = .33$), the lowest ratio was observed in TD children ($M = .068$, $SD = .12$), with the WS group falling in between ($M = .305$, $SD = .36$). A one-way between-subjects ANOVA across the three groups was conducted on these ratios, yielding a significant effect of group, $F(2, 17) = 6.59, p < .01$. To explore this effect further, post-hoc analyses (Tukey HSD test) were also conducted. The difference between children with WS and children with DS missed significance ($p < .11$), and there was also no difference between the WS group and TD control group ($p < .34$). However, the contrast between children with DS and TD children was significant ($p < .007$). In other words, for this parent report measure of sentence complexity, the group difference in the relation between telegraphic and complete utterances is coming primarily from the DS group. By contrast, children with WS were more like TD children at the same vocabulary level.

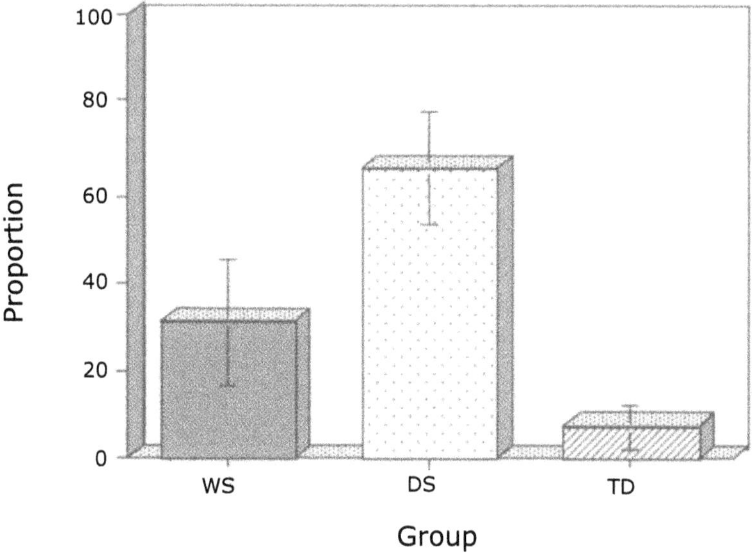

FIGURE 1 The First Child Vocabulary (PVB): Proportion of sentence pairs for which parents selected the telegraphic/incomplete option.

First Language Test (TPL)

Results on the vocabulary naming test are reported in Table 3. The numbers of correct labels, substitutions, and nonresponses are presented for each child, as well as group means and standard deviations. No significant differences were found among the groups. These results confirm that the three groups of children are matched not only for vocabulary size measured by parental report, but also on lexical production measured by a naming test in the laboratory. Furthermore, a qualitative analysis revealed no differences in the types of substitutions produced by the three groups. The number of substitutions that were not from the same semantic category (indicated in parentheses in the table) was very low in all groups. Also, the labels produced by children were similar across the three groups. Children with WS did not use rare or strange words.

Sentence Repetition Test (TRF)

Table 4 presents results for each child (as well as group means and standard deviations) for the three measures taken from the sentence repetition test: complete repetitions (e.g., the target sentence "Anna porta la torta in cucina" [Anna takes

TABLE 3
TPL: Lexical Production of Nouns

Participant Number	*Williams Syndrome Group*			*Down Syndrome Group*			*Typically Developing Group*		
	Correct Label	*Substitution*[a]	*No Response*	*Correct Label*	*Substitution*[a]	*No Response*	*Correct Label*	*Substitution*[a]	*No Response*
1	3	5 (2)	12	14	5 (0)	1	10	4 (1)	6
2	13	5 (0)	2	14	5 (1)	1	11	6 (1)	3
3	14	6 (1)	0	11	2 (0)	7	13	7 (2)	0
4	10	5 (1)	5	2	2 (0)	16	12	4 (0)	4
5	11	7 (0)	2	13	6 (2)	1	16	3 (1)	1
6	12	4 (0)	4	12	2 (0)	6	12	8 (3)	0
M	10.5	5.3	4	11	4	5	12	5	2
SD	3.9	1.0	4.2	4.6	1.9	5.9	2.1	2.0	2.4

Note. TPL = Test del Primo Linguaggio (First Language Test).
[a]Child's labels from a different semantic category are reported in parentheses (e.g., picture of an apple was labeled "ball").

TABLE 4
TRF: Types of Sentences Repeated

	Williams Syndrome Group			*Down Syndrome Group*			*Typically Developing Group*		
Participant Number	*Complete Repetitions*	*Incomplete Repetitions*	*No Response*	*Complete Repetitions*	*Incomplete Repetitions*	*No Response*	*Complete Repetitions*	*Incomplete Repetitions*	*No Response*
1	28	21	2	21	30	0	38	13	0
2	37	14	0	5	29	17	39	12	0
3	31	19	1	4	45	2	33	17	1
4	29	6	16	6	21	24	9	6	36
5	40	9	2	5	6	40	39	12	0
6	50	1	0	41	6	4	6	22	23
M	36	12	4	14	23	15	27	14	10
SD	8.4	7.7	6.2	14.9	15.2	15.6	15.6	5.4	15.7

Note. TRF = Test di Ripetizione Frasi (Sentence Repetition Test).

the cake into the kitchen] was repeated by the child as "Anna porta la torta a cucina" [Anna takes the cake at kitchen]); incomplete repetitions (e.g., the target sentence "Il gatto prende il topo piccolo" [The cat takes the little mouse] was repeated by the child as "Gatto piccolo" [Little cat]); and nonresponses (failures to reproduce any part of the target). As Table 4 shows, there was substantial variability within groups on these measures, although group differences similar to those observed with parent report are evident.

To analyze these differences statistically, we began with separate one-way between-group ANOVAs for each of the three measures in Table 3. For the nonresponse category, there was no significant group difference, $F(2, 17) = 1.04$, *ns*. The analysis of incomplete repetitions also failed to reach significance, $F(2, 17) = 2.00$, *ns*. However, there was a significant effect of group on the total number of complete repetitions produced, $F(2, 17) = 4.23$, $p < .035$. To explore this three-way group difference further, post-hoc analyses (Tukey HSD test) were conducted among the groups. In contrast with the analyses conducted earlier for parent report, in this repetition task the difference between children with WS and children with DS did reach significance ($p < .03$). However, the difference between the DS group and the TD control group was not significant ($p < .25$), nor was there a significant difference between the WS group and the TD control group ($p = .53$).

Cell means in Table 4 suggest that the relation between complete and incomplete repetitions may also differ across groups. We therefore computed the proportion of incomplete repetitions to complete plus incomplete repetitions for each child, analogous to the proportion scores reported earlier for the PVB. We again found that the proportion of telegraphic or incomplete repetitions was highest in children with DS ($M = .635$, $SD = .29$). The corresponding proportions were lower in TD children ($M = .375$, $SD = .21$) and even lower in children with WS ($M = .243$, $SD = .15$). A visual representation of these data is provided in Figure 2.

Comparing Figures 1 and 2, we note that, in contrast with results for parent report, the children with WS and the TD children have changed positions: Whereas the WS group fell between the TD children and children with DS in the parent-report proportion scores, TD children fall between children with WS and children with DS in proportion scores for sentence repetition.

Mirroring the analyses conducted earlier for parent report, we subjected these proportion scores to a one-way between-group ANOVA, yielding a significant main effect, $F(2, 17) = 4.76$, $p < .03$. Post-hoc analysis (Tukey HSD test) showed that the difference between the WS and the DS groups did reach significance in this analysis ($p < .03$), in contrast to the nonsignificant trend for parent report. The difference between children with DS and TD children missed significance in this analysis ($p < .15$), another contrast with our findings for the same children using parent report. The contrast between children with WS and TD children

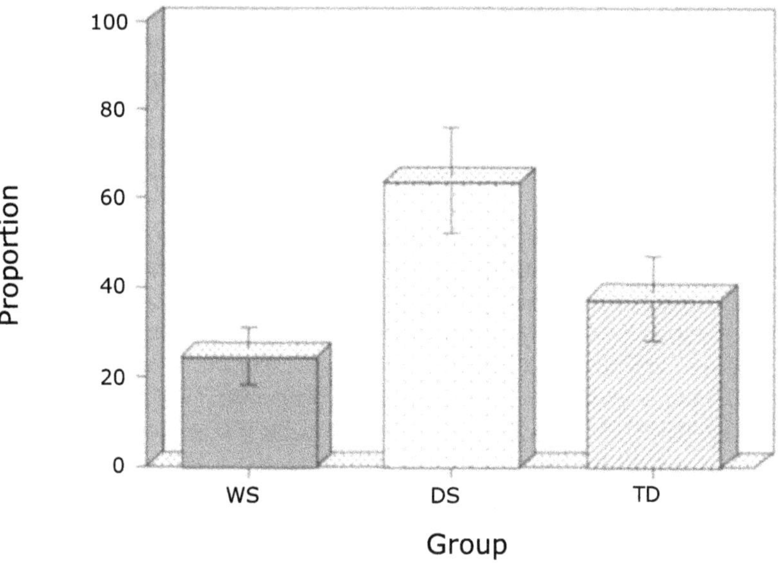

FIGURE 2 Sentence Repetition Test: Proportion of sentence repetitions that were telegraphic or incomplete.

failed to reach significance ($p = .57$), which was also true in the parent report analyses.

To summarize so far, the sentence repetition findings confirm results using parent report in two respects. First, there were significant differences among the three groups on proportion scores for both measures. Second, children with WS perform like younger TD children at the same vocabulary level on both measures. However, the two measures yield a different ranking among these three groups. On the parent reports, children with WS fell between children with DS and TD children (and the difference between the WS and the DS groups did not reach significance). On the repetition test, it was the TD children who fell between the low telegraphic proportion scores observed in children with WS and the high scores observed in children with DS. To determine whether this apparent shift in ranking is significant, we carried out a multivariate analysis of variance with proportion scores for the two measures serving as a within-subjects variable and the three groups serving as a between-subjects variable. This analysis yielded a significant main effect of group, $F(2, 15) = 6.43, p < .01$, reflecting more telegraphic speech for children with DS in both tasks. There was no significant main effect of task, $F(1, 15) = 1.71$, *ns*. However, most important for our purposes here, there was a significant interaction between task and group, $F(2, 15) = 4.06, p < .04$, confirming that the repetition task yielded an advantage for children with WS that was less apparent when sentence complexity was measured by parent report.

As a final point, we were interested in determining whether the two proportion scores were correlated across tasks (collapsing across the three groups to look at individual differences). A Pearson product–moment correlation between proportion scores for the PVB and sentence repetition was significant ($r = +.62, p < .002$). To test the limits of this relation further, the correlation was recalculated partialing out group as well as total vocabulary scores. The resulting correlation was still strong ($r = +.55, p < .03$).

We were also interested in analyzing correctness of the repetitions produced by the three groups. Table 5 presents for each child the number of repeated sentences and the number of the correct ones, in addition to means and standard deviations for each group. As shown in Table 5, most children in both the WS and the TD groups were able to repeat almost all the target sentences presented, while only three children with DS exhibited a similar performance. The DS group repeated fewer sentences ($M = 36.5$) than the WS and the TD groups ($M = 47.5$ and $M = 41$, respectively). Nevertheless, an ANOVA analysis did not show any significant difference among the three groups, $F(2, 15) = 1.12$. More evident is the difference in the mean of correct sentences repeated by children with DS ($M = 10$) and by the other two groups ($M = 28.7$ for the WS group and $M = 25.3$ for the TD group). An ANOVA approaches significance, $F(2, 15) = 3.41, p = .06$.

Sentences correctly repeated, but in which one or more words were added, were counted as correct sentences. Sentences with additions were produced by the children with WS ($M = 7.3$), but were very rarely observed in the other two groups ($M = 0.6$ and $M = 0.5$ for the DS and the TD groups, respectively). Examples of additions produced by children with WS are: the target sentence "Il bimbo va a casa" (The child goes home) was repeated with a local addition, in the middle of the sentence, as "Il bimbo va a guardare la casa" (The child goes to look the house); and

TABLE 5
TRF: Repeated and Correct Sentences

Participant Number	*Williams Syndrome Group*		*Down Syndrome Group*		*Typically Developing Group*	
	Repeated	*Correct*	*Repeated*	*Correct*	*Repeated*	*Correct*
1	49	21	51	10	51	38
2	51	23	34	4	51	38
3	50	27	49	0	50	26
4	35	20	27	4	15	9
5	49	33	11	7	51	38
6	51	48	47	35	28	3
M	47.5	29	36.5	10	41	25
SD	5.8	10.6	15.6	12.7	15.7	15.8

Note. TRF = Test di Repetizione Frasi (Sentence Repetition Test).

the target sentence "Il topo" (The mouse) was repeated as "Il topo mangia il formaggio" (The mouse eats the cheese), with a final addition at the end of the sentence. The total number of additions for children with WS was 44 (25 final additions and 19 local additions), in contrast to only 4 and 3 for the DS and the TD groups respectively. The additions provided by the children with WS were generally not consistent with the picture they were shown (e.g., in the picture presented with the target sentence "The mouse" a piece of cheese was not shown). However, in some cases the additions provided by these children reflected linguistic material presented in previous items.

Finally, we calculated the total number of errors produced by children considering only the sentences that the child attempted to repeat. We counted: each element omitted (specifying also the number of omissions in obligatory contexts) or substituted (the child repeated the target sentence, substituting one or more elements—article, name, verb, preposition, etc.); each morphological modification of a word (the child used in the repeated sentence a different morphological form of the same word—a singular form instead of a plural one, a feminine instead of a masculine form, etc.); and each repetition with word order inversion (a different order of one or more elements in the sentence repeated), without taking into account the number of inverted elements. No child made more than one modification to a word.

Table 6 presents for each child the type of errors produced, with means and standard deviations for each group. The total number of errors was 179 for children with WS, 360 for children with DS, and 174 for TD children. The mean number of errors produced was very similar for children with WS and TD children. The mean number of errors produced by children with DS, was almost twice that produced by the WS and the TD groups. Nevertheless, an ANOVA did not show any significant difference among the three groups: $F(2, 15) = 3.05$, $p = .07$. Probably, the absence of a significant difference in this analysis was due to the particular performance of two children with DS (#5 and #6), combined with the small sample size.

To analyze in more detail the types of errors produced from a qualitative perspective, Figure 3 presents the proportion of the different types of errors produced by the three groups of children: omissions, lexical substitutions, errors of bound morphology, and word inversion. Omissions were proportionally the most frequent error produced by all groups of children. For the children with WS, the percentage of omissions was lower (71%) than that for both the children with DS (87%) and the TD children (87%).

Errors in bound morphology were present in an appreciable proportion in both the WS and the DS groups (10% and 4%, respectively), but they were almost absent in the TD group (0.5%). Lexical substitutions were proportionally produced more frequently by children with WS (15%) than by children with DS (7%) or TD children (4%). The lexical substitutions produced by the TD group involve nouns,

TABLE 6
TRF: Number and Type of Errors

Participant Number	*Williams Syndrome Group* Omission[a]	Lexical Substitution	Bound Morphology	Word Order Inversion	*Down Syndrome Group* Omission[a]	Lexical Substitution	Bound Morphology	Word Order Inversion	*Typically Developing Group* Omission[a]	Lexical Substitution	Bound Morphology	Word Order Inversion
1	43 (13)	2	2	4	76 (19)	4	7	4	13 (11)	0	0	0
2	21 (11)	13	6	0	73 (18)	3	2	0	23 (9)	1	0	0
3	35 (16)	0	4	0	90 (43)	7	3	1	43 (10)	3	1	7
4	12 (7)	4	5	1	45 (22)	6	1	0	14 (3)	0	0	3
5	14 (8)	8	0	1	16 (3)	0	1	0	18 (5)	1	0	1
6	2 (1)	0	1	1	13 (1)	5	2	1	41 (28)	2	0	3
M	21	5	3	1	52	4	3	1	25	1	0	2
SD	15.3	5.1	2.4	1.5	32.6	2.5	2.3	1.6	13.4	1.2	0.4	2.7

Note. TRF = Test di Ripetizione Frasi (Sentence Repetition Test).
[a]Omissions in obligatory contexts are reported in parentheses.

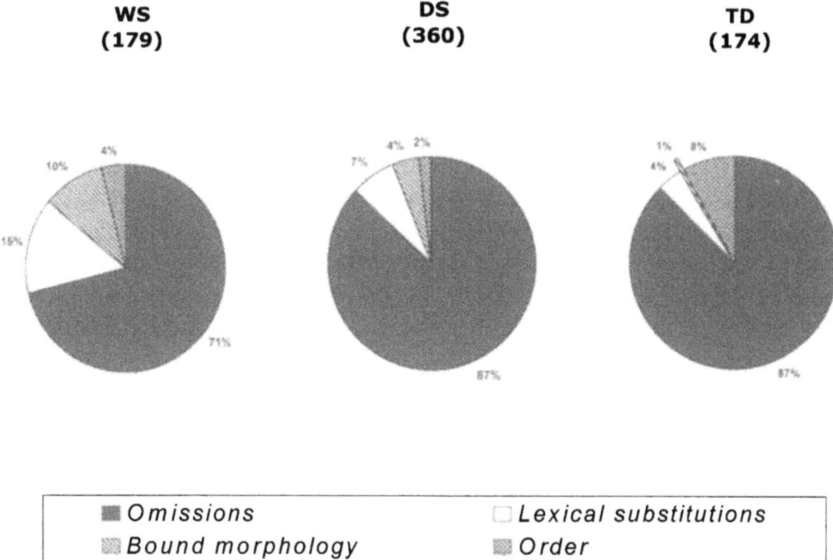

FIGURE 3 Sentence Repetition Test (TRF): Proportion of different error types (total number of errors in parentheses).

whereas the lexical substitutions produced by the WS and the DS groups involve not only nouns, but also articles, prepositions, and verbs.

Finally, word order inversions were produced in a higher proportion by TD children (8%), in an appreciable percentage by children with WS (4%), and in a lower proportion by children with DS (2%). Only the WS and DS groups produced sentences in which the order inversion generated semantically or grammatically unacceptable sentences.

SUMMARY AND DISCUSSION

In this study we explored early linguistic abilities in two genetic syndromes with cognitive impairment: children with WS and children with DS. We examined children matched for productive vocabulary size in the early stages of sentence production corresponding for them to a CA range from 3 to 6 years and to an MA range from 2 to 3 years. We considered not only data from parent report, as have other studies on the same populations of children (Mervis & Robinson, 2000; Singer Harris et al., 1997), but also data collected using a naming test and a sentence repetition test designed to investigate the children's ability to imitate specific morphological and syntactic aspects of Italian. Comparable data were collected on both measures with TD toddlers matched for vocabulary size. Results of our study confirm that most children with WS or DS evidence a consistent language delay at an early age as shown by other studies (Mervis & Robinson, 2000; Singer Harris et al., 1997). However, we underscore that the children we examined were older than the children examined by Mervis and Robinson (2000) and by Singer Harris et al. (1997), and in contrast to those studies, the groups of children with WS and DS were matched not only for CA, but also for MA and lexical repertoire. Moreover, all measures also were collected for a group of TD children matched for MA and lexical repertoire. The matching in lexical abilities is confirmed in our study by the results of the naming test: We did not find differences in the vocabulary level or in the numbers and types of lexical substitutions produced by the three groups.

Data for sentence production from parental reports also revealed interesting findings: Children with DS were reported to produce a significantly higher proportion of telegraphic sentences than TD controls and a significantly greater absolute number of incomplete sentences than both the children with WS and the TD controls. Similar findings were reported in Singer-Harris et al. (1997) and confirmed in a recent Italian study of 15 children with DS using the PVB (Vicari et al., 2000). Data on the sentence repetition test showed a similar trend: Children with WS did not differ from TD children in the number or proportion of complete repetitions, and they produced far more complete sentences (in absolute numbers and in proportion scores) than children with DS at the same CA and expressive vocabulary level.

Despite the clear similarity in results for our two tasks, it is also interesting to underline that the repetition task yielded a larger advantage for children with WS than we found when sentence complexity is measured by parent report. On parent report, children with WS fell between TD controls and children with DS in their telegraphic/complete proportion scores. On the repetition task, WS children showed the lowest telegraphic scores overall, with TD controls falling in between. We think that this difference between the two tasks may be related to the preserved phonological short-term memory ability that has been observed in children with WS. In filling out the grammar scale of the PVB, parents are asked to respond to each sentence pair by reflecting on the range of utterances that their children typically produce in spontaneous speech. Although it is likely that grammatical knowledge and short-term memory both play a role in the spontaneous speech that parents are asked to recall, it is reasonable to assume that the repetition test draws more heavily on verbal short-term memory. Hence, although it is clear that the repetition task works well with mentally handicapped children in this age range, repetition is likely to enhance differences between children with WS and children with DS matched for CA and vocabulary size. On a purely qualitative basis, we note that children with WS and children with DS are similar in the types of errors they produce: Morphological errors and word inversion errors that result in ungrammatical utterances are observed in both groups, but not in the TD group.

Nevertheless, there are intriguing qualitative differences between the WS and the DS groups at a more detailed level, including a tendency for children with WS to produce errors that are rarely observed in children with DS or in TD children at any age (e.g., the tendency for children with WS to add material that was not present in the model). In many cases the material added was not consistent with the picture shown at that time, but was present in a target sentence presented some items before. It is possible that children with WS have a spared ability to hear and store speech sounds, which permits them to acquire some aspects of language that are especially difficult for children with DS, but this ability is not enough to guarantee productive control over all grammatical aspects of language (Volterra, Capirci, & Caselli, 2001).

To summarize so far, the results reported in this study with younger children confirm and extend previous findings with older children and adolescents with WS. They confirm that language is not ahead of MA in the WS population in this early age range, in line with a revised view that has already been suggested by previous studies (Gosch, Städing, & Pankau, 1994; Mervis & Robinson, 2000; Volterra et al., 1996). Our results further suggest that the apparently spared linguistic abilities of children with WS are in part an artifact of comparisons made to children with DS, whose morphosyntactic production abilities are more compromised relative to their MA and to their lexical repertoire. Children with WS do not speak like TD peers at the same CA; they have an expressive lexical repertoire and use sentences like younger TD children, but produce types of errors rarely produced by them. Children with WS produce morphological errors like children with DS, errors almost absent in TD children. Furthermore, the word order inversions produced by children with WS or DS sometimes result in ungrammatical, unacceptable utterances for the WS and DS groups; in contrast, word order inversions produced by TD children consistently result in grammatical utterances. Thus, these differences relative to TD children could be related to cognitive impairment and not to a specific genetic syndrome.

The pattern of results that we have reported here underscores the value of direct comparisons of linguistic production in matched samples of children with WS and children with DS, as well as younger TD children. However, because the sample sizes used in this study were relatively small, we do not have enough statistical power to conduct fine-grained analyses. Nevertheless, our results underscore the importance of qualitative studies. The three groups of children we examined matched for expressive vocabulary size evidenced different profiles in their morphosyntactic abilities, showing once again that similar behavioral outcomes in one aspect of development can mask interesting differences in other aspects of the same domain (Karmiloff-Smith, 1997).

ACKNOWLEDGMENTS

The research reported here was partially supported by a Telethon–Italy Project, A Study on the Williams Syndrome: Links Between Genes, Neurobiology and Cognition (Grant No. E.C. 685). We are particularly grateful to Elizabeth Bates for her valuable advice during the revision of the manuscript, and to P. Pasqualetti for statistical consultation.

REFERENCES

Axia, G. (1995). *Il Test del Primo Linguaggio.* Florence, Italy: Organizzazioni Speciali.

Basso, A., Spinnler, H., Vallar, G., & Zanobio, M. E. (1982). Left hemisphere damage and selective impairment of auditory verbal short-term memory: A case study. *Neuropsychologia, 20,* 263–274.

Bellugi, U., Bihrle, A., Jernigan, T., Trauner, D., & Doherty, S. (1990). Neuropsychological, neurological and neuroanatomical profile of Williams syndrome. *American Journal of Medical Genetics, 1*(Suppl. 6), 15–125.

Bellugi, U., Bihrle, A., Neville, H., Jernigan, T., & Doherty, S. (1992). Language, cognition and brain organization in a neurodevelopmental disorder. In M. Gunnar & C. Nelson (Eds.), *Developmental Behavioral Neuroscience* (pp. 201–232). Hillsdale, NJ: Lawrence Erlbaum Associates, Inc.

Brunet, O., & Lezine, I. (1967). *Scala di Sviluppo Psicomotorio della Prima Infanzia.* Florence, Italy: Organizzazioni Speciali.

Capirci, O., Sabbadini, L., & Volterra, V. (1996). Language development in Williams syndrome: A case study. *Cognitive Neuropsychology, 13,* 1017–1039.

Carlesimo G. A., Marotta, L., & Vicari, S. (1997). Long-term memory in mental retardation: Evidence for a specific impairment in subjects with Down's syndrome. *Neuropsychologia, 35,* 71–79.

Caselli, M. C., & Casadio, P. (1995). *Il Primo Vocabolario del Bambino. Guida all'uso del questionario MacArthur per la valutazione della comunicazione e del linguaggio nei primi anni di vita.* Milan, Italy: Franco Angeli.

Caselli, M. C., Longobardi, E., & Pisaneschi, R. (1997). Gesti e parole in bambini con sindrome di Down. *Psicologia Clinica dello Sviluppo, 1,* 45–63.

Caselli, M. C., Vicari, S., Longobardi, E., Lami, L., Pizzoli, C., & Stella, G. (1998). Gestures and words in early development of children with Down syndrome. *Journal of Speech, Language, and Hearing Research, 41,* 1125–1135.

Chapman, R. S. (1995). Language development in children and adolescents with Down syndrome, In P. Fletcher & B. MacWhinney (Eds.), *The handbook of child language* (pp. 641–663). Oxford, England: Blackwell.

Devescovi, A., Caselli, M. C., Ossella, T., & Alviggi, F. G. (1992). Strumenti di indagine sulle prime fasi dello sviluppo linguistico: Risultati di una prova di ripetizione di frasi con bambini fra i due e i tre anni e mezzo. *Rassegna di Psicologia, 2, 9,* 29–54.

Fabbretti, D., Pizzuto, E., Vicari, S., & Volterra, V. (1997). A story description task with Down syndrome: Lexical and morphosyntactic abilities. *Journal of Intellectual Disability Research, 41,* 165–179.

Fenson, L., Dale, P. S., Reznick, J. S., Thal, D., Bates, E., Hartung, J. P. et al. (1993). *MacArthur Communicative Development Inventories: User's guide and technical manual.* San Diego, CA: Singular.

Fowler, A. E. (1990). Language abilities in children with Down syndrome: Evidence for a specific delay. In D. Cicchetti & M. Beeghly (Eds.), *Children with Down syndrome: A developmental perspective* (pp. 302–328). Cambridge, England: Cambridge University Press.

Fowler, A. E. (1995). Language variability in persons with Down syndrome: Research and implications. In L. Nadel & D. Rosenthal (Eds.), *Down syndrome: Living and learning in the community* (pp. 121–131). New York: Wiley-Liss.

Gosch, A., Städing, G., & Pankau, R. (1994). Linguistic abilities in children with Williams–Beuren syndrome. *American Journal of Medical Genetics, 52,* 291–296.

Karmiloff-Smith, A. (1985). Language and cognitive processes from a developmental perspective. *Language and Cognitive Processes, 1,* 61–85.

Karmiloff-Smith, A. (1997). Crucial differences between developmental neurosciences and adult neuropsychology. *Developmental Neuropsychology, 13,* 513–524.

Karmiloff-Smith, A., Grant, J., Berthoud, I., Davies, M., Howlin, P., & Udwin, O. (1997). Language and Williams syndrome: How intact is "intact"? *Child Development, 68,* 246–262.

Klein, B. P., & Mervis C. B. (1999). Cognitive strength and weaknesses of 9- and 10-year-olds with Williams syndrome or Down syndrome. *Developmental Neuropsychology, 16,* 177–196.

Leiter, R. G. (1980). *Leiter International Performance Scale.* Chicago: Stoelting.

Maratsos, M., & Matheny, L. (1994). Language specificity and elasticity: Brain and clinical syndrome studies. *Annual Review of Psychology, 45,* 487–516.

Mervis, C. B., Morris, C.A., Bertrand, J., & Robinson, B. F. (1999). Williams syndrome: Findings from an integrated program of research. In H. Tager-Flusberg (Ed.), *Neurodevelopmental disorders: Contribution to a new framework from the cognitive neurosciences* (pp. 65–110). Cambridge, MA: MIT Press.

Mervis, C. B., & Robinson, B. F. (2000). Expressive vocabulary ability of toddlers with Williams syndrome or Down syndrome: A comparison. *Developmental Neuropsychology, 17,* 111–126.

Miller, J. F. (1992). Development of speech and language in children with Down syndrome. In J. Y. Lott & E. E. Mc Loy (Eds.), *Clinical care for persons with Down syndrome* (pp. 39–50). Cambridge, MA: MIT Press.

Pezzini, G., Vicari, S., Volterra, V., Milani, L., & Ossella, M. T. (1999). Children with Williams syndrome: Is there a single neuropsychological profile? *Developmental Neuropsychology, 15,* 141–155.

Pinker, S. (1994). *The language instinct: How the mind creates language.* New York: Morrow.

Pinker, S. (1999). *Words and rules.* London: Weidenfeld & Nicholson.

Reilly, J. S., Klima, E. S., & Bellugi, U. (1991). Once more with feeling: Affect and language in atypical populations. *Development and Psychopathology, 2,* 367–391.

Rondal, J. A. (1995). *Exceptional language development in Down syndrome.* Cambridge, England: Cambridge University Press.

Shallice, T., & Warrington, E. K. (1970). Independent functioning of verbal memory stores: A neuropsychological study. *Quarterly Journal of Experimental Psychology, 22,* 261–273.

Singer Harris, N., Bellugi, U., Bates, E., Jones, W., & Rossen, M. (1997). Contrasting profiles of language development in children with Williams and Down syndromes. *Developmental Neuropsychology, 13,* 345–370.

Udwin, O., & Dennis, J. (1995). Psychological and behavioural phenotypes in genetically determined syndromes: A review of research findings. In G. O'Brien & W. Yule (Eds.), *Behavioural phenotypes* (pp. 90–208). London: MacKeith.

Vallar, G., & Papagno, C. (1993). Preserved vocabulary acquisition in Down's syndrome children: The role of phonological short-term memory. *Cortex, 29,* 467–483.

Vicari, S., Brizzolara, D., Carlesimo G. A., Pezzini, G., & Volterra, V. (1996). Memory abilities in children with Williams syndrome. *Cortex, 32,* 503–514.

Vicari, S., Carlesimo, G., Brizzolara, D., & Pezzini, G. (1996). Short-term memory in children with Williams syndrome: A reduced contribution of lexical-semantic knowledge to word span. *Neuropsychologia, 34,* 919–925.

Vicari, S., Carlesimo, A., & Caltagirone, C. (1995). Short-term memory in persons with intellectual disabilities and Down syndrome. *Journal of Intellectual Disability Research, 39,* 532–537.

Vicari, S., Caselli, M. C., & Tonucci, F., (2000). Asynchrony of lexical and morphosyntactic development in children with Down syndrome. *Neuropsychologia. 38,* 634–644.

Volterra, V., Capirci, O., & Caselli, M. C. (2001). What atypical populations can reveal about language development: The contrast between deafness and Williams syndrome. *Language and Cognitive Processes, 16,* 219–239.

Volterra, V., Capirci, O., Pezzini, G., Sabbadini, L., & Vicari, S. (1996). Linguistic abilities in Italian children with Williams syndrome. *Cortex, 32,* 663–677.

Volterra, V., Longobardi, E., Pezzini, G., Vicari, S., & Antenore, C. (1999). Visuo-spatial and linguistic abilities in a twin with Williams syndrome. *Journal of Intellectual Disability Research, 43,* 294–305.

Wang, P., & Bellugi, U. (1993). Williams syndrome, Down syndrome and cognitive neuroscience. *American Journal of Diseases of Children, 147,* 1246–1251.

Morphological Abilities of Hebrew-Speaking Adolescents With Williams Syndrome

Yonata Levy
Psychology Department and
Hadassah–Hebrew University Medical School
Jerusalem, Israel

Shula Hermon
Weinberg Child Development Center
Sheba Medical Center
Tel-Hashomer, Israel

In recent years research has focused on the exact nature of the linguistic skills that individuals with Williams syndrome (WS) exhibit. This work has resulted in controversial positions, with an increasing number of studies casting doubt on previous claims of superior linguistic competence for individuals with WS. This study investigated morphosyntactic knowledge in Hebrew-speaking adolescents with WS. The participants' performance was compared to 2 groups of typically developing mental age-matched controls. Participants and controls were tested on experimental tasks designed to investigate knowledge of morphology. The findings suggest that individuals with WS have good control over the basic consonantal root structure of Hebrew words. However, rather poor performance was evident on other morphological paradigms. We conclude that there is little evidence from Hebrew to support a selective preservation of grammatical competence in individuals with WS.

The cognitive profile of individuals with Williams syndrome (WS) has been characteristically described as composed of spared auditory short-term memory and spared linguistic and face recognition abilities together with serious deficits in number skills,

---

Requests for reprints should be sent to Yonata Levy, Psychology Department, Hadassah–Hebrew University Medical School, Jerusalem, Israel. E-mail: msyonata@mscc.huji.ac.il

visuospatial cognition, motor behavior, planning, and problem-solving (Bellugi, Marks, Bihrle, & Sabo, 1993; Bellugi, Mills, Jernigan, Hickock, & Galaburda, 1999; Bellugi, Wang, & Jernigan, 1994; Gosch, Städing, & Pankau, 1994; Mervis, Morris, Bertrand, & Robinson, 1999; Udwin & Yule, 1991; Udwin, Yule, & Marin, 1987). Studies of language in individuals with WS in the 1980s and early 1990s often presented WS as the prime example within developmental disorders of the dissociation of language from other cognitive skills, particularly from visuomotor skills.

In recent years research has focused on the exact nature of the linguistic competence that individuals with WS exhibit. This work has resulted in controversial positions, with an increasing number of studies casting doubt on the claim of superior linguistic performance of individuals with WS. At the focus of this debate are studies of morphosyntax and lexical semantics. In the review of the literature that follows we focus on the former because this is the area of linguistic knowledge to which studies of Hebrew are uniquely relevant.

In her seminal work on the cognitive profile of adolescents and adults with WS, Bellugi et al. (1994) argued that the WS linguistic profile shows a sparing of syntax both in comprehension and in production, which extends to tests of metalinguistic abilities. Morphological markers are generally used correctly, including markers for tense and aspect, as well as auxiliaries and articles. In most of these studies, the achievements of participants with WS were compared to those of individuals with Down syndrome. Udwin and Dennis (1995) agreed with the view expressed by Bellugi and colleagues. They, too, concluded that mature individuals with WS have an unusual command of language: their comprehension is usually far more limited than their expressive language, which tends to be grammatically correct, complex, and fluent at a superficial level, but verbose and pseudo-mature (but see Udwin & Yule, 1991).

Investigations of language in individuals with WS that have used standardized tests consistently yield an advantage of performance on verbal tasks over performance on visuomotor tasks. However, achievement on verbal tasks is not superior in any sense. Although performance varies considerably among individuals with WS, it typically does not reach chronological age (CA) level. Auditory memory more often reaches the expected CA level.

Mervis et al. (1999) studied the cognitive profile of individuals with WS, children as well as adults. They concluded that the language abilities of individuals with WS as measured on standardized tests are significantly delayed relative to CA controls. Delay was evident on receptive vocabulary, receptive grammar, semantic fluency, and syntactic measures (see also Karmiloff-Smith et al., 1997). However, syntactic abilities as well as mean length of utterance (MLU) were at the expected level for mental age (MA). Furthermore, whereas achievements on visuospatial tasks were significantly lower than scores on verbal tasks, performance on these two types of tasks was strongly correlated. The existence of such correlations suggests that language in individuals with WS is not independent of other cognitive skills.

Jarrold, Baddeley, and Hewes (1998) reported a large discrepancy between verbal and nonverbal abilities seen in the group of WS participants they studied as a whole, as measured by MAs obtained from standardized tests. However, they argued that this discrepancy is a function of the performance of only some of the participants in the study. The authors suggested that these results may be explained as a function of verbal ability developing at a faster rate than nonverbal ability in WS. Larger discrepancies between verbal and nonverbal abilities are thus expected in adolescents than, for example, in young children. Udwin and Yule (1990) reached a similar conclusion. They observed that one third of the group they studied produced significantly more speech output, with more complex syntactic structure, more social phrases, and more clichés than seen for the rest of the group.

Studies of Italian-speaking individuals with WS are of particular relevance to this work because Italian, like Hebrew, has complex morphology, although these languages are typologically different. Volterra, Capirci, Pezzini, Sabbadini, and Vicari (1996) investigated 17 children and adolescents with WS, with CA ranging from 4 years, 10 months (4:10) to 15:3. MA ranged from 3:8 to 6:8 and IQ from 38 to 90. Typically developing (TD) children whose CAs corresponded to the MA of the individuals with WS served as controls. Results showed that the two groups did not differ on tests of lexical comprehension or semantic fluency or on MLU. However, the participants with WS obtained significantly lower scores than the TD controls on receptive syntax, vocabulary, and sentence repetition. When individual scores were considered, most of the participants with WS performed below the lowest levels achieved by the TD controls on all of the these tasks.

Recent investigations of the cognitive profiles of Italian children with WS lend further support to these findings. Studies show impaired visuospatial abilities along with linguistic performance that did not exceed MA expectations. Linguistic knowledge was characterized by very good phonological abilities along with specific deficiencies in syntax as well as in lexical semantics (Volterra et al., 1996).

Along with assessments on standardized tests, individuals with WS have been tested on experimental, nonstandardized tasks. Such tasks are particularly important when specific claims concerning preserved linguistic abilities are at stake. Karmiloff-Smith et al. (1998) studied a group of individuals with WS, of CA 14:9 to 34:8, with a mean Performance IQ of 58 and a mean Verbal IQ of 71. Participants were given online tasks of monitoring for target words and an offline picture-matching task. Results from the online tasks show sensitivity to the violation of auxiliary markers and phrase structure rules, but significantly less sensitivity to violations of subcategorization rules. Performance on the offline task was overall poorer than that of the controls.

Testing individuals with WS on online tasks is important because these offer ways of dealing with two major difficulties that plague the other two most common methods of investigation of linguistic knowledge, analysis of naturalistic productions and explicit testing. Whereas the first provides limited data, which may be biased in crucial ways, the second requires a level of awareness that is likely to complicate the task for individuals with cognitive impairments. The results from the online task are therefore particularly interesting and informative. However, the choice of control group in this particular study—18 normal adults ranging in age between 19 and 29 years—is problematic because neither MA nor CA served as matching criterion.

Few studies have been concerned with the early phases of language development in children with WS. Capirci, Sabbadini, and Volterra (1996) reported on a longitudinal follow-up of an Italian girl with WS. Observations of this child began when she had about 20 words and no syntax. The study reported similarities between the acquisitional course followed by this child and the developmental course observed in TD children. However, some differences were noted as well. In particular, although the child with WS had good vocabulary and proficient syntax, she made agreement errors and errors of pronominalization not documented for TD Italian children. By the age of 4:10, the child's cognitive profile as measured on standardized tests was typical of WS, with linguistic abilities better than visuospatial ones, although the latter were less impaired than often seen in children with WS.

Levy (2002) followed 2 Hebrew-speaking children with WS from the beginning of two-word combinations, when their MLU was 1.8, until MLU reached 2.8, 18 months later. The children's progress on 12 different linguistic variables was documented. The course of development was compared to the course observed in TD children of similar MLU. The linguistic profile of the children with WS differed from that of the controls in every phase observed. Interestingly, this finding is very different from what has been observed in children with other neurodevelopmental disorders (Levy, Tennebaum, & Ornoy, 2000). In the latter, development in the early phases, when MLU barely reached 3.00, was very similar to that observed in TD children. Thus, similar to the early development of the Italian child studied by Capirci et al. (1996), the Hebrew-speaking children seem to differ in interesting ways from what has been observed in TD children.

Pezzini, Vicari, Volterra, Milani, and Ossella (1999) argued that individual profiles of children with WS vary considerably and thus one cannot argue that there exists a single neuropsychological profile of individuals with this syndrome. The Italian study argues against the findings of Frangiskakis et al. (1996) and Mervis et al. (1999), who reported a characteristic cognitive profile for individuals with WS. In a recent study of the cognitive profile of Hebrew-speaking adolescents with WS, we were able to replicate the results of Frangiskakis et al. (1996) and Mervis et al. (1999), both for the group overall as well as in the individual profiles (Levy & Bechar, in press). There was no evidence in the Hebrew data for the variability seen in the Italian group.

Three recent studies (Clahsen & Almazan, 1998; Clahsen & Temple, 2003; Karmiloff-Smith et al., 1997) are of particular relevance to the work on Hebrew reported here. These studies focused on morphology and morphosyntax in children with WS. Karmiloff-Smith et al. (1997) studied gender agreement between article and noun in French-speaking adolescents and young adults with WS. Whereas the participants performed well with familiar nouns, they seemed unable to apply gender agreement between the definite article and novel nouns that were presented to them. MA controls, however, performed well on this task. Karmiloff-Smith et al. (1997) concluded that knowledge of morphosyntactic rules is impaired in WS and suggested that the impressive spontaneous language of individuals with WS is a consequence of their good auditory memory.

The findings of Clahsen and Almazan (1998) and Clahsen and Temple (2003) are in direct opposition to those of Karmiloff-Smith et al. (1997). Past tense formation, noun plurals, and compounding were investigated in 4 English-speaking children with WS. Results showed that children with WS overregularize the past tense –ed and the plural –s significantly more often than MA controls; knowledge of the irregular past and the irregular plural forms was relatively poor. The children overapplied the –s plural to the internal nominal elements within lexical compounds (yielding, for example, the ungrammatical compound "*rats-eater" instead of "rat-eaters"). Similarly, the children overapplied the regular comparative affix –er to cases in which a comparative "more" was required. Clahsen and colleagues interpreted these findings as evidence of a preserved grammatical rule system along with considerable deficits in lexical knowledge such as is implicated in knowledge of irregular forms.

In this work we investigated knowledge of Hebrew morphology in 10 adolescents with WS. Of particular relevance to the current debate concerning the nature of the linguistic knowledge of individuals with WS is the participants' performance on tasks that involve strictly formal morphological systems. If indeed the grammatical rule system is preserved in WS, as argued by Clahsen and his colleagues, then performance on those tasks should reflect such knowledge. One of the tasks that was used to this end was a replication of Karmiloff-Smith et al.'s (1997) study of gender agreement with minor modifications due to the differences between French and Hebrew. As for knowledge of other morphological systems in which change of forms affects meaning, those may be more directly affected by the participants' cognitive impairments and thus less informative with respect to their grammatical competence.

BRIEF DESCRIPTION OF HEBREW MORPHOLOGY AND RELATED ACQUISITIONAL FACTS

Hebrew has the characteristics of Semitic languages, that is, words are composed of consonantal roots cast in vocalic word patterns. The roots are usually tri-consonantal, whereas the patterns are in the form of vocalic infixes, prefixes, and suffixes. There are seven verb patterns (*binyanim*) and about three dozen noun patterns (*mishkalim*).

All verbs are analyzable into root + pattern. With respect to nouns, however, this generalization is only partial because some nouns do not have a recognizable root.

It is generally the case in Hebrew that the roots convey core meanings, whereas *binyanim* and *mishkalim* are essentially derivational paradigms that may partially introduce meaning modulations. However, although the formal paradigms are highly systematic, the semantics that they convey is only partially predictable from their forms. For example, the verb patterns (*binyanim*) may serve to express a set of predicate relations such as transitivity, reciprocity, reflexivity, passive, and causative. However, the same function may be expressed by more than one pattern, whereas the same pattern may serve to express more than one meaning or be "basic" for a given root (see examples that follow). Derivational paradigms for nouns are often strictly formal and do not convey meanings at all although some noun patterns do have a productive semantics. Thus, one can consider well-formedness of verbs and nouns that is independent of the meanings that these formal manipulations may convey. Hebrew has a rich inflectional morphology. Generally, verbs are inflected for tense, number, person, and gender.

The following are examples of verbs and nouns from the root *G-D-L* (root consonants are in capitals; verbs are in third person, masculine, singular, past tense; nouns are in singular form):

1. *GaDaL*, "grew," intransitive verb
2. *GiDeL*, "*grew*," transitive verb
3. *GuDaL*, "was grown," passive verb
4. *hiGDiL*, "made bigger," active causative verb
5. *huGDaL*, "made bigger," passive causative verb
6. *GDiLa*, "growing up," noun
7. *GiDuL*, "tumor, growth," noun
8. *GaDLut*, "grandeur," noun
9. *haGDaLa*, "enlargement," noun
10. *miGDaL*, "tower," noun

Berman (1994) argued that early verb use is rote-learned and thus item-based. It is characterized by one verb form per root. Once the child begins to vary verb forms, there will be many more forms for each root, for roots will occur in different *binyanim* bearing different inflectional endings. The expectation is, therefore, that with development, there will be an increase in the proportion of verb forms to verb roots (Levy, 1996).

Hebrew-speaking children start out with semantically unanalyzed forms of verbs, yet at the same period they can effectively control the morphological manipulations of the various root + pattern combinations. Two-year-old Hebrew speakers differentiate between the consonantal roots and the vocalic word patterns, although they are still unable to use those to modulate meaning (Levy,

1988a). For quite some time children continue to use a rich variety of verb forms in morphosyntactically appropriate contexts, not knowing that these formal manipulations may be systematically used to achieve modulations of meanings. It is only around age 4 years, a long time after they have been using most verb patterns productively, that children's errors indicate that they begin to appreciate the semantics of the system (Berman, 1985, 1994).

Hebrew nouns are classified for gender and this classification determines forms of agreement. Although gender is correlated with noun endings, the correlation is not perfect. Typically, nouns ending with a stressed /***a***/ or in /***t***/ are feminine. Such nouns take the suffix /***-ot***/ for plural. All other nouns are in general masculine and take /***-im***/ for plural. Importantly, however, although the system is rather regular, exceptions do exist. Thus, not all feminine nouns take /***-ot***/ for plural and similarly not all masculine nouns take /***-im***/ for plural. Because ultimately gender is a lexical property of nouns, despite the high correlation between morphological endings and gender, the infallible clue to noun gender is syntactic agreement, which is marked on adjectives and on verbs.

The following are examples of noun + adjective combinations in Hebrew in the singular and in the plural. Examples 1 to 4 are of cases of concordant combinations, in which the ending on the noun matches the agreement marker on the adjective, whereas examples 5 to 10 are of discordant cases, in which there is a mismatch between the ending on the noun and the agreement marker on the adjective. These examples are important because they illustrate the paradigm that was used to replicate Karmiloff-Smith et al.'s (1997) study of gender agreement in French:

1. *agala-**a*** + *ktan-**a***
   cart (fem.) + little (fem.): small cart
2. *agal-**ot*** + *ktan-**ot***
   carts (fem.) + little (fem. pl.): small carts
3. *bakbuk* + *katan*
   bottle (masc.) + small (msc.): small bottle
4. *bakbuk-**im*** + *ktan-**im***
   bottles (masc.) + little (masc. pl.): small bottles
5. *zipor* + *levan-**a***
   bird (fem.) + white (fem): white bird
6. *zipor-**im*** + *levan-**ot***
   birds (fem.) + white (fem. pl.): white birds
7. *beic-**a*** + *kash-**a***
   egg (fem.) + hard (fem.): hard-boiled egg
8. *beic-**im*** + *kash-**ot***
   eggs (fem.) + hard (fem. pl.): hard-boiled eggs
9. *kir* + *shaxor*
   wall (masc.) + black (masc.): black wall

10. *kir-**ot*** + *shxor-**im***
    walls (masc.) + black (masc. pl.): black walls

Finally, notice that feminine nouns may be derived from masculine nouns by adding one of the familiar feminine endings, as in the following examples:

11. *yeled* → *yald-**a***
    boy girl
12. *tarnegol* → *tarnegol-**et***
    rooster hen

Previous studies of the acquisition of gender in Hebrew have shown that children master the formal–morphological parts of this system relatively early (Berman & Armon-Lotem, 1996; Levy, 1983, 1988b). Thus, by age 3 years, errors of linguistic gender on inanimate nouns as well as errors of gender agreement across noun phrase and sentence constituents are infrequent. In cases of animate nouns, in which the linguistic gender is determined by the semantic notion of gender, learning is a more protracted process. These findings hold cross-linguistically for all languages studied so far (Levy, 1988b; Mulford & Morgan, 1983; Smoczynska, 1985).

In sum, Hebrew has a very rich morphology with a few paradigms that are strictly formal, whereas others serve to introduce meaning modulations. There is considerable knowledge concerning the acquisition of these different systems in TD children. Data from Hebrew-speaking individuals with WS may therefore provide additional insights into the nature of linguistic abilities of people with WS.

METHOD

Participants

Ten adolescents (6 girls, 4 boys) with a firm genetic diagnosis of WS who are monolingual, native speakers of Hebrew participated in the study. The participants were living at home with their families and were in good health. They were recruited through the Israeli Williams Syndrome Association. All were given the full Wechsler Intelligence Scale for Children–Revised. Mental ages were derived from performance on this test. Table 1 provides information on the participants' CA and IQ. The participants were similar in CA, with a mean of 14 years, 8 months (14:8) and a range from 12:8 to 17:7.

As can be gleaned from Table 1, despite their closeness in CA, there is a large disparity in MA among the participants. Consequently, averaging over the participants to select a control group appeared problematic. We therefore decided to have two groups of controls each with 10 TD children (and an equal number of boys and

TABLE 1
Chronological Age, IQ, and Mental Age as Measured by the WISC–R for Participants with Williams Syndrome

Participant	*CA*	*IQ*	*MA*	*VIQ*	*VA*	*PIQ*	*PA*
1	12:8	76	9:6	79	10:0	77	9:9
2	14:6	92	13:4	96	14:0	88	12:9
3	13:5	52	7:0	52	7:0	61	8:2
4	12:11	45	5:8	47	6:0	55	7:1
5	13:3	40	5:0	45	5:11	45	5:11
6	17:7	43	7:6	47	8:3	49	8:7
7	14:11	69	10:3	74	11:0	68	10:1
8	15:8	46	7:3	51	8:0	50	7:9
9	17:2	53	9:1	58	10:0	56	9:7
10	17:1	50	8:6	56	9:6	52	8:9

Note. CA = chronological age; MA = mental age; WISC–R = Wechsler Intelligence Scale for Children–Revised; VIQ = Verbal IQ; VA = verbal age; PIQ = Performance IQ; PA = performance age.

girls), whose CA was at or close to the ends of the distribution of MA of the individuals with WS. The younger group (henceforth, Group I) was the same CA as the control group in Karmiloff-Smith et al.'s (1997) study. The mean CA of Group I was 5:7 (range 5:3–5:11). The mean CA of the older group (henceforth, Group II) was 11:7 (range 10:3–12:6).

Procedure

Participants with WS were tested in their homes during two or three visits. Sessions lasted over 1 hr, during which there was much play and conversation as well as testing. Each task was preceded by four familiarization items modeled after the stimuli in the task (discussed later). During the administration of the familiarization items, the investigator provided feedback as well as the correct reply, whenever necessary. The tasks were administered in the order given in the following. The investigator kept a complete protocol of the participant's behavior and of his or her comments during the sessions. This was important for coding the participants' understanding of the tasks (see later discussion). Group I was tested at school, whereas Group II was tested at home.

Noun derivations and gender inflection of animate nouns. Recall that most Hebrew words are in fact derived. Thus, if one is given a word from which the root can be extracted, that root may be cast into existing word patterns and new lexical items will be created. Hebrew nouns are marked for gender and number.

Nonce words were introduced through presentation of drawings or unfamiliar objects. The child was asked to repeat the nonce word before any question was asked. The participant was expected to use the nonce form in a noun pattern that has a clear semantics as well as give its form in the feminine. Half the novel words that the participant was expected to coin had existing roots, whereas the other half were novel words from nonexisting roots.

For example, the participant was shown a picture of a man who is ironing and was asked what he or she would call a man whose occupation is to iron clothes. The participant was then asked what he or she would call a woman whose occupation is to iron clothes. In replying to this question the participant needed to cast the root *G-H-Z* (the root for the verb *le-GaHeZ*, "to iron") in the nominal pattern for agent and coin the novel word for "a man who irons," **GHaZan* or **GHaZ*. This novel noun could also be put in a feminine form to refer to "a woman who irons," **GHaZanit* or **GHaZana*. Four questions with existing roots were presented. Each drawing included one male character. The participant had to coin a novel agent noun to refer to the male character in the picture as well as provide the novel form used to refer to a female individual.

The following procedure was used to introduce nonce nouns with novel roots: The experimenter produced a movement with his hand. The child was told that producing this movement is called **leCaKeR* (this is a morphologically well-formed infinitive of a nonexistent root, **C-K-R*). The child was asked what he or she would call a man who repeatedly did such movements. A correct (nonce) agent form in the masculine is **CiKuRan* or **CiKuR*. A correct (nonce) agent in the feminine is **CiKuRanit* or **CiKuRana*. Four such questions with novel roots were asked and the participant was required to produce a masculine as well as a feminine noun.

In sum, the test of noun derivation required that the participant coin agent nouns out of existing or nonce roots that the participant had to extract from the verb produced by the experimenter. Whereas root extraction is a formal operation, coining agent nouns requires familiarity with the appropriate word patterns that designate agents. Providing the feminine form of these newly coined nouns requires at least some conceptual understanding of the referential implications of gender-marked forms.

Production of verb forms. The procedure used to elicit verb forms was similar to the one described for nouns. The focus, however, was exclusively on the formal well-formedness of the verbs produced. The experimenter presented a picture in which a familiar action was shown. The participant was asked to describe the action. The participant was then shown another picture with a different action that required the use of the same root in a causative pattern. In this case, too, the participant was expected to reply with an existing Hebrew verb.

For example, the participant was shown a picture of a baby eating and was expected to use the verb *OXeL*, "eat," to describe the picture. The participant was then shown a picture of the father feeding the baby and was expected to say *mAXiL*, "feeding." The form *mAXiL* is the causative form of that same root, *O-X-L*. Four questions with familiar verbs were asked. Questions were in present tense, masculine, singular.

A similar procedure was used with novel roots. The participant was shown a picture in which there is an unfamiliar action. He or she was given a novel verb in a basic form and was told that this describes the novel action. The participant was then shown a different picture that could be appropriately described through the use of the same novel root, cast in a causative pattern. Four questions with novel verbs were asked. In this case, too, verbs were presented in the present tense, masculine, singular.

Note that although the questions were directed toward production of causative forms, replies were coded as correct whenever the child produced a morphologically correct verb, disregarding the specific pattern. Thus, if the child gave a form that was not causative yet was a morphologically well-formed verb, the response was scored as correct. The focus of this task was therefore on formal well-formedness rather than on the causative verb form.

Gender agreement. This test was a replication of Karmiloff-Smith et al.'s (1997) study of gender agreement in French. Whereas the French study focused on article–noun agreement, our procedure focused on agreement between nouns and adjectives. This change was necessary because Hebrew does not have agreeing articles. Our study used the same drawings that were used in the French study.[1]

Recall that agreement is a syntactic phenomenon, which is reflected in the form of the *agreeing* words, that is, articles in French and adjective endings in Hebrew. Thus, in Hebrew one knows what the gender of the noun is by observing the form of the adjective, without necessarily relying on the noun ending. This is crucial because the latter is not a fool-proof cue to the noun gender.

The procedure was the following: The participant was shown a colored drawing that had two or more identical unfamiliar objects. The experimenter said:

13. *ele* + **xashur-**im*** + *cehub-**im***
    those + *nonce noun (pl.) + yellow (pl. masc.):
    those are yellow (pl.) *nonce (pl.)

The participant was asked to repeat what the experimenter said. As can be gleaned from the example, the noun and the color adjective share the same plural ending, ***-im***. This therefore is a concordant noun–adjective combination (Karmiloff-Smith et al., 1997).

The experimenter then showed the participant another card, which had a single object that was identical to the objects shown on the previous card except for its color. The participant was asked to close his or her eyes while the experimenter hid a small ring under one of the cards. Although the participant could not see

[1]We thank Annette Karmiloff-Smith for the use of her stimuli.

where the ring was, given the bulge under the drawing of the single object, it was rather obvious where the ring had been placed. The participant then opened his or her eyes and was asked to tell the experimenter where he or she thought the ring was. In the case of statement 13, the gender of the singular nonce noun had to be masculine because the agreeing adjective had a masculine ending. The correct answer was therefore:

14. *mitaxat + la-xishur + ha-adom*:
    under definite-*nonce (masc. sing.) definite-red (masc. sing.)

Note that when the combination is concordant, that is, the plural form of the noun and the plural form of the adjective share the same ending, the form of the adjective singular can be determined on the basis of phonological cues. Such cues, however, will not resolve the problem presented by discordant combinations. The following example presents such a case. Crucially, in discordant combinations it is the ending of *the plural adjective* that informs the child what the gender of the noun is and hence what the form of the adjective singular should be. For the example:

15. *ele + *mikdon-**im** + vrud-**ot***
    those + *nonce noun (pl.) + pink (pl. fem.):
    those [are] pink *nonce (pl.)

the expected response is:

16. *mitaxat + la-mikdon-**a** + ha-yeruk-**a***
    under definite-*nonce (fem.) definite-green (fem. sing.):
    under the green *nonce

Thus, although the task has concordant as well as discordant noun + adjective combinations, the focus is on discordant combinations because those are the cases in which knowledge of the agreement rule is required and phonological matching of endings will not suffice. Altogether there were eight questions with discordant combinations, four in which the adjective was in the masculine plural and four in which the adjective was in the feminine plural.

RESULTS

Understanding Task Requirements

Based on participants' performance on the familiarization items preceding each task, it was clear that none of the participants had to be excluded from the study on the basis of lack of understanding of the tasks. However, some participants failed to understand specific questions. It was therefore felt that prior to any analysis, the proportion of cases of lack of understanding among the groups had to be compared to see whether, as a group, the participants with WS and the controls had similar proportions of such instances. Unless this is the case, differences among the groups will be difficult to interpret.

Instances of lack of understanding included cases in which the participant did not know that he or she had to refer to the size or the color of the drawing (as in the gender agreement task), or when the participant asked the investigator to repeat the question time and again. Refusal to answer was not considered an instance of lack of understanding. In such cases testing was discontinued and tried again on another day. Because there were no instances of lack of understanding of the tasks in the Group II controls, coding for participants' understanding of the task demands was carried out for the participants with WS and for Group I controls. Two investigators who did not participate in the collection of the data coded the files. Between-coder agreement was .92. Cases for which agreement could not be reached were excluded from the analysis.

Figure 1 gives box plots for percentages of instances of lack of understanding of task requirements for the WS group and Group I. The mean percentage of lack of understanding task requirements was 13.4% for the WS group and 6.43% for Group I. The difference between the two groups with respect to understanding of the tasks was not significant (median test; $Z = 0$).

For both Group I and the WS group, difficulty understanding task requirements was weakly and nonsigificantly negatively correlated with success on the tests

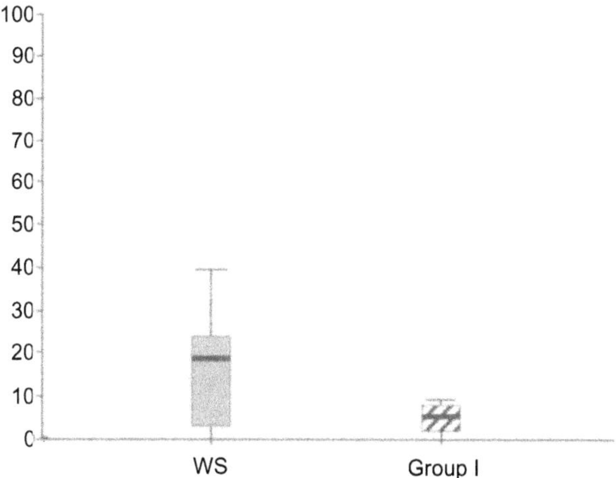

FIGURE 1 Percentage of instances of failure to understand task requirements.

(WS group: Spearman $r = -.33$; Group I: Spearman $r = -.16$). Note that the variability among individual participants in both groups was great, with some of the participants having no difficulty in understanding task requirements and others having serious difficulties. Consequently, discriminant analysis did not predict group membership.

Knowledge of Morphology

Recall that the morphological systems of interest were either meaning-related, such as noun inflections (plurality and linguistic gender on animate nouns) and noun derivations, as well as systems that are strictly formal, such as verb form, root extraction, and gender agreement on inanimate nouns.

Figure 2 presents box plots for noun derivations and for gender marking on animate nouns. Both tasks required morphological manipulations that introduced meaning modulations. Participants with WS were not significantly different from Group I, but significantly worse than Group II on gender marking on animate nouns (median test for gender on animate nouns: WS and Group II, $z = 1.96$; $p = .05$; WS and Group I, $z = 1.84$; $p < .07$). Participants with WS were significantly worse than Group II on noun derivations, but did not differ significantly from Group I on this same task (median test for noun derivations: WS and group I, $z = 1.84$; $p < .07$; WS and group II, $z = 2$; $p < .03$).

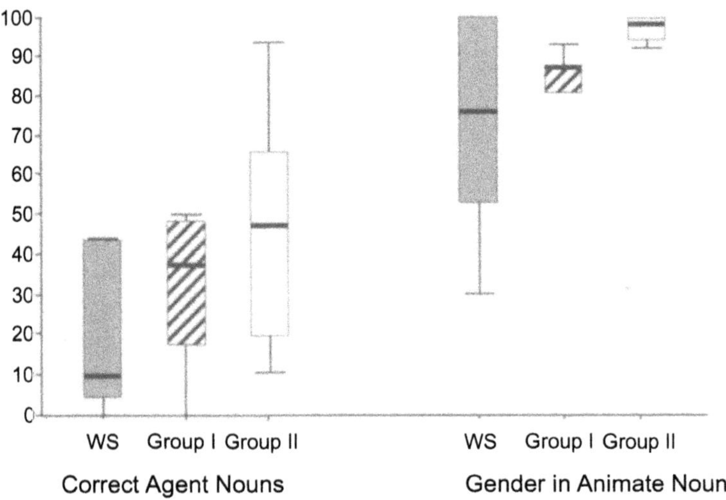

FIGURE 2 Percentage correct for coining agent nouns and gender marking on animate nouns.

Figure 3 presents box plots for two morphological systems that can be considered unrelated to meaning: root extraction and verb forms. Recall that given the systematic morphophonological structure of Hebrew words, sensitivity to roots could be evident even in cases in which the participant failed to give a correct response to the specific question asked. For example, in responding to a question concerning verb derivation the participant could use the root that he or she correctly extracted from the verb form given in the question, yet the form of the pattern might be erroneous. This would count as correct with respect to root extraction despite the fact that it would result in an incorrect verb form. Altogether, 17 of the questions asked in the different tasks required uncovering the root structure of the stimuli. For verb forms, the percentages reported in Figure 3 are for morphophonological well-formedness disregarding the semantics of the verb form.

No statistically significant difference was found between the groups with respect to ability to extract roots (WS group and Group I: $z = 0$; WS group and Group II, $z = .68$). There were no significant differences between the WS group and Group I in verb derivations ($z = 0.92$). The difference between the WS group and Group II, however, was statistically significant ($z = 3.00$, $p < .003$).

Figure 4 presents box plots related to participants' performance on the discordant combinations of noun + adjective in the gender agreement task. Recall that this task was a replication of that of Karmiloff-Smith et al. (1997). Knowledge of agreement was necessary to handle discordant combinations of nonce

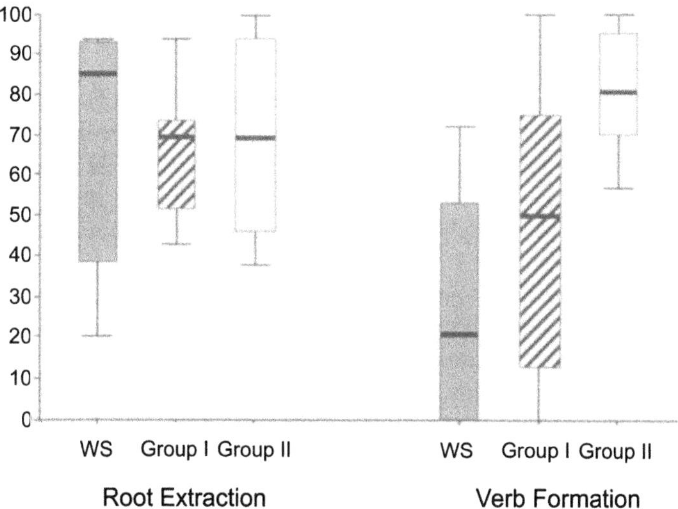

FIGURE 3 Percentage correct for root extraction and verb formation.

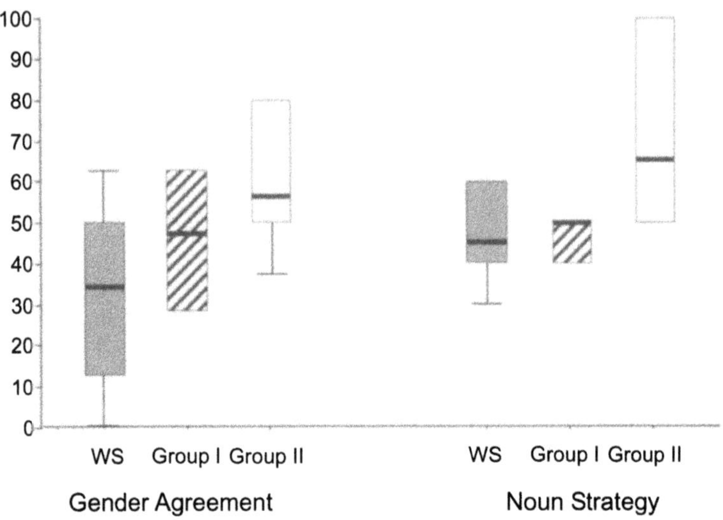

FIGURE 4 Percentage correct for gender agreement for discordant noun–adjective combinations (left) and percentage of responses that conform to application of a "noun strategy" (right).

nouns + adjectives. Differences in performance on the gender agreement task were statistically significant between the WS group and Group II (Mann–Whitney U, $Z = 2.07$; $p = .038$), but not between the WS group and Group I ($Z = 0.557$). Surprisingly, however, performance with respect to discordant combinations was poor in all the groups. Thus, contrary to our expectations, and unlike the participants in the Karmiloff-Smith et al. (1997) study, neither TD children nor participants with WS could handle the task.

In view of the poor performance on this task, we considered the possibility that the participants used a "noun strategy," namely, that replies were based on the plural ending of the noun with complete disregard of the form of the agreeing adjective. Note that such a strategy would lead to erroneous replies in the case of discordant combinations, as explained earlier. A speaker who follows such a strategy in fact ignores agreement.

The right side of Figure 4 presents box plots for the percentage of responses that conform to a noun strategy. Importantly, the performance of all three groups remains low even under the assumption of a noun strategy. Statistical comparisons between the groups were not significant. It remained to be seen whether the participants were using any strategy at all when performing this task. Figures 5 through 7 give the distribution of replies for individual participants in the different groups. Recall that there were equal numbers of questions in the masculine and in the feminine. Consideration of these figures suggests that most participants settled on a default reply, which is either masculine or feminine, ignoring agreement as well as

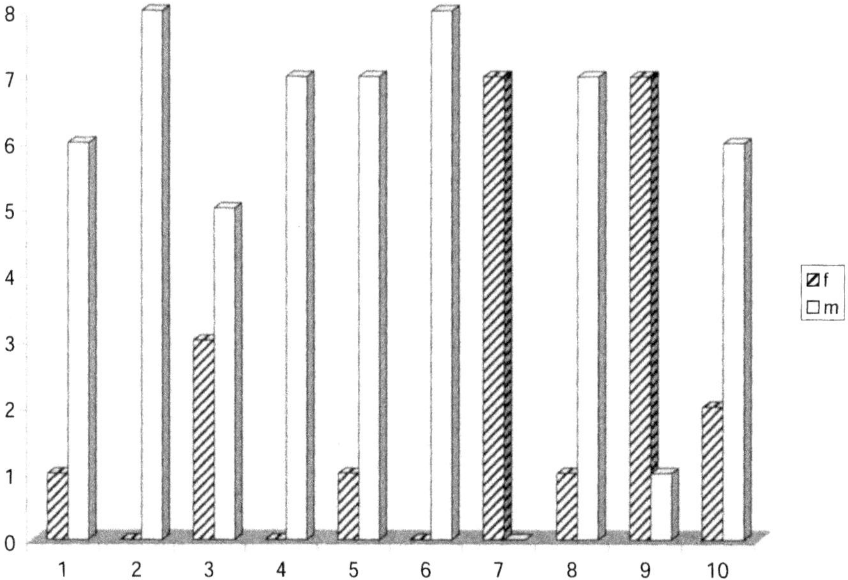

FIGURE 5 Distribution of replies to discordant noun + adjective in individual children of Group I controls.

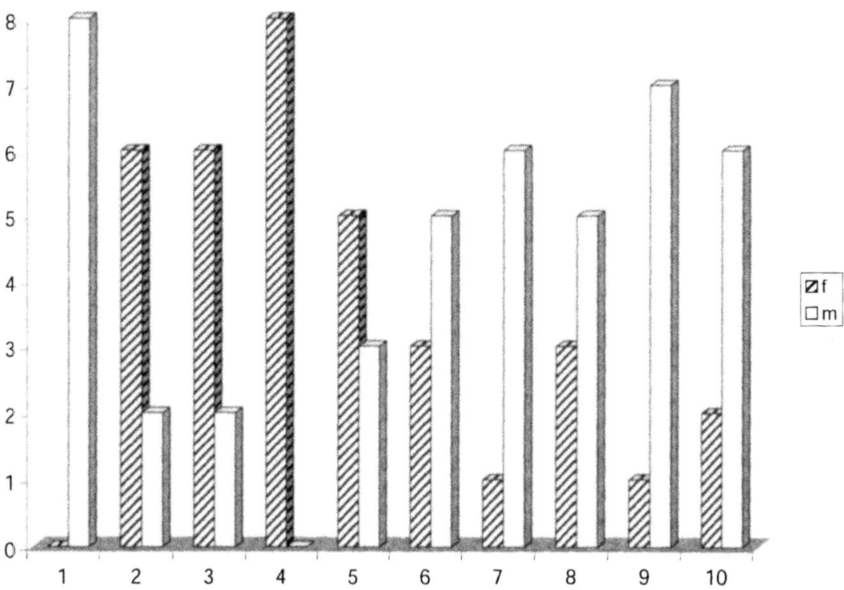

FIGURE 6 Distribution of replies to discordant noun + adjective in individual children of Group II controls.

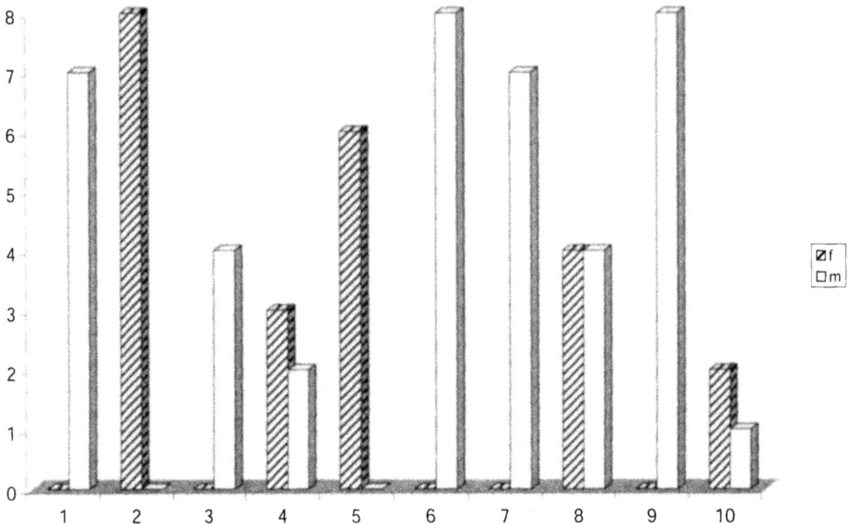

FIGURE 7 Distribution of replies to discordant noun + adjective in individual participants with Williams Syndrome.

noun ending. This is the case for the participants with WS as well as for the control groups.

Profile Analysis

Profile analysis was done through the use of partial order scalogram analysis by base coordinates (POSAC; Shye, 1985; Shye, Elizur, & Hoffman, 1994). POSAC is a technique for measuring individuals with respect to multivariate attributes. The information that can be drawn from plots produced through POSAC concerns the comparability among individual profiles that make up the groups. Rather than separating variables, POSAC considers the individual's whole linguistic profile, placing each profile in a space relative to other profiles in the sample. We may then ask the following questions: Do participants with WS resemble the controls and hence their profiles cluster such that a separation in the space is not evident? Alternatively, do the groups differ in such a way that each group occupies its own space on the POSAC plot?

POSAC (Shye, 1985; Shye et al., 1994) works in the following way: When a sample of participants is observed on certain variables (or test items) a data matrix can be produced in which each column represents a variable and each row represents a participant. The program works on a minimum of four variables with four data points but can take into consideration more variables. The data points in each row constitute the participant's profile. If the items all have a common range (i.e., they are ordered with respect to the measured attribute) order relations can be defined among profiles. Profiles are mapped onto a two-dimensional Cartesian coordinate plane preserving order relations.

Once the two-dimensional map has been plotted, the goal is to find an interpretation for the scales such that the original meaning of the common range is retained. The interpretation of these scales can be helped by observing the role of specific variables in the organization of the plotted space. Note that the axes represent general aspects of the content world rather than any individual variable. By saying that the meaning of the two coordinate scales is determined by certain variables we are not saying that the axes can be thus labeled, because the analysis is done post hoc and is based on the distribution of the profiles in the multidimensional space. The researcher may further look for a single variable that is the best predictor of the partial order among the profiles. Such a variable may or may not exist.

POSAC has the following advantages over other nonparametric analyses: All variables are simultaneously considered. Variables are not represented by other, more central variables and there are no weights given. Each variable is equally important in the analysis. Combination of variables, whether linear or nonlinear, is not attempted. POSAC is the only technique in which all of these properties coexist.

POSAC may be used for a discriminant analysis as well. That is, one can observe the extent to which a certain variable divides the space into meaningful sections. While exploring the possibility of a separation line along the POSAC space, two considerations have to be respected: (a) The line should be parsimonious, that is, as straight as possible with a minimal number of curves, and (b) the number of deviant profiles should be as small as possible.[2]

In sum, the variable of interest in this study was the group to which a participant (i.e., a profile) belongs. Do the profiles of participants with WS cluster in certain areas of the plotted space or are they indistinguishable from the profiles of either Group I or Group II of the controls? Can we predict the group from which a given profile has been drawn on the basis of its position within the POSAC space?

Figure 8 plots the POSAC profiles for the participants with WS and the controls. Each profile included four variables: root extraction and verb form, which are strictly formal systems, and noun derivations and gender on animate nouns, which are morphological systems that correlate with meaning.

---

[2]The procedure used to create POSAC plots maps the profiles into two-dimensional Cartesian coordinate space, so any separation procedure among profiles (i.e., profiles that belong to different groups) must take into account the coordinates on both axes. Also, theoretically the POSAC partition lines must run along the coordinate grid and must be a monotone nonincreasing curve that is looked upon as describing a function of one of the axes on the other (Shye, 1985).

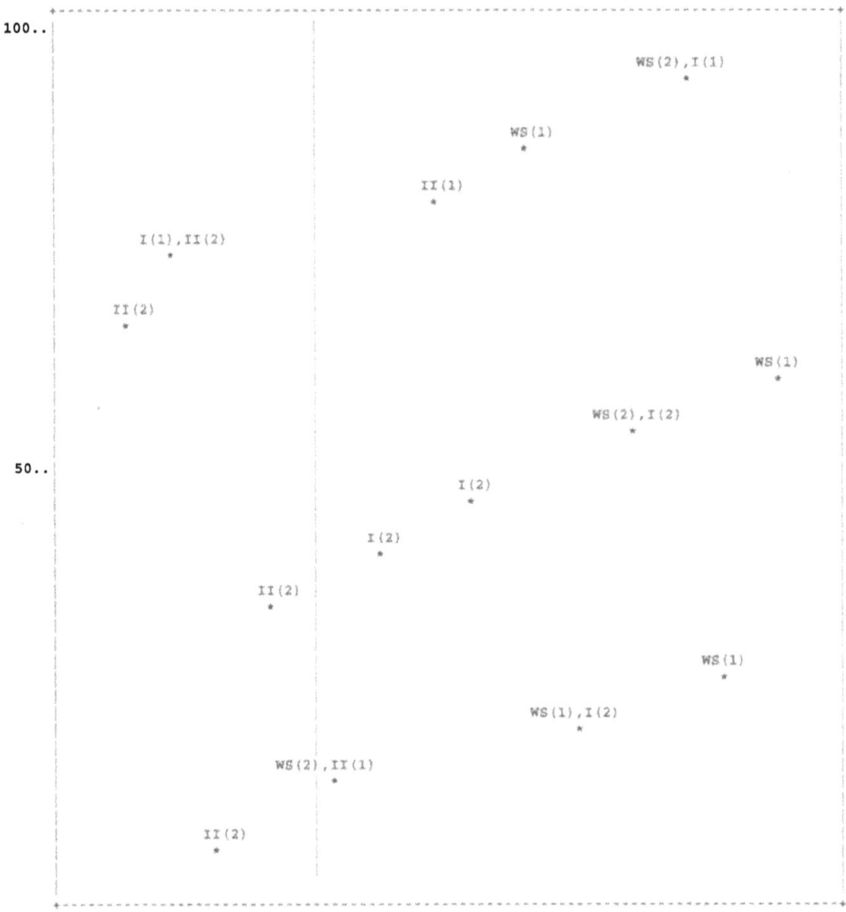

FIGURE 8 Linguistic profiles (POSAC space) of participants with WS and Groups I and II of controls.

The two-dimensional mapping in space was perfect. Although the axes are not determined by any single variable, the distribution of the profiles along the two coordinate scales in Figure 8 is correlated with percentage of correct use of roots and verb forms. No single variable that was the best predictor of the order among the profiles was found.[3]

As shown in Figure 8, the individuals with WS cannot be separated on the POSAC plot from Group I of the controls. However, none of the WS participants

[3]Recall that by saying that the meaning of the two coordinate scales is determined by certain variables we are not saying that the axes can be thus labeled, because this is a post hoc analysis.

appears to the left of the orthogonal line, that is, none of them is close in space to the Group II of the controls. Thus, when participants' fuller profiles are taken into consideration, the participants with WS are indistinguishable from the younger control group but quite separate from the older control group.

SUMMARY AND DISCUSSION

This article focuses on knowledge of Hebrew morphology in adolescents with WS and the current controversy concerning the nature of the grammatical system underlying the excellent conversational skills attributed to individuals with WS. In view of the great variability in MA seen in the WS group, we decided not to average over participants and instead chose two control groups that were at the lower and the upper ends of the distribution of MA seen in the individuals with WS.

Although no participant had to be excluded from the study due to difficulty in understanding task requirements, there were sporadic cases of lack of understanding of specific questions in both the participants with WS and the younger controls. However, level of understanding of task requirements did not differ significantly between these two groups. There were no instances of lack of understanding of task requirements in the older controls. Thus, on the face of it, difficulties in understanding task requirements may account, at least in part, for the differences in the linguistic performance among participants with WS and the older controls. A consideration of the findings to be summarized in what follows—the fact that the results are not unidirectional as they would be if this were the correct explanation—suggests that the differences among the groups reflect differences in the participants' underlying linguistic knowledge rather than problems having to do with understanding the tasks.

We studied both strictly formal morphosyntactic systems—gender agreement within noun phrases, verb forms, and root extraction—as well as morphological paradigms that serve to introduce meaning modulations—gender marking of animate nouns and derivation of agent nouns. It is the former systems that offer the strongest test for the hypothesis originally raised by Bellugi and colleagues and recently supported in the work of Clahsen and colleagues, arguing for a relative preservation of grammar in WS. Evidence against this hypothesis was brought forth by Karmiloff-Smith et al. (1997) and by Mervis et al. (1999) as well as others.

There were no significant differences among the groups in this study in ability to extract roots. Previous work on Hebrew has shown that this is a key grammatical feature of the Hebrew lexicon, to which TD children are sensitive rather early and continue to be so throughout their mature years (Levy, 1988a). Our results show that this is an aspect of the language to which participants with WS are also very sensitive. Whereas root extraction is an early acquisition with TD children, it is important to note that one may envisage alternative ways of learning the language that will not implicate high sensitivity to roots. In other words, good spontaneous Hebrew might have been present without sensitivity to the compositional structure of Hebrew words and to the grammatical status of consonantal roots. For example, a full lexicon could have been learned, aided by the participants' good auditory phonological memory (Karmiloff-Smith et al., 1997). Apparently, this is not the road taken.

Another aspect that concerns basic typological features of Hebrew is verb forms. We refer to the morphophonological alterations rather than to the semantic modulations that may be introduced through changes in verb patterns. Participants with WS performed as well as the younger controls, yet significantly less well than the older control group. Although we completely disregarded erroneous aspects of verb meaning in the coding of replies, we cannot rule out the possibility that because changes in verb forms affect meaning, this might have limited the children's success on this task. The results with respect to other morphological manipulations that involve a change in meaning, summarized in what follows, suggest that this could have been the explanation.

Contrary to our expectations, all three groups performed poorly on the gender agreement test. This was surprising, given the early age at which Hebrew-speaking children as well as children learning other languages with rich morphologies acquire linguistic gender and agreement (Berman, 1985; Levy, 1983, 1988b). A consideration of performance of individuals in the groups suggests that in all three groups participants in fact did not encode the gender information that was given in the stimuli. Agreement did not seem to be a rule with which the children worked when they performed this task. We conclude that the gender agreement task failed to test knowledge of this system in either the participants with WS or in the controls.

The interest in reporting those "nonresults" lies in the fact that despite the analogical nature of our tasks, including the fact that we used the identical stimuli and the same-age TD participants, we did not succeed in replicating Karmiloff-Smith et al.'s (1997) findings on gender agreement in French. Recently we failed to replicate the results from French in three additional groups of 7-year-old TD Hebrew speakers as well as in 6-year-old TD Spanish children (Levy & Tolchinsky, in preparation).[4] Given that Spanish is very similar to French, in that both languages have agreeing articles and consequently the procedure was identical in both studies, this failure to replicate is troublesome. More work is needed to account for the discrepancies.

A comparison of the performance of the participants with WS and the controls on the morphological paradigms that introduce meaning modulations indicated that the older control group performed significantly better than the WS group on

[4]In a series of experiments we tried to impute a meaning to the nonce words in the hope that children would apply agreement rules to them. Preliminary results do not show any improvement on the task, that is, 7-year-old Hebrew speakers still fail to apply agreement to mismatched pairs of nonce noun + adjective combinations.

both gender marking of animate nouns and coinage of agent nouns. The difference in performance between the WS group and the younger control group was not significant. Note that sensitivity to the typological features of Hebrew along with difficulties in morphology that involve meaning is not characteristic exclusively of individuals with WS. A similar language profile can be seen at an earlier developmental phase in individuals with other neurological syndromes who have similar levels of intellectual handicaps (Levy et al., 2000).

A comparison among the groups based on children's fuller morphological profile, produced in the form of a POSAC plot, suggests the direction that these results are taking. The mapping of individual profiles in a two-dimensional space did not show a separation between profiles of the participants with WS and those of the younger control group. A separation in space did exist, however, between the WS group and the older control group. Thus, when a more comprehensive morphological profile of a child is considered, involving morphological manipulations that are exclusively formal as well as those that involve aspects of meaning, the profiles of participants with WS are more like those of TD children who are at the lower end of the MA range for the participants with WS than those of TD children who are at the upper end of the MA range for the participants with WS.

In sum, with respect to the debate between Karmiloff- Smith et al. (1997; Karmiloff-Smith et al., 1998) and Clahsen and Almazan (1998) and Clahsen and Temple (2003), the findings relating to knowledge of word structure in Hebrew-speaking adolescents with WS are inconclusive. Although knowledge of the root structure of the Hebrew lexicon is at MA level, other features of morphology seem less preserved. Given how central a typological feature this is for Semitic languages (Hebrew as well as Arabic), the fact that children with WS are sensitive to roots is perhaps not so surprising.

Still, information is needed relating to gender agreement before one can argue that the data from Hebrew support the idea of preservation of grammar in WS. Gender agreement is particularly important in this regard because it is a formal syntactic rule that has morphological consequences but no meaning attached to it. Furthermore, as shown in the discussion of the task analysis, in the absence of an agreement rule, it is possible to predict a pattern of errors that may turn out to be very revealing, for example, if there was evidence for the adoption of a noun strategy.

With respect to the other systems studied, the WS group performed mostly at the lower end of their MA range. We conclude therefore that there is little evidence from Hebrew to support a selective preservation of grammatical competence in individuals with WS.

ACKNOWLEDGMENT

This work was supported by a grant to Y. L. from the Israel Science Foundation.

REFERENCES

Bellugi, U., Marks, S., Bihrle, A., & Sabo, H. (1993). Dissociations between language and cognitive functions in Williams syndrome. In D. Bishop & K. Mogford (Eds.), *Language development in exceptional circumstances* (pp. 177–189). Hillsdale, NJ: Lawrence Erlbaum Associates, Inc.

Bellugi, U., Mills, D., Jernigan, Y., Hickock, G., & Galaburda, A. (1999). Linking cognition, brain structure and brain function in Williams syndrome. In H. Tager-Flusberg (Ed.), *Neurodevelopmental disorders* (pp. 111–136). Cambridge, MA: MIT Press.

Bellugi, U., Wang, P. P, & Jernigan, T. L. (1994). Williams syndrome: An unusual neuropsychological profile. In S. H. Broman & J. Grafman (Eds.), *Atypical cognitive deficits in developmental disorders: Implications for brain functions* (pp. 23–56). Hillsdale, NJ: Lawrence Erlbaum Associates, Inc.

Berman, R. A. (1985). The acquisition of Hebrew. In D. I. Slobin (Ed.), *The cross-linguistic study of language acquisition.* Hillsdale, NJ: Lawrence Erlbaum Associates, Inc.

Berman, R. A. (1994). Developmental perspectives on transitivity: A confluence of cues. In Y. Levy (Ed.), *Other children, other languages* (pp. 189–242). Hillsdale, NJ: Lawrence Erlbaum Associates, Inc.

Berman, R., & Armon-Lotem, S. (1996). How grammatical are early verbs? *Annales Littéraires de l'Université de Besancon, 1996,* 17–59.

Capirci, O., Sabbadini, L., & Volterra, V. (1996). Language development in Williams syndrome: A case study. *Cognitive Neuropsychology, 13,* 1017–1039.

Clahsen, H., & Almazan, M. (1998). Syntax and morphology in Williams syndrome. *Cognition, 68,* 167–198.

Clahsen, H., & Temple, C. (2003). Words and rules in Williams syndrome and SLI. In Y. Levy & J. Schaeffer (Eds.), *Language competence across populations—Toward a definition of SLI* (pp. 323–352) Mahwah, NJ: Lawrence Erlbaum Associates, Inc.

Frangiskakis, J. M., Ewart, A. K., Morris, C. A., Mervis, C. B., Bertrand, J., Robinson, B. F., et al. (1996). LIM-kinase1 hemizygosity implicated in impaired visuospatial constructive cognition. *Cell, 86,* 59–69.

Gosch, A., Städing, G., & Pankau, R. (1994). Linguistic abilities in children with Williams–Beuren syndrome. *American Journal of Medical Genetics, 52,* 291–296.

Jarrold, C., Baddeley, A., & Hewes, A. K. (1998). Verbal and nonverbal abilities in the Williams syndrome phenotype: Evidence for diverging developmental trajectories. *Journal of Child Psychology and Psychiatry, 39,* 511–523.

Karmiloff-Smith, A., Grant, J., Berthoud, I., Davies, M., Howlin, P., & Udwin, O. (1997). Language and Williams syndrome: How intact is "intact"? *Child Development, 68,* 274–290.

Karmiloff-Smith, A., Tyler, L. K., Sims, K., Udwin, O., Howlin, P., & Davies, M. (1998). Linguistic dissociations in Williams syndrome: Evaluating receptive syntax in on-line and off-line tasks. *Neuropsychologia, 36,* 343–351.

Levy, Y. (1983). It's frogs all the way down. *Cognition, 12,* 75–93.

Levy, Y. (1988a). The nature of early language knowledge: Evidence from the development of Hebrew morphology. In Y. Levy, I. M. Schlesinger, & M. D. S. Braine (Eds.), *Strategies and processes in language acquisition.* Hillsdale, NJ: Lawrence Erlbaum Associates, Inc.

Levy, Y. (1988b). On the early learning of formal grammatical systems: Evidence from studies of the acquisition of gender and countability. *Journal of Child Language, 15,* 179–187.

Levy, Y. (1996). On the early development of morphology and syntax in children with congenital brain pathology. *Journal of Reproductive and Infant Research, 14,* 255–270.

Levy, Y. (2002). Longitudinal study of language acquisition in two children with Williams syndrome. In B. Skarabela, S. Fish, & A. H.-J. Do (Eds.), *BUCLD 26: Proceedings of the 26th Annual Boston University Conference on Language Development* (pp. 348–358). Ithaca, NY: Cascadilla.

Levy, Y., & Bechar, T. (in press). Cognitive, lexical and morphological profile of Israeli adolescents with Williams syndrome. *Cortex*.

Levy, Y., Tennebaum, A., & Ornoy, A. (2000). Spontaneous language of children with specific neurological syndromes. *Journal of Speech, Language and Hearing Research, 43*, 351–365.

Levy, Y., & Tolchinsky, L. (in preparation). Constraints on the use of tests with nonce words.

Mervis, C. B., Morris, C. A., Bertrand, J., & Robinson, B. F. (1999). Williams syndrome: Findings from an integrated program of research. In H. Tager-Flusberg (Ed.), *Neurodevelopmental disorders* (pp. 65–110). Cambridge, MA: MIT Press.

Mulford, R., & Morgan, J. L. (1983, May). *On learning to assign gender to new nouns in Icelandic*. Paper presented at the Ninth Annual Minnesota Regional Conference on Language and Linguistics, Minneapolis, MN.

Pezzini, G., Vicari, S., Volterra, V., Milani, L., & Ossella, M. T. (1999). Children with Williams syndrome: Is there a single neuropsychological profile? *Developmental Neuropsychology, 15*, 141–155.

Shye, S. (1985). *Multiple scaling: The theory and application of partial order scalogram analysis*. Amsterdam: North Holland.

Shye, S., Elizur, D., & Hoffman, M. (1994). *Introduction to facet theory*. Thousand Oaks, CA: Sage.

Smoczynska, M. (1985). The acquisition of Polish. In D. I. Slobin (Ed.), *The cross linguistic study of language acquisition*. (Vol. 1, pp. 595–686). Hillsdale, NJ: Lawrence Erlbaum Associates, Inc.

Udwin, O., & Dennis, A. (1995). Psychological and behavioral phenotype in genetically determined syndromes: A review of research findings. In G. O'Brien & W. Yule (Eds.), *Behavioral phenotypes* (pp. 90–208). London: MacKeith.

Udwin, O., & Yule, W. (1990). Expressive language of children with Williams syndrome. *American Journal of Medical Genetics Supplement, 6*, 108–114.

Udwin, O., & Yule, W. (1991). A cognitive and behavioral phenotype in Williams syndrome. *Journal of Clinical and Experimental Neuropsychology, 13*, 232–244.

Udwin, O., Yule, W., & Martin, N. (1987). Cognitive abilities and behavioral characteristics of children with idiopathic infantile hypercalcaemia. *Journal of Child Psychology and Psychiatry, 28*, 297–309.

Volterra, V., Capirci, O., Pezzini, G., Sabbadini, L., & Vicari, S. (1996). Linguistic abilities in Italian children with Williams syndrome. *Cortex, 32*, 663–677.

Can Adolescents With Williams Syndrome Tell the Difference Between Lies and Jokes?

Kate Sullivan
Eunice Kennedy Shriver Center
University of Massachusetts Medical Center

Ellen Winner
Boston College and Harvard Project Zero

Helen Tager-Flusberg
Boston University School of Medicine

A group of adolescents with Williams syndrome (WS) was compared to matched groups of adolescents with Prader–Willi syndrome and nonspecific mental retardation on a task that tested the ability to distinguish different forms of nonliteral language. Participants listened to stories that ended in either a lie or an ironic joke. They were asked to decide the form of the nonliteral utterance and justify their responses. Almost none of the participants in any of the groups were able to correctly classify the ironic jokes, instead judging them to be lies because they did not correspond to reality. Their errors were similar to those made by younger normally developing children, but contrasted with those made by brain-damaged adults. These data are taken as further evidence that neurodevelopmental disorders are quite different from acquired brain disorders and require different neuropsychological models. The findings from this study also have important implications for considering the difficulties that adolescents with WS and other disorders will have in everyday social situations, especially among peers.

Effective communication entails the capacity to handle both literal and nonliteral forms of language. The essence of communication is the ability to interpret the

Requests for reprints should be sent to Helen Tager-Flusberg, Lab of Developmental Cognitive Neuroscience, Boston University School of Medicine, 715 Albany Street L-814, Boston, MA 02118. E-mail: htagerf@bu.edu

speaker's intended meaning, whether the speaker uses literal language, where intended meaning matches surface structure, or nonliteral language, where form does not match intended meaning. Our everyday discourse incorporates both forms, including metaphor, irony, sarcasm, and indirect or elliptical utterances, and speakers often use a variety of cues, especially nonverbal cues, to convey intended meaning. Current theories of pragmatics emphasize that the capacity to interpret intended meaning in both literal and nonliteral utterances lies at the intersection between language and social cognition, specifically theory of mind (e.g., Sperber & Wilson, 1986). This perspective highlights the fact that only when the mental states of the speaker and the listener are clearly understood can one make an accurate interpretation of intended meaning in nonliteral utterances. An inability to decipher the communicative intent of the speaker would seriously compromise one's ability to make sense of much of our everyday conversation.

Thus far there has been little research exploring the use or interpretation of nonliteral language in individuals with Williams syndrome (WS). Given their unique cognitive and personality phenotype, one might hypothesize that people with WS would have little difficulty with nonliteral language. We know that language itself is a relative strength (Bellugi, Mills, Jernigan, Hickok, & Galaburda, 1999; Mervis, Morris, Bertrand, & Robinson, 1999), and that children with WS are effective in conversation with others, especially adults (Bellugi, Jones, Harrison, Rossen, & Klima, 1995; Kelley & Tager-Flusberg, 1995). Anecdotal reports of their discourse skills, especially narratives, indicate that their language is often filled with colorful descriptions including metaphors and idioms (Bellugi, Bihrle, Neville, Jernigan, & Doherty, 1992), and they are skilled at using prosodic features to express speaker attitude (Reilly, Klima, & Bellugi, 1990). People with WS are also known for their warm empathic personality and keen interest in other people (Gosch & Pankau, 1997; Udwin & Yule, 1991). Thus the WS profile seems to incorporate the main characteristics—good language and social interest—that would be needed to interpret speakers' intended meaning in both literal and nonliteral forms of language.

In normally developing children, the ability to distinguish between literal and nonliteral forms of language emerges between 5 and 8 years of age (Andrews, Rosenblatt, Malkus, Gardner, & Winner, 1988; Happé, 1993; Leekam, 1991; Sullivan, Winner, & Hopfield, 1995; Winner, 1988; Winner & Leekam, 1991; Winner, Windmueller, Rosenblatt, Bosco, & Best, 1987). By 5 years of age, children are able to distinguish between metaphor and irony (Happé, 1993), and between ironic jokes and lies (Leekam, 1991). Somewhat later, children begin to distinguish between sarcasm and other forms of falsehood (Winner et al., 1987).

Research has also shown that children's ability to distinguish among various forms of falsehood is related to their theory of mind abilities, namely, their ability to understand the mental states of the speaker and listener. To distinguish between forms of nonintentional and intentional falsehoods (e.g., mistakes vs. lies), one must be able to conceptualize the speaker's first-order mental state. For example, a mistaken speaker believes what he or she says is true, and thus intends to be truthful. On the other hand, a liar does not believe what he or she says is true, and thus intends to deceive. To distinguish between forms of intended falsehood (e.g., lies vs. irony), one must be able to conceptualize more complex or higher order mental states (e.g., what the speaker knows the listener knows [second-order knowledge], what the speaker intends the listener to believe [second-order intention], what the speaker believes the listener believes [second-order belief]). In the case of an ironic joke, the speaker knows that the listener knows the truth, and thus does not intend to deceive, whereas the liar believes that the listener does not know the truth, and thus intends to deceive. Thus, the ability to distinguish among different forms of nonliteral and literal language rests on the ability to understand the intentions and related knowledge states of the speaker.

Early studies demonstrated that by the time children are able to understand a speaker's first-order false belief (4 years of age), they are also able to distinguish mistakes from lies (Wimmer & Perner, 1983; Wimmer, Gruber, & Perner, 1984, 1985) and are able to comprehend metaphor (Happé, 1993). More recently, several studies have demonstrated a strong association between understanding of various complex mental states and intentional falsehood (Happé, 1994; Leekam, 1991; Sullivan et al., 1995; Winner & Leekam, 1991). For example, Sullivan et al. (1995) showed that the ability to conceptualize the second-order knowledge state of the speaker (e.g., she knows that he knows) is necessary to distinguish lies from ironic jokes, suggesting that certain mental states may be more relevant than others for these types of linguistic distinctions. In the majority of these studies, children's mental state understanding precedes lie/joke comprehension by approximately 2 years, which suggests that understanding of complex mental states is necessary but not sufficient.

This relationship between theory of mind and nonliteral language has also been demonstrated for atypical and brain-damaged populations. Happé (1993) found that whereas individuals with autism passing first-order theory of mind tasks understood metaphor, only those passing second-order tasks understood irony. Winner, Brownell, Happé, Blum, and Pincus (1998) found that in adults with right-hemisphere brain damage (RHD), who have known difficulties with discourse interpretation, the ability to distinguish lies from jokes was also strongly correlated with measures of second-order belief. Their study, which used a task based on one developed by Sullivan et al. (1995) for children, found that although the relation between higher order mental states and lie/joke discrimination was present in the RHD individuals, their error pattern was quite different from what had been found in normally developing children. Thus, children who fail to distinguish between lies and jokes tend to judge all the nonliteral utterances as lies. In contrast, the RHD individuals who failed the task were as likely to judge the lies as jokes as they were to judge the jokes as lies. This suggests that these individuals do not use a developmentally primitive strategy (to take all nonliteral utterances as lies) and highlights the differences between how children and adult brain-damaged individuals process socially relevant stimuli. Nevertheless across all the groups that have been studied thus far, the ability to distinguish between various forms of intended falsehood rests on the ability to conceptualize the second-order mental states of the speaker.

Only one study has examined the ability of adolescents and adults with WS to interpret nonliteral language. Karmiloff-Smith, Klima, Bellugi, Grant, & Baron-Cohen (1995) conducted a series of experiments with a group of individuals with WS demonstrating their relatively spared theory of mind abilities, including their ability to interpret intended meaning. Their work, however, has been criticized for not including appropriately matched comparison groups, especially other groups of individuals with mental retardation (e.g., Sullivan & Tager-Flusberg, 1999), and for including small samples of participants varying widely in age. Karmiloff-Smith et al. (1995) used a task designed by Happé (1993) to test the participants' ability to understand metaphor and sarcasm. Half of the participants with WS in their study succeeded on both the metaphor and the sarcasm statements, though it is not clear whether these were the same participants who passed their second-order knowledge task.

In contrast to the findings reported by Karmiloff-Smith et al. (1995), other studies have not found theory of mind abilities to be spared in either children (Tager-Flusberg & Sullivan, 2000; Tager-Flusberg, Sullivan, & Boshart, 1997) or adolescents with WS (Sullivan & Tager-Flusberg, 1999). When compared to other groups of retarded individuals, matched on age, IQ, and language level, children and adolescents do not perform better on either first-order or second-order tasks that require them to attribute knowledge and belief states to story characters. Given these findings, we hypothesize that adolescents with WS would not be able to distinguish between different forms of nonliteral language, especially those that entail the attribution of higher order mental states to other people.

The goal of this study was to test this hypothesis, using the task designed by Sullivan et al. (1995). As in our previous research on theory of mind in WS, in this study we compared adolescents with WS to age-matched individuals with Prader–Willi syndrome (PWS), another rare genetic disorder, and children with nonspecific mental retardation. Neither of these groups has the striking cognitive or personality phenotypes that are typical of WS. At the same time, the IQ distribution in these groups is fairly comparable to the range found in WS, making it easy to identify participants who are matched on IQ. Moreover, given the variation in language levels across all these groups, it is possible to select groups that are well matched across all these variables.

METHOD

Participants

Three groups participated in this experiment: children and adolescents with WS, PWS, and nonspecific mental retardation (MRU). Table 1 presents the main characteristics of these groups. The first group included 16 adolescents with WS (9 girls and 7 boys) all of whom had previous confirmed clinical diagnoses of WS. Participants were either tested at the 1996 National Williams Syndrome Association Family Conference (11 participants) or referred from the New England Williams Syndrome Association and the National Williams Syndrome Association for local children and tested in their homes (5 participants).

The second group included 11 adolescents with PWS (2 girls and 9 boys), all of whom had received clinical diagnoses of PWS. Most of the adolescents with PWS (9 participants) were tested at the 19th Annual Prader–Willi Syndrome National Conference in 1997. The other 2 participants were referred by the Prader–Willi Association of New England and tested in their homes. Although participants in the WS and PWS groups were not required to provide documented evidence of genetic

TABLE 1
Participant Characteristics

	Williams Syndrome[a]	*Prader–Willi Syndrome*[b]	*Nonspecific Mental Retardation*[c]
Chronological age			
M	12.3	12.8	12.00
SD	1.1	2.9	2.7
Range	8.4–16.7	10.1–17.1	9.0–15.2
PPVT–R mental age			
M	9.0	9.7	7.9
SD	2.7	2.9	2.7
Range	4.8–15.6	3.3–13.1	5.0–11.8
PPVT–R standard score			
M	77.2	78.5	64.4
SD	14.6	15.2	18.8
Range	46–107	55–101	34–86
Full-scale IQ			
M	65.7	75.1	66.5
SD	12.2	12.7	5.7
Range	52–96	55–97	60–76

Note. PPVT–R = Peabody Picture Vocabulary Test–Revised.
[a]$n = 16$. [b]$n = 11$. [c]$n = 12$.

testing, only those with confirmed clinical diagnoses (through parental report and medical documentation) were included in the study. Unclear cases were excluded.

The third group included 12 adolescents with MRU (7 girls and 5 boys), drawn from special education classes in local public schools. In all cases the etiology of the mental retardation was unknown.

All participants were administered Form M of the Peabody Picture Vocabulary Test–Revised (PPVT–R; Dunn & Dunn, 1981), a receptive one-word vocabulary test. The majority of participants also received the Kaufman Brief Intelligence Test (K–BIT; Kaufman & Kaufman, 1990) as a general measure of cognitive level. The K–BIT yields verbal and nonverbal domain scores, as well as an overall IQ score. Three (19%) of the WS and 2 (18%) of the PWS participants were administered the Differential Abilities Scales (DAS; Elliot, 1990). The DAS yields verbal, nonverbal, and spatial domain scores, as well as an overall composite score (GCA), which is equivalent to a Full-Scale IQ score. The full-scale equivalents yielded by these two IQ measures have been shown to be highly correlated (Kaufman & Kaufman, 1990). Analyses of variance (ANOVA) confirmed that at a group level there were no statistically significant differences among the groups on chronological age ($p < .69$), PPVT–R mental age ($p < .40$), PPVT–R standard score ($p < .32$), or Full-Scale IQ ($p < .14$). However, because the p value of the IQ variable was somewhat low, we have treated IQ as a covariate in the relevant analyses.

Materials

Participants were presented with four stories based on the task developed by Sullivan et al. (1995). The stories described situations in which an adult knows that a child has not completed a required chore. In all stories, the child utters a literal falsehood that the adult knows is false (e.g., "I did a great job cleaning up my room"); in two of the stories the false statements were lies, in two they were ironic jokes. In the lie stories, the child does not know that the adult knows the truth. The liar intends for the listener to believe him and thus be deceived. In the joke stories, the child does know that the adult knows the truth and thus does not intend to deceive the listener. Thus, the only structural difference between the lie and the joke stories was the child's second-order belief about the adult's knowledge of the truth. The Appendix presents both the lie and the joke versions of one of the stories.

Procedure

Participants were first given a training session to ensure that they understood the correct usage of the terms "lie" and "joking or just kidding." One experimenter (E1) showed the participant the contents of a small box (a tiny doll) without letting a second experimenter (E2) look inside. E2 then asked E1 what was in the box. E1 replied in a sincere tone of voice that the box was empty, and then asked the participant whether the answer was a lie or a joke. After a correct response, participants were told, "That's right, I was lying. I knew that she couldn't see what was in the box, so I lied and told her it was empty." Following an incorrect response, E1 said, "Well, really, I was lying. I knew that she couldn't see what was in the box, so I lied and told her it was empty." Next, E1 showed both the participant and E2 a small box containing a small dog and said in a joking intonation, "Hey look, this dog is really big." The participant was again asked if the answer was a lie or a joke. After a correct response, participants were told, "That's right, I was just kidding or joking. I knew that she could see the tiny dog, so I was just kidding when I said it was really enormous!" Following an incorrect response, E1 said, "Well, really, I was just kidding or joking. I knew that she could see the tiny dog, so I was just kidding when I said it was really enormous!"

The four stories were then presented. For each story, five test questions were asked. The questions are discussed using the story presented in the Appendix.

Perceptual access question. "Does the grandfather see that Frank did not clean up his dishes?" This question was asked to ensure that participants understood that the adult in the story had perceptual access to the actual state of affairs. Understanding that a character has perceptual access to relevant story facts is critical for making inferences about that character's knowledge state. Corrective feedback was given to participants who answered this question incorrectly.

First-order knowledge question. "Does Frank know that his grandfather saw the dirty dishes?" The purpose of this question was to explore participants' understanding of the main character's (Frank) first-order mental state. The correct answer was "no" for the lie stories and "yes" for the joke stories. To succeed on this question, participants had to override their own knowledge of the truth (i.e., that the grandfather did see the dirty dishes) and report on Frank's knowledge.

Second-order knowledge question. "Does Frank know that his grandfather knows he did not clean up the dishes?" The purpose of this question was to explore participants' understanding of Frank's second-order knowledge state. It required participants to comment on what one character knew about the other character's knowledge state. As in the previous question, the correct answer was no for the lie stories and yes for the joke stories.

Lie/joke question. At the conclusion of each story, participants were asked to classify the final utterance, which was presented with neutral intonation, as follows: "Was Frank lying or just kidding." The presentation order of the response choices was counterbalanced both within and across participants. We asked this question to determine whether participants could judge the difference between the two forms of literally false statements.

Justification question. "How can you tell that Frank was_____(lying or just kidding)?" Following the lie/joke question, we asked participants to explain their responses.

The four stories were presented in counterbalanced order across participants and each was accompanied by four colored drawings depicting the main characters and story events. Story root by ending (lie vs. ironic joke) was counterbalanced such that each story root appeared an equal number of times as a lie and as a joke. Participants were tested individually by two experimenters. Responses were audiotaped and later transcribed and checked by a second coder.

Response Coding

Responses to the test questions were coded as correct or incorrect. Responses to the justification question were coded into the following categories:

- *Explicit second-order reasoning*: The participant explicitly refers to the knowledge states of both story characters. For example, "Because he doesn't know that his grandfather knows he didn't clean up the dishes."
- *Perceptual information*: The participant refers to the perceptual access of the story character. For example, "Because his grandfather saw that she didn't clean up the dishes."
- *Reality response*: The participant refers to the actual state of affairs. For example, "Because he didn't clean up the dishes."
- *Story facts*: The participant states accurate but irrelevant story facts. For example, "Because he wanted to play with his friends."
- *Reiteration of response*: The participant simply repeats his or her response. For example, "Because he was not telling the truth. Because he was just lying/joking."
- *Other*: No response, or a nonsensical response.

RESULTS

Preliminary analyses revealed that there were no gender differences on any of the test questions. Table 2 shows the means (and standard deviations) for each group on the test questions. A series of one-way ANOVAs, carried out to test for differences among the groups on each of the test questions, revealed that there were no significant group differences on any of the questions. A second set of analyses using Full-Scale IQ as a covariate also revealed no significant group differences on any of the test questions.

We also analyzed the number of participants passing each of the test questions; the data are presented in Table 3. For this analysis, passing consisted of scoring correctly on at least three of four trials for the perceptual-access, first-order and second-order questions. For the lie/joke question there were two questions for which the correct answer was lie, and two for which the correct answer was just kidding. We used two different criteria for this question. The first considered success as the ability to discriminate between lies and jokes, judging this across two pairs of lie/joke stories. Thus, on this criterion, passing the lie/joke discrimination question was defined as answering correctly on all the stories. Passing the lie stories only and the joke stories only was defined as scoring correctly on both trials of these stories.

As shown in Table 3, almost all the participants in the three groups passed the perceptual access question, showing that they understood that the adult character had perceptual access to the story facts. On the first-order knowledge question a majority adolescents in all groups passed at least three of four trials, showing that

TABLE 2
Mean Scores and Standard Deviations on Test Questions

	Williams Syndrome		*Prader–Willi Syndrome*		*Nonspecific Mental Retardation*	
	M	*SD*	*M*	*SD*	*M*	*SD*
Perceptual access	3.44	1.36	3.91	0.30	3.83	0.39
First-order knowledge	2.81	0.98	3.09	1.04	3.17	1.27
Second-order knowledge	2.63	0.96	3.18	1.17	2.75	1.06
Total lie/joke score	2.13	0.34	2.36	0.81	2.42	0.90

Note. Maximum score for all questions = 4.

TABLE 3
Number and Percentage of Participants Passing Test Questions

	Williams Syndrome[a]		*Prader–Willi Syndrome*[b]		*Nonspecific Mental Retardation*[c]	
	Number	%	*Number*	%	*Number*	%
Perceptual access[d]	14	88	11	100	12	100
First-order knowledge[d]	9	56	8	73	8	67
Second-order knowledge[d]	7	44	7	64	8	67
Pass lie/joke[e]	0		2	18	2	17
Pass lie question[f]	14	88	11	100	10	83
Pass joke question[f]	0		2	18	2	17

[a]$n = 16$. [b]$n = 11$. [c]$n = 12$. [d]Passing at least three of four trials. [e]Passing both story pairs. [f]Passing two of two trials.

they were able to override their own knowledge of the story facts and correctly report the knowledge state of the main character. Overall, participants did somewhat less well on the second-order knowledge question. Although a majority of PWS and MRU adolescents passed at least three of four trials of this question (64% and 67%, respectively), only 44% of the WS adolescents passed. Chi-square analyses revealed that this difference was not significant. Adolescents in all three groups performed extremely poorly on the lie/joke discrimination question. Whereas 18% of the PWS and 17% of the MRU were able to correctly distinguish the lies from the jokes, none of the WS adolescents were able to do so, although this difference was not significant.

Looking at performance on the lie and the joke questions separately helps to clarify adolescents' difficulty in distinguishing these two forms of nonliteral utterance. As can be seen in Table 3, nearly all of the adolescents across all groups passed both trials of the lie question. That is, they correctly classified the lies as lies. However, only 2 of the PWS, 2 of the MRU, and none of the WS groups were able to correctly classify both of the joke statements. Of these adolescents, 14 (88%) of the WS, 10 (91%) of the PWS, and 11 (92%) of the MRU groups misclassified the jokes as lies. In contrast, none of the adolescents in any group misclassified the lies as jokes. To summarize, almost all the participants in this study judged all nonliteral statements as lies.

Correlations were computed for each group between performance on the second-order knowledge question, the lie/joke discrimination, and chronological age, Full-Scale IQ, PPVT–R mental age, and PPVT–R standard score. For the WS group, none of these correlations was significant. For the PWS group, performance on the second-order knowledge question was significantly correlated with PPVT–R mental age, $r(11) = .62$, $p < .04$. For the MRU group, performance on the lie/joke discrimination question was significantly correlated with Full-Scale IQ, $r(12) = .63$, $p < .03$. However, because our sample is quite small, the results of these analyses would need to be replicated on a much larger sample of children to determine the reliability of the relations found.

Justifications

The frequencies of different responses to the justification question are presented in Table 4. There were no differences between the lie and the joke stories in the use of the various justification responses. As can be seen, for both the lie and the joke stories, the majority of the justifications either referred to reality or to explicit second-order reasoning. Adolescents in the PWS and the MRU groups gave significantly more explicit second-order justifications than did WS adolescents: $\chi^2(1) = 5.07$, $p < .02$, and $\chi^2(1) = 9.28$, $p < .002$, for the lie stories, and $\chi^2(1) = 5.40$, $p < .02$, and $\chi^2(1) = 6.39$, $p < .01$, for the joke stories,

TABLE 4
Frequency of Justification Responses to the Lie/Joke Test Questions

	Williams Syndrome	*Prader–Willi Syndrome*	*Nonspecific Mental Retardation*
Lie stories			
Explicit second-order	1 (3.1%)	5 (22.7%)	8 (33.3%)
Perceptual information	2 (6.3%)	2 (9.1%)	2 (8.3%)
Reality response	18 (56.3%)	13 (59.1%)	10 (41.7%)
Story facts	4 (12.5%)	2 (9.1%)	2 (8.3%)
Reiteration of response	3 (9.4%)	0 (0.0%)	0 (0.0%)
Other	4 (12.5%)	0 (0.0%)	2 (8.3%)
Joke stories			
Explicit second-order	1 (3.1%)	5 (23.8%)	6 (25.0%)
Perceptual information	5 (15.6%)	3 (14.3%)	4 (16.7%)
Reality response	21 (65.6%)	11 (52.4%)	8 (33.3%)
Story facts	0 (0.0%)	2 (9.5%)	2 (8.3%)
Reiteration of response	0 (0.0%)	0 (0.0%)	0 (0.0%)
Other	5 (15.6%)	0 (0.0%)	4 (16.7%)

respectively. For the joke stories only, the WS adolescents provided significantly more reality justifications than did PWS and MRU adolescents: $\chi^2(1) = 8.87$, $p < .002$, and $\chi^2(1) = 9.52$, $p < .003$, respectively. This suggests that despite the lack of group differences on the lie/joke discrimination question, on the joke stories the adolescents with PWS and MRU were more likely to focus on the mental states of the story characters, whereas the adolescents with WS were more likely to justify their lie/joke decisions by judging the statement against what really happened.

Contingency Between Second-Order Knowledge and Lie/Joke Test Question

Because the ability to distinguish between lies and jokes rests on the ability to conceptualize second-order knowledge states (i.e., what the speaker knows about what the listener knows), we would expect to find a relationship between these two abilities (Sullivan et al., 1995). To test this hypothesis, we looked at the contingency between performance on the lie/joke discrimination and the second-order knowledge questions. Table 5 shows the contingency between passing the second-order knowledge questions and the lie/joke questions, where *passing* was defined as scoring correct on at least three trials of the second-order question and passing at least three of the lie/joke test questions. As can be seen, in all three groups, adolescents were more likely to pass the second-order knowledge question and fail

TABLE 5
Contingency Between Passing Lie/Joke and Second-Order Questions

Group	*Pass Both*	*Pass Lie/Joke Only*	*Pass Second-Order Only*	*Fail Both*
Williams syndrome	0	0	7 (44%)	9 (56%)
Prader–Willi syndrome	2 (18%)	0	4 (36%)	4 (36%)
Non-specific mental retardation	2 (17%)	0	6 (50%)	4 (33%)

the lie/joke discrimination than the reverse: McNemar's test, WS: $\chi^2(1) = 5.15$, $p < .02$, PWS: $\chi^2(1) = 2.25, p < .15$; and MRU: $\chi^2(1) = 4.16, p < .05$.

Finally, to see to what extent adolescents who can conceptualize second-order knowledge states go on to use this knowledge in their explanations of other's behavior, we looked at the number of justifications that included explicit references to complex mental states following correct responses on the second-order knowledge question. Both the PWS (38%) and the MRU (45%) adolescents provided significantly more explicit references to complex mental states in their justifications than did the WS adolescents (5%): $\chi^2(1) = 12.54$, $p < .001$, and $\chi^2(1) = 15.67, p < .001$, respectively. This suggests that even those WS participants who were able to conceptualize second-order knowledge states were not as likely to use that information in their justifications as adolescents in the other two groups.

DISCUSSION

The results of this study demonstrate that adolescents with WS have great difficulty distinguishing lies from jokes. Despite anecdotal reports of good language skills, particularly with conversational discourse, and their intense social investment in others, the WS adolescents in this study were no better at telling the lies from the jokes than matched comparison groups of PWS and mentally retarded adolescents. Thus, the assumption that there is a link among good language, social interest, and theory of mind is erroneous. None of the WS adolescents and only two adolescents in each of the PWS and mentally retarded groups could correctly identify both pairs of lie/joke stories. Nearly all the participants in the three groups misclassified the jokes as lies (88% WS, 91% PWS, and 92% MRU), whereas none of the adolescents in any group misclassified the lies as jokes. This error pattern mirrors what has been found in much younger normally developing children (Sullivan et al., 1995). Given that we know that normally developing children are able to distinguish between lies and other forms of intentional falsehood by middle childhood (Andrews et al., 1988; Leekam, 1991; Winner et al., 1987), the strikingly poor performance of the developmentally disordered adolescents in this study suggests serious impairment in this critical social–cognitive ability in these populations.

Adolescents in all three groups were much more successful at attributing perceptual access and first- and second-order knowledge states. Nearly all participants in all three groups understood the story characters' access to relevant perceptual information, and the majority of participants were also able to correctly report the main characters' first-order knowledge states. Thus, in the lie stories, participants were able to override their own knowledge of the story facts and correctly report on the main character's inaccurate knowledge of the truth. On the more complex second-order knowledge question, a majority of PWS and MRU adolescents and nearly half of the WS adolescents were able to attribute second-order knowledge states on at least three of four trials. Although many of the participants in all three groups had the prerequisite underlying knowledge of the characters' complex mental states, the vast majority was unable to tell lies from jokes.

These findings demonstrate that for adolescents with a variety of developmental disorders, the ability to distinguish lies from jokes depends in part on the prerequisite ability to attribute second-order mental states, specifically second-order knowledge. Adolescents in the three disordered groups were all more likely to pass the second-order knowledge question and fail the lie/joke discrimination than the reverse. Again, this is consistent with findings in the developmental literature (Happé, 1993; Leekam, 1991; Sullivan et al., 1995; Winner & Leekam, 1991). At the same time, it is important to note that among normally developing children there is a strong connection between the acquisition of second-order mental state knowledge and the ability to distinguish lies and other forms of nonliteral language; the timing between these developments is within a couple of years.

In contrast, among the developmentally disordered populations, although more than half passed the second-order knowledge questions, only 10% successfully discriminated between the lies and the jokes. Furthermore, many of the adolescents justified their responses by comparing the false statement to reality, rather than considering the second-order knowledge of the speaker. This is a strikingly immature response, suggesting that many adolescents had considerable difficulty integrating their understanding of other minds with their interpretation of speakers' nonliteral utterances. Further, whereas a substantial proportion of PWS and MRU participants who evidenced an understanding of second-order knowledge states referred to those states in their justifications, only 5% of the participants with WS did so. This suggests that adolescents with WS may have particular difficulty grasping the underlying connection between mental states and nonliteral language. Overall, the connection between acquiring a theory of mind and nonliteral language may not be as close in disordered populations as it is in normally developing children. However, longitudinal data would be needed to distinguish whether the gap is greater for children with mental retardation than for children who are developing normally.

The findings reported here on adolescents with WS contrast with those reported by Karmiloff-Smith et al. (1995), who found that 50% of WS participants were able to interpret sarcastic statements, which, like lie/joke discrimination, require an understanding of higher order mental states. One possible explanation for this discrepancy may be in the way in which the stimuli were presented. In our study, the critical lie/joke statement was purposefully delivered in neutral prosody to rule out the possibility that participants could discriminate the lies and jokes on the basis of prosodic features alone. The sarcastic statements in the Karmiloff-Smith et al. study may have been presented with natural prosody; the description of the methods used in their study does not preclude this possibility. If prosodic cues were provided, this could have allowed the WS participants to ignore the speaker's stated attitude to an internally represented thought (higher order understanding) and solve the task by interpreting the social–affective meaning of the statement via the prosodic features of the utterance. Although no studies have directly investigated whether people with WS are good at interpreting the social–affective aspects of prosody, their natural expressiveness in both conversational and narrative discourse contexts suggests that this may be the case (Reilly et al., 1990).

Recently we proposed that in WS, there is an important distinction in theory of mind abilities between a social perception component and a social cognitive component (Tager-Flusberg & Sullivan, 2000). The social perceptual component, which we argue is relatively spared in WS, refers to the capacity to make online immediate judgments of mental states on the basis of perceptual information available in facial expressions, vocal prosody, or body gesture. In contrast, the social cognitive component of theory of mind, which is not spared in WS, encompasses more complex cognitive reasoning about the mind, as tapped in more classic theory of mind tasks, such as false belief. Thus, on this view, adolescents with WS might be particularly adept at using prosodic cues to distinguish lies and jokes because this would draw on their relatively spared social perceptual component of theory of mind. On the other hand, this model of theory of mind fits with our findings that adolescents with WS would not perform well on tasks that entailed complex cognitive reasoning required for distinguishing between lies and jokes solely on the basis of information in the stories, which was required in the task we presented.

Despite the relatively good performance of all three groups on the theory of mind test questions, none of the groups performed well on the lie/joke discrimination. What is the social relevance of this poor performance? The inability to distinguish between intentionally false utterances intended as jokes versus those intended to deceive would seriously impair one's ability to relate to others in everyday social situations. Not being able to tell, for example, when someone is making a joke at your expense (e.g., "I just love your new haircut") or always being in the dark about a deceptive plan meant to hurt you would lead to severe problems with peers. It is not hard to imagine why children with developmental disabilities often find themselves the objects of teasing and cruel jokes by other children (Guralnick, 1984; Kasari & Bauminger, 1998). Simply keeping up with everyday discourse on the playground, which is littered with lies, jokes, ironic statements, and sarcastic remarks, would be an overwhelming if not impossible task for many of these children. Difficulties with peers would be the inevitable outcome of this sort of communicative incompetence. Indeed, we know that despite their social interest, people with WS have great difficulty forming and maintaining peer relationships throughout childhood (Davies, Udwin, & Howlin, 1998; Einfield, Tonge, & Florio, 1997; Udwin & Yule, 1991). Interestingly, children and adolescents with WS often have very positive relationships with adults, which do not seem to be affected by their lack of understanding of the differences between literal and nonliteral language. One possible explanation is that adults are more understanding of the limitations of individuals with WS and other developmental disorders, and simply do not use these types of intended falsehoods or other forms of nonliteral language in their conversations with these individuals.

Finally, the results of this study also provide some interesting evidence that neurodevelopmental disorders are fundamentally different from acquired disorders in adulthood. (Karmiloff-Smith, 1997; Paterson, Brown, Gsodl, Johnson, & Karmiloff-Smith, 1999). The participants in this study who were unable to discriminate between lies and ironic jokes all made the same kind of error: They systematically called all the jokes lies, and many of their justifications were comparisons between what was said with the reality. Thus the adolescents with WS, PWS, and MRU who failed the task considered nonliteral utterances to be lies, without reference to the speaker's mental state. This error pattern is similar to what has been reported among normally developing children (Sullivan et al., 1995; Winner & Sullivan, 1999). In contrast, Winner et al. (1998) found that adults with RHD had a very different error pattern, confusing lies and jokes. In their study, the adults with RHD were as likely to say that lies were jokes as they were to say that jokes were lies (the typical pattern.) Thus, whereas normally children and the atypical children in the present study have a default strategy to take nonliteral utterances as lies, the individuals with RHD do not. Winner et al. attribute the RHD adults' difficulty with nonliteral language to acquired impairments in higher order theory of mind. Because the patients in their study had once been capable of distinguishing among different types of falsehood, they were more likely to mix up the different nonliteral forms rather than resort to a developmentally primitive strategy (Brownell, Griffin, Winner, Friedman, & Happé, 2000; Winner & Sullivan, 1999). Thus, individuals with neurodevelopmental disorders, including those with WS, process nonliteral language in quite different ways from adults with acquired brain damage. We cannot take the parallel difficulties both groups have with distinguishing between lies and jokes as evidence that people with WS have a form of right hemisphere damage. Clearly the source of their difficulties lies elsewhere, and it is too simplistic and theoretically naive to equate the neuropsychological deficits associated with acquired RHD and WS, or even other neurodevelopmental disorders. Future research may provide insights into the underlying neurocognitive mechanisms that can explain why individuals with neurodevelopmental disorders, including WS, have such difficulty interpreting speakers' intended meaning in nonliteral discourse.

ACKNOWLEDGMENTS

This research was supported by a grant from the National Institute of Child Health and Human Development (RO1 HD 33470) to Helen Tager-Flusberg. We express our sincere thanks to the New England chapters and national organizations of the Williams Syndrome and Prader–Willi Syndrome associations for their help in recruiting participants, and to all the families who participated. We are also grateful to the students in the Plymouth public schools who participated in this project and to Robert Sherman for his continued support of our research.

REFERENCES

Andrews, J., Rosenblatt, E., Malkus, U., Gardner, H., & Winner, E. (1988). Children's abilities to distinguish metaphoric and ironic utterances from mistakes and lies. *Communication and Cognition, 19,* 281–298.

Bellugi, U., Bihrle, A., Neville, H., Jernigan, T., & Doherty, S. (1992). Language, cognition, and brain organization in a neurodevelopmental disorder. In M. Gunnar & C. Nelson (Eds.), *Developmental behavioral neuroscience: The Minnesota symposium* (pp. 201–232). Hillsdale, NJ: Lawrence Erlbaum Associates, Inc.

Bellugi, U., Jones, W., Harrison, D., Rossen, M. L., & Klima, E. (1995, March). *Discourse in two genetically-based syndromes with contrasting brain anomalies*. Paper presented at the meeting of the Society for Research in Child Development, Indianapolis, IN.

Bellugi, U., Mills, D., Jernigan, T., Hickok, G., & Galaburda, A. (1999). Linking cognition, brain structure, and brain function in Williams syndrome. In H. Tager-Flusberg (Ed.), *Neurodevelopmental disorders* (pp. 111–136). Cambridge, MA: MIT Press.

Brownell, H., Griffin, R., Winner, E., Friedman, O., & Happé, F. (2000). Cerebral lateralization and theory of mind. In S. Baron-Cohen, H. Tager-Flusberg, & D. J. Cohen (Eds.), *Understanding other minds: Perspectives from developmental cognitive neuroscience* (2nd ed., pp. 306–333). Oxford, England: Oxford University Press.

Davies, M., Udwin, O., & Howlin, P. (1998). Adults with Williams syndrome: Preliminary study of social, emotional and behavioural difficulties. *British Journal of Psychiatry, 172,* 273–276.

Dunn, L. E., & Dunn, L. E. (1981). *Peabody Picture Vocabulary Test-Revised*. Circle Pines, MN: American Guidance Services.

Einfield, S. L., Tonge, B. J., & Florio, T. (1997). Behavioral and emotional disturbance in individuals with Williams syndrome. *American Journal on Mental Reatardation, 102,* 45–53.

Elliott, C. D. (1990). *Differential Ability Scales*. San Diego, CA: Harcourt Brace.

Gosch, A., & Pankau, R. (1997). Personality characteristics and behavior problems in individuals of different ages with Williams syndrome. *Developmental Medicine and Child Neurology, 39,* 327–533.

Guralnick, M. J. (1984). The peer interaction of young developmentally delayed children in specialized and integrated settings. In T. Field, J. L. Roopnarine, & M. Segal (Eds.), *Friendships in normal and handicapped children* (pp. 139–152). Norwood, NJ: Ablex.

Happé, F. G. E. (1993). Communicative competence and theory of mind in autism: A test of Relevance theory. *Cognition, 48,* 101–119.

Happé, F. G. E. (1994). An advanced test of theory of mind: Understanding of story characters' thoughts and feelings by able autistic, mentally handicapped, and normal children and adults. *Journal of Autism and Developmental Disorders, 24,* 129–154.

Karmiloff-Smith, A. (1997). Crucial differences between developmental cognitive neuroscience and adult neuropsychology. *Developmental Neuropsychology, 13,* 513–524.

Karmiloff-Smith, A., Klima, E., Bellugi, U., Grant, J., & Baron-Cohen, S. (1995). Is there a social module? Language, face processing and theory of mind in individuals with Williams syndrome. *Journal of Cognitive Neuroscience, 7,* 196–208.

Kasari, C., & Bauminger, N. (1998). Social and emotional development in children with mental retardation. In J. A. Burack, R. M. Hodapp, & E. Zigler (Eds.), *Handbook of mental retardation and development* (pp. 411–433). Cambridge, England: Cambridge University Press.

Kaufman, A. S., & Kaufman, N. L. (1990). *Kaufman Brief Intelligence Test.* Circle Pines, MN: American Guidance Service.

Kelley, K., & Tager-Flusberg, H. (1995). Discourse characteristics of children with Williams syndrome: Evidence of spared theory of mind abilities. *Genetics Counseling, 6,* 169–170.

Leekam, S. (1991). Jokes and lies: Children's understanding of intentional falsehood. In A. Whiten (Ed.), *Natural theories of mind* (pp. 159–174). Oxford, England: Blackwell.

Mervis, C. B., Morris, C. A., Bertrand, J., & Robinson, B. F. (1999). Williams syndrome: Findings from an integrated program of research. In H. Tager-Flusberg (Ed.), *Neurodevelopmental disorders* (pp. 65–110). Cambridge, MA: MIT Press.

Paterson, S. J., Brown, J. H., Gsodl, M. K., Johnson, M. H., & Karmiloff-Smith, A. (1999). Cognitive modularity and genetic disorders. *Science, 286,* 2355–2358.

Reilly, J., Klima, E., & Bellugi, U. (1990). Once more with feeling: Affect and language in atypical populations. *Development and Psychopathology, 2,* 367–391.

Sperber, D., & Wilson, D. (1986). *Relevance: Communication and cognition.* Cambridge, MA: Harvard University Press.

Sullivan, K., & Tager-Flusberg, H. (1999). Second-order belief attribution in Williams syndrome: Intact or impaired? *American Journal on Mental Retardation, 104,* 523–532.

Sullivan, K., Winner, E., & Hopfield, N. (1995). How children tell a lie from a joke: The role of second-order mental attributions. *British Journal of Developmental Psychology, 13,* 191–204.

Tager-Flusberg, H., & Sullivan, K. (2000). A componential view of theory of mind: Evidence from Williams syndrome. *Cognition, 76,* 59–89.

Tager-Flusberg, H., Sullivan, K., & Boshart, J., (1997). Executive functions and performance on false belief tasks. *Developmental Neuropsychology, 13,* 487–493.

Udwin, O., & Yule, W. (1991). A cognitive and behavioral phenotype in Williams syndrome. *Journal of Clinical and Experimental Neuropsychology, 13,* 232–244.

Wimmer, H., & Perner, J. (1983). Beliefs about beliefs: Representation and constraining function of wrong beliefs in young children's understanding of deception. *Cognition, 13,* 103–128.

Wimmer, H., Gruber, S., & Perner, J. (1984). Young children's conception of lying: Lexical realism–moral subjectivism. *Journal of Experimental Child Psychology, 37,* 1–30.

Wimmer, H., Gruber, S., & Perner, J. (1985). Young children's conception of lying: Moral intuition and the denotation and connotation of "to lie." *Developmental Psychology, 21,* 993–995.

Winner, E. (1988). *The point of words: Children's understanding of metaphor and irony.* Cambridge, MA: Harvard University Press.

Winner, E., Brownell, H., Happé, F., Blum, A., & Pincus, D. (1998). Distinguishing lies from jokes: Theory of mind deficits and discourse interpretation in right hemisphere brain-damaged patients. *Brain and Language, 62,* 89–106.

Winner, E., & Leekam, S. (1991). Distinguishing irony from deception: Understanding the speaker's second-order intention. *British Journal of Developmental Psychology, 9,* 257–270.

Winner, E., & Sullivan, K. (1999, April). *Children's understanding of nonliteral statements and actions: Pretense, disguise, jokes and lies.* Paper presented at the meeting of the Society for Research in Child Development, Albuquerque, NM.

Winner, E., Windmueller, G., Rosenblatt, E., Bosco, L., & Best, E. (1987). Making sense of literal and nonliteral falsehood. *Metaphor and Symbolic Processes, 2,* 13–32.

APPENDIX
Script for Lie/Joke Task

Lie Version

This is a story about a boy named Frank and his grandfather. They are in the living room. Frank really wants to go to the mall with his friends, but his grandpa says he must first clean up his dishes. Frank hates cleaning up.

Grandpa goes out of the room to make a phone call. Frank does not clean up his dishes. See the dishes on the table? Now Frank goes into his room. While he is gone, Grandpa comes back into the living room and looks at the table covered with dishes. Frank does not see Grandpa looking at the dishes because he is in his room.

Perceptual access question. Does Grandpa see that Frank did not clean up his dishes? (If correct: That's right! Grandpa is looking right at the table covered with dishes; If incorrect: But look, Grandpa is looking right at the table covered with dishes.)

First-order knowledge question. Does Frank know that Grandpa saw the dirty dishes? Grandpa says to himself, "Frank did not clean up the dishes!"

Second-order knowledge question. Does Frank know that Grandpa knows that he did not clean up the dishes?

Now, Grandpa goes to Frank's room. Frank says to Grandpa, "I did a really good job cleaning up my dishes!" Now remember, Frank does not know that Grandpa saw the dishes on the table.

Lie/Joke discrimination question. Was Frank just kidding or lying (lying or kidding)?

Justification. How can you tell that Frank was (lying/just kidding)?

Joke Version

This is a story about a boy named Frank and his grandfather. They are in the living room. Frank really wants to go to the mall with his friends, but his grandpa says he must first clean up his dishes. Frank hates cleaning up.

Grandpa goes out of the room to make a phone call. Frank does not clean up his dishes. See the dishes on the table? Now Grandpa comes back. He looks right at the table covered with dishes.

Perceptual access question. Does Grandpa see that Frank did not clean up his dishes? (If correct: That's right! Grandpa is looking right at the table covered with dishes; If incorrect: But look, Grandpa is looking right at the table covered with dishes.)

First-order knowledge question. Does Frank know that Grandpa saw the dirty dishes? Grandpa says to himself, "Frank did not clean up the dishes!"

Second-order knowledge question. Does Frank know that Grandpa knows that he did not clean up the dishes?

Frank says to Grandpa, "I did a really good job cleaning up my dishes!" Now remember, Frank knows that Grandpa saw the dirty dishes.

Lie/joke discrimination uestion. Was Frank just kidding or lying (lying or kidding)?

Justification. How can you tell that Frank was (lying/joking)?

Objects, Motions, and Paths: Spatial Language in Children With Williams Syndrome

Barbara Landau
Johns Hopkins University

Andrea Zukowski
University of Maryland

The acquisition of spatial language is often assumed to be built upon an early-emerging system of nonlinguistic spatial knowledge. We tested this relationship by examining spatial language in children with Williams syndrome (WS), a rare genetic disorder that gives rise to severe nonlinguistic spatial deficits together with relatively spared language. Twelve children with WS, 12 normally developing mental-age matched children, and 12 normal adults described 80 videotaped motion events. Children with WS showed substantial control over key linguistic components of the motion event, including appropriate semantic and syntactic encoding of Figure and Ground objects, Manner of Motion, and Path. The expression of Path, although surprisingly spared, was more fragile among children with WS in contexts plausibly related to their nonlinguistic spatial deficit. The results show strong preservation of the formal aspects of spatial–linguistic knowledge and suggest that the nonlinguistic spatial deficits shown by children with WS have, at most, limited effects on their spatial language. These findings have implications for the relationship between spatial language and other aspects of spatial cognition.

One of our most fundamental capacities is the ability to talk about the objects and events around us. Even during early language learning, children take delight in commenting on objects and their motions through space. The privileged nature of the motion event in language learning stems, no doubt, from the salience and

Requests for reprints should be sent to Barbara Landau, Department of Cognitive Science, Krieger Hall, Johns Hopkins University, Baltimore, MD 21218. E-mail: landau@cogsci.jhu.edu

interest that such events hold for young children. However, equally important is the fact that languages are well designed to capitalize on this salience, with universal means of encoding objects, their motions, and the paths along which they move. The early emergence of such aspects of language has traditionally been viewed as evidence that language builds on nonlinguistic representations: Because children can and do perceive and represent objects, motions, and paths, they naturally tend to express these notions linguistically. In fact, the character of children's spatial language has often been taken as a clue to the nature of their underlying nonlinguistic representation of space (Brown, 1973; Clark, 1973; Bowerman, 1996).

From this perspective, severe impairment in the child's nonlinguistic representation of space would predict corresponding impairments in spatial language. Must this necessarily be true? In this article, we address this question by examining the linguistic expression of motion events among children with Williams syndrome (WS)—a rare genetic defect which results in severe spatial deficits together with relatively spared language. The striking difference in profile between the two systems of knowledge—spatial cognition and language—raises the question of the extent to which spatial deficits in WS have an impact on the acquisition of spatial language. At the extremes lie two possibilities: Spatial language in children with WS might show severe deficits, like other aspects of their spatial cognition. Alternatively, their spatial language might be relatively spared, like other aspects of their language. Between these extremes lies the intriguing possibility that spatial language may be selectively impaired in ways that closely reflect the nature of the nonlinguistic spatial deficit. In this case, examining spatial language in children with WS should shed light on how nonlinguistic representations of space support spatial language and what consequences for spatial language follow from a deficit in nonlinguistic spatial representations. The results of such an investigation can, more generally, be brought to bear on considerations of the relationships between spatial language and spatial cognition.

BACKGROUND AND GENERAL ISSUES

WS is a neurodevelopmental disorder caused by a hemizygous microdeletion on the long arm of chromosome 7 (7q11.32). The syndrome gives rise to a variety of characteristics, including pathology of the heart and other internal organs, a characteristic facial profile (often referred to as *elfin facies*), and mild to moderate mental retardation. Of particular interest to cognitive scientists, however, is the unusual cognitive profile typical of individuals with WS: They show severe spatial deficits accompanied by surprisingly spared language. The unique developmental profiles of space and language naturally suggest the possibility that the two systems may be developmentally modular, emerging independent of each other (Bellugi, Bihrle, Neville, Doherty, & Jernigan, 1992).

The spatial deficits of individuals with WS have been documented in a range of studies, but the most widely cited evidence comes from tasks which require that people observe a spatial configuration and then reconstruct it, either by drawing a copy of a pictured object or array or by putting together a set of blocks to duplicate an existing multiblock spatial design. The spatial performance of individuals with WS is typically far inferior to normally developing children of the same chronological age (Bellugi et al. 1992; Mervis, Morris, Bertrand, & Robinson, 1999) and it is even inferior to normally developing children of the same mental age (Hoffman, Landau, & Pagani, in press; Mervis et al., 1999). For example, Bellugi et al. (1992) reported that individuals with WS performed in the bottom percentile of their age group in a standardized block construction task, and Mervis et al. (1999) reported the same. Importantly, the performance of these individuals in these construction tasks is qualitatively different from that shown by individuals with comparable retardation of different etiology. For example, when copying a multiblock design, children with WS tend to duplicate the local elements at the expense of the global form, but children of the same mental age with Down syndrome tend to do the reverse (Bellugi et al., 1992; see also Birhle, Bellugi, Delis, & Marks, 1989). The pattern of spatial deficit appears early in development, and although there is some developmental growth in the ability to solve spatial construction tasks, the severe deficit persists into adulthood (Mervis et al., 1999).

In contrast to this impairment in the spatial domain, individuals with WS typically show language capabilities that meet or exceed expectations based on mental age. The relative advantage of linguistic over nonlinguistic abilities appears quite early, within the first several years (Mervis & Bertrand, 1997), and thereafter, children with WS have language that is surprisingly fluent, with rich modulation of tone and expression (Bellugi et al., 1992). Despite this strength, recent research indicates that language in individuals with WS may not be entirely intact. For example, mastery of morphological rules and aspects of lexical learning may be impaired (Clahsen & Almazan-Hamilton, 1999; Karmiloff-Smith et al., 1997) and the semantics underlying certain lexical items in individuals with WS may not be as in conceptually rich as in normally developing children (Johnson & Carey, 1998). Nevertheless, vocabulary measures show performance generally above overall mental age (Bellugi et al., 1992) and, to the casual ear, the children's spontaneous vocabulary and overall language skills are strong (Bellugi, Wang, & Jernigan, 1994). It is safe to say that the contrast between their profound spatial deficit and their relatively spared language is striking.

What do these profiles predict for the acquisition of spatial language? Because spatial language sits at the intersection of spatial cognition and language, it affords us an unusual opportunity to understand the degree to which the two systems of knowledge emerge independently and/or interact with each other. In particular, it can help us to understand what aspects of spatial cognition might be crucial support for the acquisition of spatial language. At one extreme, if spatial language in WS is severely compromised, the details of its breakdown could provide insight about which aspects of spatial cognition are impaired. At the other extreme, if spatial language in WS is completely preserved, the details regarding preserved structure would provide insight about what aspects of spatial cognition might be intact. Each of these broad possibilities raises further questions. If spatial language is selectively impaired, does the nature of the impairment closely reflect the nature of the nonlinguistic spatial impairment? What do the selectively preserved aspects of spatial language suggest about mechanisms of acquisition?

To test these broad possibilities, we examined the language produced by children with WS when they were asked to describe on-going motion events. The motion events depicted a wide range of objects undergoing a variety of motions and moving along a variety of paths (see Materials for details). Motion events are of particular interest because languages universally encode them in terms of a small but specific set of components, which can plausibly be viewed as corresponding to the nonlinguistic components that guide our perception and understanding of such events. The question arises whether children with WS can represent these components and whether they can correctly encode them using language in order to describe the entire motion event.

SPATIAL COGNITION AND THE LINGUISTIC ENCODING OF THE MOTION EVENT

In an influential analysis, Talmy (1975) showed that the linguistic expression of motion events is universally encoded by a small set of key components, which are then assembled somewhat differently in different languages. Many linguists have suggested that these components may be reflections of the nonlinguistic representation of events (Fillmore, 1997; Gruber, 1976; Jackendoff, 1983; Langacker, 1987; Pustejovsky, 1991; Talmy, 1975).

The linguistic components represent the objects participating in the event, the types of motions that they undergo, and the paths along which the objects travel. Talmy uses the following example in English:

The bottle	floated	into	the cave.
Figure object	Motion + Manner	Path	Ground object

In Talmy's (1975) terms, the Figure object is that which normally undergoes motion, and in English, this is typically encoded as a noun phrase, in this case "the bottle." The Motion is represented by the verb in English, which may represent a simple motion such as "come," "go," or "move," but may also include a semantic element encoding the "manner of motion," in this case, resulting in the Motion + Manner verb "float." The Path along which the Figure object moves is usually encoded in English by a spatial preposition, as "into" in the example, and this is often combined with the Ground object, encoded in English as a noun phrase (in this case, "the cave"). Thus, the basic pattern in English encodes the Figure and Ground objects, Manner of Motion, and Path in separate terms, yielding what Talmy calls a "satellite" language, one in which the Path term is encoded separately from the Motion.

Although all languages encode the same set of components, they vary in how these components are packaged. For example, English possesses many Manner of Motion verbs, often packaging Manner together with Motion and expressing Path separately. In contrast, French and Spanish tend to package Path together with Motion (resulting in numerous verbs such as "exit" or "descend," which are relatively rare in English), and encode the Manner in a separate form, such as the adverb (e.g., La bottella *entra* en la cueva *flotando*/The bottle *moved into* the cave *floating*).

How might the linguistic expression of the motion event be affected by the spatial deficit characteristic of individuals with WS? Each component of the motion event might be affected somewhat differently because each encodes a different spatial element and because these elements differ somewhat in their linguistic requirements. This means that different patterns of preservation and sparing might follow from deficits in spatial cognition versus deficits in knowledge of language. We therefore consider the components separately, describing the requirements for appropriate conceptual/spatial and linguistic use of each. These are summarized in Table 1.

TABLE 1
Conceptual and Linguistic Components of the Motion Event

Component	*Nonlinguistic Representation*	*Linguistic Coding*
Figure object	Object kind (e.g., dog, woman, truck)	Noun phrase
	Spatial role (object that moves)	Theme/subject of sentence
Motion and Manner	Motion (and specific kind)	Verb (Manner of Motion)
Path	Path of travel	Preposition
	Bounded TO	TO prepositions
	Bounded FROM	FROM prepositions
	VIA	VIA prepositions
Ground object	Object kind (e.g., dog, woman, truck)	Noun phrase
	Spatial role (reference object)	Goal/object of the preposition
	Path-relevant properties	Semantic match to
	Container-type	IN/OUT prepositions
	Surface-type	ON/OFF prepositions

Note. The linguistic components listed here are appropriate to simple English sentences such as the ones described in the text. Most of the sentences produced by participants in our study were of this type.

Figure and Ground Objects

These require representation of the objects involved, their respective semantic/thematic roles in the event (i.e., Figure or Ground object), and correct assignment of each to its syntactic position. Figure and Ground objects are typically encoded in simple English sentences as the subject of the sentence and the object of the preposition, respectively.

The evidence on object representation in Williams syndrome is meager. However, the early emergence of object terms among children with WS does not appear to be seriously impaired (Mervis & Bertrand, 1997; Stevens & Karmiloff-Smith, 1997), and experimental evidence suggests no severe impairment in the object recognition system (see also Hoffman & Landau, 2000; Wang, Doherty, Rourke, & Bellugi, 1995). Furthermore, the early vocabulary of children with WS is comprehensive enough that one would not expect profound deficits in naming common objects. Beyond this, however, children with WS may or may not be able to understand the spatial/thematic roles of the Figure and Ground, respectively. If they have difficulties in understanding these roles or difficulty in mapping these roles into language, they might show problems in assigning the corresponding nouns to their semantic roles and to their proper syntactic positions. For example, correct assignment of Figure "the bottle" and Ground "the cave" to theme/sentential subject and goal/object of the preposition, respectively, requires accurate perception of which object serves each role (Figure/theme; Ground/goal) and how these are encoded syntactically. It is possible, therefore, that the children might name the objects correctly, but show errors in assigning the nouns to their proper thematic roles and syntactic positions.

Motion and Manner of Motion

These require that the child accurately perceive the motion that an object undergoes and encode it in the verb. To our knowledge, there is no evidence on knowledge of motion verbs among children with WS. However, there is some evidence regarding motion perception. In one study, individuals with WS were found to have abnormal motion perception, specifically showing raised thresholds for the detection of motion (Atkinson et al., 1997). In a different study, children with WS were found to have preserved perception of biological motion, showing the capacity to judge the direction of motion under a variety of noise conditions (Jordan, Reiss, Hoffman, & Landau, 2002). Neither study permits a straightforward prediction for whether children with WS should experience difficulty with the motion component of motion events because the stimuli and task requirements in studies of motion perception differ considerably from those in language tasks. What we can say, however, is that if children with WS have significant deficits in motion perception, this could result in difficulties naming specific motions, some of which require perception of direction (e.g., come vs. go/jump vs. fall). Furthermore, the encoding of specific Manners of Motion could be affected, since this requires perception of particular Manners and encoding by the proper Manner of Motion verb. It is possible, therefore, that children with WS might show impairment in the ability to use motion verbs appropriately, especially specific Manner of Motion verbs.

Path

Paths play a major role in the linguistic encoding of motion events (Jackendoff, 1983). In English, verbs of motion typically can accept a Path expression, although this is not obligatory. For example, verbs such as roll, spin, fly, walk, and move are grammatical with or without an accompanying specification of the Path (e.g., both "John flew" and "John flew to the moon" are grammatical). If the Path is expressed, this is accomplished using a "Path-function" term that encodes the Path itself, and in English, this is usually a spatial preposition. Some prepositions are intransitive, that is, they do not require that a Ground object be specified (e.g., both "John went up/down" and "John went up/down the street" are grammatical); others are transitive, requiring the presence of a noun phrase expressing the Ground object for grammaticality (e.g., "John went into the house" is grammatical, whereas *"John went into" is not). Thus, the structure of Path expressions requires accurately perceiving the Path, linguistically encoding it, and, in some cases, also encoding the Ground object, which must be placed in its proper syntactic position as object of the preposition.

Path expressions show further complexity, as they can be divided into three broad types, which code different kinds of spatial relationships (Jackendoff, 1983[1]; see Figure 1). In TO Paths, the Ground object is the goal, lying at the end of the path, for example, John ran *to* the *house*. In contrast, in FROM Paths, the Ground object is the source, lying at the beginning of the path, for example, John ran *from* the *house*. Both of these are Bounded Paths (i.e. they have definite origins or endpoints) and each can be encoded using a variety of prepositions (e.g., *on, to, in*, and *into* all encode TO Paths and *off, away/from*, and *out* all encode FROM Paths). In the third broad type, VIA Paths, the Ground object lies somewhere along the Path, but not at its beginning or end, for example, John went *by* the *house*). VIA paths can be encoded by terms such as *by, along, through*, or *over*. Thus, properly encoding the Path requires perceiving and representing the

[1]Jackendoff (1983) also discusses Directional Paths, which code Paths in which the Ground object does not lie at either beginning or end, but somewhere more distant along the Path, if it were to continue, for example, John went *toward* the house. *Toward* and *away from* encode this Path type; these two illustrative terms differ in polarity, just like the TO/FROM Path types discussed in the text.

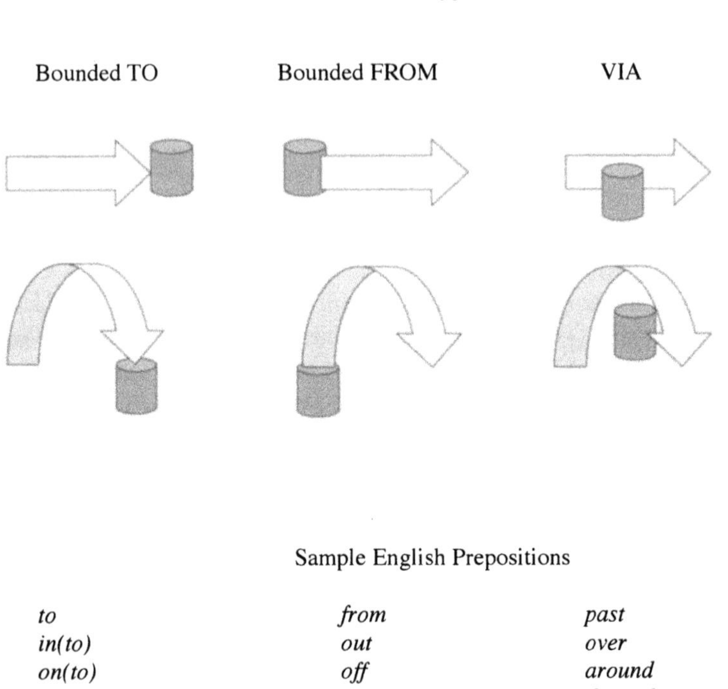

FIGURE 1 Three types of Paths that are distinguished in English by the sets of spatial prepositions that can encode them.

particular type of Path (Bounded TO, FROM, or VIA), each of which specifies a different spatial role for the Ground object. This representation of the Path must be used to select an appropriate spatial preposition.

A final complexity of Path expressions stems from the conceptual constraints that some prepositions place on their accompanying Ground objects (Herskovits, 1986; Jackendoff, 1983; Landau & Jackendoff, 1993; Talmy, 1983). We have already observed that encoding the Ground object requires representing the particular kind of object as a noun phrase, which is the object of the preposition. In addition, however, the meanings of some prepositions restrict the type of Ground object they can accept. Violations of these restrictions lead to oddities of expression in some cases, and in other cases to downright inaccuracies. Several prominent examples include the prepositions *in*(to), *out* (of), *on*(to), and *off* (of; see Figure 2). The first two terms are restricted to geometric types that, in some abstract sense, function like "containers": Because the semantics of in and out

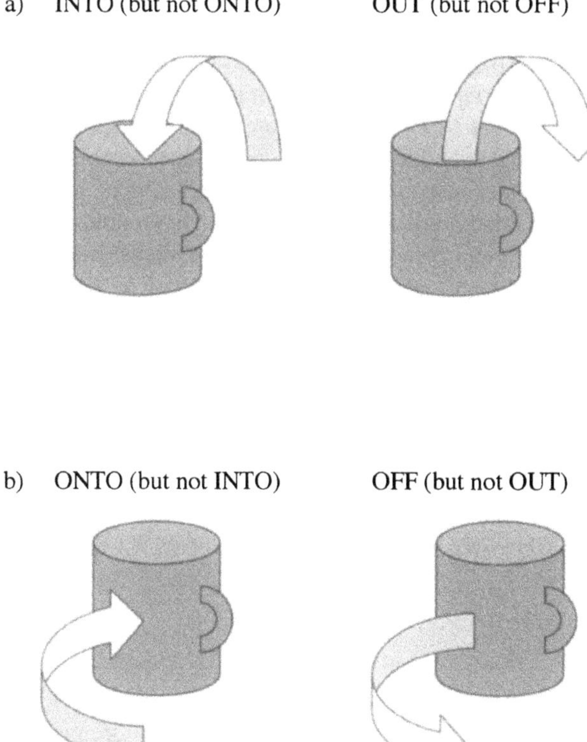

FIGURE 2 Certain spatial prepositions place geometric constraints on the Ground objects they can accept. See text for discussion.

refer, respectively, to the interior and exterior regions of containers, these prepositions can only occur with "container-type" Ground objects. Paths that lead from the inside to the outside of a container (or vice versa) must encode this "containerness" by using *into* (or *out of*) rather than *onto* (or *off of*). For example, given a bug that jumps from a table to the inside of a coffee cup, one can sensibly say, "The bug jumped *into* the coffee cup," but not "*onto*" the coffee cup. Similarly, because the semantics of on and off refer to the external surface and the exterior region of "surfaces," respectively, these prepositions can only occur with "surface-type" objects. Given a bug that flies from a table to the external surface of a cup, one can say "The bug jumped *onto* the cup," but not "*into*" the cup.

Properly encoding the Path therefore requires perceiving and representing the Path type, selecting an appropriate Path term, matching this Path term to an appropriate Ground object, and placing them in an appropriately structured prepositional phrase. Although, to our knowledge, nothing is known about the linguistic encoding of Paths by children with WS, it seems possible that this element of the motion event would be quite vulnerable to the effects of their nonlinguistic spatial deficit. Because Paths encode spatial relationships over time, and because the linguistic expression of Paths incorporates such rich spatial information, it seems quite possible that children with WS could show impairment in encoding different types of Path, selecting appropriate prepositions, and observing the selection restrictions that prepositions impose on their Ground objects.

In sum, the motion event encodes rich spatial information including the Figure object, its Motion and Manner-of-Motion, and the Path along which it travels with respect to a Ground object. Each of these components requires selection of an appropriate semantic element and placement of this element in the appropriate syntactic position. Spatial language in children with WS might be impaired overall or impaired selectively, reflecting breakdown in particular aspects of spatial representation. Conversely, spatial language in these children might be spared, either overall or selectively. In either case, the character of spatial language in WS is bound to shed light on which aspects of spatial representation are vulnerable and which are robust when they coexist with a severely impaired system of nonlinguistic spatial representation.

METHOD

To examine these issues, we elicited descriptions of simple motion events from children with WS and compared their performance to that of normally developing children matched for mental age as well as normal adults. The question was what pattern of sparing and deficit would be shown in this rich domain of spatial language.

Participants

Twelve children with WS (median age 9 years, 7 months [9:7], range 7:0–14:0) participated as well as 12 normally developing children who served as mental age matches (median age 5:0, range 3:6–6:9). Twelve undergraduates also participated to provide a ceiling against which the children's data could be compared. All groups were roughly balanced for gender. The children were given the Kaufman Brief Intelligence Test (Kaufman & Kaufman, 1990), which yields an overall IQ score as well as scores for two components, Verbal and Matrices. The Verbal component requires the child to name a series of objects portrayed by black and white line drawings. The Matrices component taps conceptual abilities, requiring judgments of which objects go together in pairs or form complete sets, but there are very few items that require spatial representation. With this measure, the children with WS are not penalized for their spatial deficit, and therefore their scores represent a fair measure of nonverbal (but nonspatial) intelligence. The children with WS were individually matched to controls, resulting in excellent matching for the component scores (*M* Verbal scores = 30.2 and 30.6, *SE*s = 2.2 and 1.9, ranges = 18–46 and 21–39, respectively; *M* Matrices scores = 17.3 and 17.6, *SE*s = 1.3 and 1.1, ranges = 10–24 and 13–21, respectively). The corresponding composite IQ scores were *M* = 77.3 (*SE* = 2.8, range 61–92) and 116.7 (*SE* = 2.8, range 102–139), respectively. The scores of the children with WS are similar to those of other groups studied by other researchers (e.g., Mervis et al., 1999).

On a variety of measures, the children with WS were severely impaired in their nonlinguistic spatial capacity, as would be expected. For example, their drawings of simple figures revealed the lack of spatial organization that is characteristic of people with WS (e.g., Hoffman & Landau, 2000). As part of a larger research program, the children were tested on the Pattern Construction subtest of the Differential Abilities Scale (Elliot, 1990). This requires the child to reconstruct a complex design composed of individual blocks, and is widely regarded as a hallmark task for diagnosing the spatial deficit in WS. Nine of the children with WS scored in the 1st percentile for their age, and the remaining three performed at the 4th, 8th, and 10th percentiles, respectively; the mean age equivalent for the group was 4 years, 2 months. These scores are similar to those reported in other studies of individuals with WS (Bellugi et al., 1992; Mervis et al., 1999) and indicate severely impaired spatial cognition. At the time of this study, only 4 of the normally developing controls were tested on the Pattern Construction test. They scored in the 60th percentile for their age (*SE* = 15.8), with a mean age equivalent of 6 years, 11 months. These scores are similar to those of our larger sample of normally developing controls (*n* = 9), who are also matched for mental age to the same children with WS, but are participating in other studies of spatial cognition in our lab. These children scored in the 51st percentile for their age (SE = 7.6), with a mean age equivalent of 6 years.

The children with WS were recruited with the assistance of the National Williams Syndrome Association and the A. I. DuPont Hospital for Children. They all lived within a 2.5-hr travel range of the University of Delaware. Normally developing control children were recruited from parent groups and preschools local to the University of Delaware. Undergraduates were students at the University of Delaware, who participated for class credit.

Design, Materials, and Procedure

Each participant viewed a set of 80 brief (5 sec) animated videoclips, one at a time, and described the simple motion events that occurred in them. This yielded a corpus of 2,880 sentences, which formed the basis for all analyses. The stimulus battery, the Verbs of Motion Production Test, was created and used by Supalla and Newport to evaluate mastery of the morphology of motion verbs in American Sign Language

(ASL; Newport, 1990; Singleton & Newport, in press; Supalla, 1982). The motion events were designed to elicit contrasts relevant in ASL, and many of these contrasts are also encoded in English, as discussed later; hence the battery was appropriate for use with English speakers. There was a broad range of motion events, which elicited a broad range of object, Motion, and Path terms in English (see Appendix for a complete list of events).

Participants were told that they were going to watch some short movies and that after each one they would be asked to tell the experimenter what happened. Our goal was to elicit sentences that included as many of the relevant components of the motion event as possible (Figure, Ground, Motion and Manner, Path). To maximize performance, and following Newport (1990), practice trials were given prior to showing the test events. The experimenter praised the sentences produced in these trials and, if necessary, encouraged more detail. For example, one practice event showed a chicken jumping off of a fence. If a child said, "It's a chicken," then the experimenter would say, "Right—and what happened?" Participants then generally produced more complete descriptions. Before moving to the next practice trials, the experimenter said, "Good—that's right, the chicken jumped off of the fence. Say it nice and complete, like that." Five practice trials were given just before the beginning of the task. During the test, children occasionally commented only on the existence of the Figure object; in these cases, they were prompted for more complete sentences as during the practice trials. Test sessions were videotaped and all of the responses were later transcribed for analysis.

The 80 events in the battery vary in the participating objects, the motions they undergo, and the paths along which they move. The objects include toy people, animals, vehicles, and common everyday objects. Forty of the scenes involve just a single moving object (the Figure object, which moves against an unmarked background) and the other 40 involve both a moving Figure object and a stationary Ground object. The events differ in Manner of Motion (e.g., rolling, flying, falling, jumping) and Path type. For the 40 events including a Ground object, Path type was determined by inspecting the videotaped event to ascertain the role of the Ground object. Of the 40 events, 12 involved Bounded TO Paths, 16 involved Bounded FROM Paths, and 12 involved VIA Paths. The Paths were executed in a variety of ways, including along a straight line, with a turn, or zigzagging. The categorization of Path types was confirmed by later analysis of the Path terms that were used by adults to describe each event. Path terms used by adults conformed perfectly to the initial categorizations of Path type.

RESULTS

The transcribed sentences were analyzed for quantitative and qualitative differences among the participant groups in the expression of the central components of the motion event. Participants in all three groups produced coherent, grammatical sentences and syntactically well-formed sentence fragments.

Figure Objects

Both quantitatively and qualitatively, the encoding of Figure objects was remarkably similar across the adults, normally developing children, and children with WS. Quantitatively, participants encoded the Figure object for almost every event (1% omission among children with WS, 2% among control children), and the Figure was almost always encoded as a subject noun phrase in full grammatical sentences. Of the 960 descriptions produced by each group (80 events × 12 participants), 480 involved a Ground object; of these, there were only 3 instances of reversal in syntactic assignment between Figure and Ground object, all produced by 2 children with WS. Among all participants, the preferred means for encoding the Figure was to use a specific noun. Across the 80 events, adults used a specific noun to name the Figure object 97% of the time ($SE = 0.9$), with the remaining 3% accounted for by more general noun phrases (e.g., "the thing"). The WS children used specific nouns 85% of the time ($SE = 5.5$), general noun phrases 5% of the time, and pronouns 6% of the time. The corresponding percentages for control children were 88% ($SE = 2.9$), 4%, and 6%, respectively.

The qualitative nature of the specific nouns used was also quite similar across the participant groups, reflecting considerable consensus in what the objects were and what they should be called. To quantify this, the modal adult response was listed for each of the events, and the children's responses were analyzed in terms of percentage that matched these adult-produced nouns. Across the 80 events, there were four different categories of Figure object: People, Animals, Vehicles, and Other types of object (*ns* = 8, 9, 17, 46, respectively). Across all categories, the adult modal responses accounted for 95% of their data; children with WS matched these 67% of the time ($SE = 2.8$), and control children 72% of the time ($SE = 2.8$). The remaining responses were semantically plausible alternatives to the modal adult responses. All Figure objects produced by the children were evaluated for semantic anomaly by two independent coders, blind to participant group. Semantic anomalies were defined as terms that incorrectly named the Figure in the context of each event, and only items scored as anomalies by both coders were further considered. Out of the 960 descriptions produced by each group, anomalous Figure objects were produced less than 1% of the time in either group.

The percentage of children's matches to the adult modal term for each category of Figure object were entered into a 2 (Group) × 4 (Category of Figure object) analysis of variance (ANOVA), resulting in a main effect of Figure object Category, $F(3, 66) = 9.07$, $p < .01$, and an interaction between Group and Figure Category, $F(3, 66) = 3.13$, $p < .05$. The control children matched the adult responses more frequently than did the children with WS on all Figure types except People, where the reverse was true, but none of the pairwise comparisons between controls and children with WS reached significance (Tukey's HSD = 21, critical $p = .05$, in this and all further comparisons). In sum, Figure objects were encoded at ceiling levels by all groups, and responses were syntactically well-formed and semantically coherent.

Ground Objects

Across the 40 events in which a specific Ground object was present, adults produced a pertinent term 99% of the time; these were almost always as object of the preposition. Of these, 93% were specific nouns (*SE* = 1.5) and 4% were general noun phrases. Thus, for adults, the Ground object was considered to be an obligatory element of their descriptions. In contrast, both groups of children omitted the Ground object relatively frequently, with controls omitting it approximately12% of the time and WS children 26% of the time (*SE*s = 2.0, 3.5), a difference considered at more length later. When they included the Ground object, control children produced specific nouns 77% of the time (*SE* = 4.4), and general noun phrases 6% of the time; children with WS produced specific nouns 60% of the time (*SE* = 6.5) and general noun phrases 4% of the time. The remaining responses fell into the following categories. Ground objects were coded by pronouns 1% of the time (each group of children) and were supplied by the experimenter 1% of the time (WS only). The remaining 4% of the controls and 8% of the responses from WS children were somewhat ambiguous with respect to whether they coded the Ground object, as they appeared to code it implicitly by using impact verbs such as crash (whose semantics assumes a goal, 1.4% controls, 3% WS) or specific Path terms such as off or out for events where the Ground object was a surface or container, respectively (thus suggesting a specific kind of Ground, 2.6% controls, 5% WS). Two different sets of analyses were conducted, one including and one excluding these ambiguous items in the category of Omissions. The results did not differ. Therefore, the results reported here used the more conservative estimate of Omissions; that is, without these ambiguous items.

Considering the children's specific nouns against the adults' modally produced Ground objects for each event, control children matched the adult choices 62% of the time (*SE* = 3.0), and children with WS matched 68% of the time (*SE* = 2.9). The rest of the nouns were plausible alternatives to the adult choice. Using the same criteria for semantic anomaly as for Figure objects, we found that anomalous Ground objects were produced less than 1% of the time by either group of children.

Inspection of the contexts of the Ground object omissions revealed that certain types of events—specifically, those involving certain types of Paths—were especially vulnerable (see Table 2). Recall that there were 12 Bounded TO Paths, 16 Bounded FROM Paths, and 12 VIA paths. A 2 (Group) × 3 (Path type) ANOVA was conducted on the percentage of omissions made by children over different

TABLE 2
Mean Percentages and Standard Error of Ground Object Omissions as a Function of Path Type in the 40 Figure–Ground Events

	Adults		*Controls*		*Williams Syndrome Group*	
Path Type	*M*	*SE*	*M*	*SE*	*M*	*SE*
Bounded TO[a]	0.0	0.0	6.9	1.7	14.6	4.1
Bounded FROM[b]	1.0	0.7	12.0	3.8	35.9	7.2
Via[c]	2.1	1.5	16.0	4.2	22.9	5.1
Total[d]	1.0		11.7		25.6	

[a]$n = 12$. [b]$n = 16$. [c]$n = 12$. [d]$n = 40$.

Path types. The results showed a main effect of Group, $F(1, 22) = 5.5$, $p < .05$, and Path type, $F(2, 44) = 8.9$, $p < .01$, and an interaction between the two, $F(4, 44) = 4.6$, $p = .01$. Children with WS omitted more Ground objects overall than control children. Moreover, the omissions by the children with WS were reliably related to Path type. Post-hoc comparisons revealed no reliable differences across Path type for the control children, but the children with WS omitted reliably more Ground objects in events with FROM Paths than events with either TO or VIA Paths (critical difference = 13). We return to this fact when we discuss the results for Path terms.

Motions

As with the naming of Figure and Ground objects, there are many options for naming the motion: Each could be encoded using a simple motion verb such as go or move; most could also be encoded using more specific verbs that express Manner of Motion, such as jump or fly. Some of the events could be plausibly described without using a motion verb at all. Nevertheless, all groups of participants encoded most events using Motion verbs (adults 92%, control children 89%, and WS children 89%, *SE*s = 1.4, 1.7, and 1.7, respectively), and these were produced in syntactically correct contexts. The remaining nonmotion verbs will not be considered further in any analyses.

A first analysis was conducted to determine whether, across all 80 scenes, there were quantitative differences across the groups in the use of simple verbs of motion, compared to more specific ones. All verbs were classified as Simple (including the verbs go, come, and move) or Specific (including all remaining verbs, most of which were Manner of Motion). Adults used Specific Motion verbs 72% of the time, whereas controls did so 64% of the time and children with WS 57% of the time (*SE*s = 2.5, 3.0, and 5.4, respectively). An ANOVA was conducted on the proportion of Specific Motion verbs used by different participant groups. There was a reliable effect of Group, $F(2, 33) = 3.5$, $p < .05$; post-hoc tests showed a reliable difference only between adults and children with WS (critical difference = 13.4). Thus children with WS used fewer Specific Motion verbs than adults, but were not reliably different from their mental age matches.

Remarkably, the Specific verbs used by the participants were very similar. Table 3 shows the 12 most frequent Specific verbs of motion and their relative frequency. The top 7 verbs—all Manner of Motion verbs—were identical and are ranked identically across the three groups. These verbs account for approximately 71% of the uses of adults and WS children and 78% of the uses of the control children (*SE*s = 3.2, 2.8, and 2.5, respectively). The remaining verbs include additional Manner of Motion verbs and Path verbs (e.g., turn, zigzag), and bring the total up to roughly 84% for adults, 86% for control children, and 88% for children with WS (*SE*s = 2.2, 2.2, and 2.5, respectively). Verbs were coded for semantic anomaly, as with Figure and Ground objects. Control children produced anomalous verbs 1% of the time and children with WS did so 3% of the time.

Given the inherent ambiguity of any motion event, we find it remarkable that the three groups of participants converged so closely on their choice of motion verbs to describe the main motion. Although the children with WS did use simple verbs of motion reliably more often than adults, the absolute difference was not large.

Paths

The three groups of participants produced broad corpora of Path terms, which overlapped each other considerably. The complete corpus produced over the 80 events by each group is shown in Table 4. The high degree of overlap indicates that the bulk of

TABLE 3
Twelve Most Frequent Specific Verbs of Motion

Adults		*Controls*		*Williams Syndrome Group*	
Verb	%	*Verb*	%	*Verb*	%
Fall	26.6	Fall	31.0	Fall	28.1
Jump	14.7	Jump	17.2	Jump	12.7
Fly	9.1	Fly	11.3	Fly	11.5
Hop	7.1	Hop	7.5	Hop	5.6
Walk	5.6	Walk	4.5	Walk	7.3
Roll	4.4	Roll	5.5	Roll	4.2
Drive	4.2	Drive	1.5	Drive	1.9
Slide	3.8	Slide	1.9	Flip	4.4
Make a turn	2.6	Run	1.4	Turn	3.8
Spin	1.5	Go in "L"	1.5	Zigzag	3.5
Back up	2.3	Ride	1.4	Run	2.9
Bounce	1.8	Bump	1.4	Bounce	1.9
Totals	83.7		86.1		87.9

TABLE 4
Percentage Production of All Path Terms over All 80 Events

Terms	*Adults*	*Controls*	*Williams Syndrome Group*
Simple path terms			
Across	22.2	5.3	2.9
Against	0.1	0.2	—
Along	0.8	0.2	—
Around	3.1	2.5	2.5
At	0.3	0.7	—
Away	—	3.6	2.7
Back	0.2	0.7	1.7
Backwards	2.7	3.3	1.5
Behind	0.7	0.7	0.2
Beside	—	0.2	—
By	1.3	0.5	0.6
Down	5.2	8.3	10.1
Downhill	0.3	—	—
Downward	0.1	—	—
Forwards	—	0.4	—
From	1.2	0.8	0.4
In	1.6	5.1	4.8
Inside	0.2	—	—
Into	3	1	3.4
Near	—	0.5	—
Off	13.7	18	15.2
On	3.8	9.4	5.3
Onto	1.2	1.3	0.8
Out	3.9	3.8	1.7
Over	9	10.6	26.9
Past	1.7	3	0.8
Through	6.7	6.3	2.3
To	3.1	2.6	5
Toward(s)	1.7	—	—
Under	0.1	0.2	—
Up	2.5	3.6	2.5
Uphill	0.3	—	—
Other simple	—	—	0.4
Around and Around	—	0.7	0.8
Away from	2.3	1.2	0.8
Back of/back to	—	0.3	0.2
Close to	—	0.2	—
Down from/down off	0.1	0.2	0.4
From x to y	1.2	0.7	—
In back of/in front of	0.2	0.4	0.2

(*continued*)

TABLE 4 (*Continued*)

Terms	*Adults*	*Controls*	*Williams Syndrome Group*
In front of	—	0.2	—
In and out	—	0.2	0.8
In his way	—	0.5	—
In the middle	—	—	0.2
In through	—	—	0.2
Left to right	0.1	—	—
Next to	—	0.2	0.2
On left side of	0.1	—	—
On over	—	—	0.2
On top of	2	0.2	0.4
Out around	—	—	0.2
Over and over	—	—	1.3
Over to	0.6	0.2	1.5
Over towards	0.1	—	—
Perpendicular to	0.1	—	—
Right in front	—	—	0.2
Up and down	0.1	2.8	1.1
Up to	2	0.2	0.2

the Path terms available to adults are also part of the vocabulary of both children with WS and their mental-age matches. However, there were differences across groups in both the tendency to encode Path for different kinds of events and in the qualitative nature of the Path terms used.

To quantify these differences, Path terms were coded in terms of four categories: Correct terms, Incorrect terms, Ambiguous Intransitives (terms *over, around, away*, and *back/backwards* when used intransitively), and Omissions. Correct terms were those that were acceptable descriptions of the Path in adult usage. These included terms that were the same as the term used modally by the adults as well as other terms that accurately represented the path, though not with the modal adult term. Incorrect terms were those that were not accurate representations of the path (e.g., "jumped *over*" to express the motion of a cup "jumping" *onto* a frog's head). Ambiguous intransitives were included as a separate category because the children sometimes used these terms in a fashion that made it unclear whether they were encoding a distinct path, for example, "He flew over" or "It hopped around." Omissions were responses that included no Path term at all. Coding of all responses was done by the second author. In addition, 20% of the corpus of sentences coded as "Other Correct" or "Incorrect" (i.e., those that required a subjective judgment for coding) were also coded by Barbara Landau to compute reliability, which was above 90%.

Initial inspection of the Path terms revealed that events portraying motion of a Figure object alone (n = 40) elicited a very different pattern among both adults and children than Figure–Ground events ($n = 40$). In particular, the Figure-only events tended to elicit a very broad range of Path terms. This is understandable: Because there is no specific Ground object, speakers have free choice as to whether they describe the path as moving TO some point or moving FROM some point. This means that, for these events, a wide variety of Path terms could be used sensibly, for example, X moved FROM the left, X moved TO the right, and X moved ACROSS the screen. In contrast, the Figure–Ground object events tended to elicit a much more constrained range of Path terms, which varied systematically across the different Path types (TO, FROM, VIA). Therefore, the Figure–only events were analyzed separately from the Figure-Ground events.

Figure-Only Events

Table 5 presents the results for 34 of the 40 Figure-only events. These portrayed an object moving either across the ground (grass, floor, etc.), through the air, or up/down a hill. The remaining 6 events portrayed a single object falling over, and all groups of participants described this correctly with either "fall *over/down*" or "fall" (adults, 86%, 14%, *SE*s = 7.1, 7.1; control children, 69%, 31%, *SE*s = 11.8, 11.8; children with WS 57%, 33%, *SE*s = 9.7, 8.9). For the 34 events summarized in Table 5, adults encoded the Path roughly 87% of the time ($SE = 3.8$), including the background as Ground object, saying, for example, "The bunny hopped downhill" or "The knife moved across the screen." In contrast, both controls and children with WS tended to omit mention of the Path in these events, producing a Path term only 37% and 38% of the time (*SE*s = 7.6 and 4.9), respectively. Note that describing these events without a Path term is perfectly grammatical, as when one reports only the Manner of Motion of the Figure object (e.g., "The bunny was hopping" or "The knife moved").

The children's uses of Path terms were often Correct (25.2% controls, 15.9% WS over all 40 events), with modest proportions of Incorrect terms (3.6% controls, 7.3% WS) and Ambiguous Intransitives (8.4%, 14.3%, respectively). Adults'

TABLE 5
Mean Percentges and Standard Errors of Classified Path Expressions in 34 Figure-Only Events

	Percent Correct		*Percent Incorrect*		*Percent Ambiguous Intransitives*		*Percent Omissions*	
	M	*SE*	*M*	*SE*	*M*	*SE*	*M*	*SE*
Adults	80.0	6.2	0.5	0.3	6.8	0.4	12.7	3.9
Controls	25.2	8.3	3.6	1.0	8.4	2.3	62.8	7.6
Williams syndrome group	15.9	3.6	7.3	2.7	14.3	3.6	62.4	4.9

modal term for these events was *across* (52% of all terms used, $SE = 7.9$). The most frequently produced term for control children was *up* or *up and down* (32%, $SE = 5.1$). The modal term for the children with WS was *over* (24%, $SE = 8.8$), one of the Ambiguous Intransitives (e.g., "The knife went *over*" to describe a knife moving along the ground). The percentages of the children's responses were entered into a 2 (Group) × 2 (Response type: Correct vs. Incorrect and Ambiguous Intransitive) ANOVA which showed no reliable main effects, $F(1, 22) = 1.1$, *ns*, or interactions, $F(1, 22) = 2.4$, $p = .13$. Thus although the children with WS produced fewer correct responses than controls, the difference was not reliable.

In sum, for events portraying the Figure object moving alone with respect to a background, children in both groups omitted the Path term frequently, but their remaining responses were roughly comparable.

Figure and Ground Object Events

These events elicited a constrained set of Path terms among all participant groups, and the terms corresponded quite well to the three Path types that were portrayed: Bounded TO, Bounded FROM, and VIA. The top five terms produced by the different participant groups for each of these event types are shown in Table 6.

Inspection of the table reveals several notable facts. First, the Path terms were well suited to the nature of the Path portrayed in the videos, suggesting that all participant groups generally organized their corpus of Path words in terms of these distinct Path types. Second, there was considerable overlap across participant groups in the Path terms produced for events corresponding to the different Path types. Nevertheless, there were also several apparent differences.

For Bounded TO paths, participants in all three groups used terms describing motion to a surface (*on/onto/on top of*), to a container (*in/into*), and to a point (*to/up to*). There were no violations of the semantic restrictions for the two sets of terms, that is, no uses of *in* to describe motion to a surface or *on* for motion to a container. In addition to these terms, adults alone used the term *towards* (indicating motion that is not bounded), control children alone used *backwards* (to describe the orientation of the Figure as it approached the Ground), and children with WS alone used *over*. The latter was produced frequently as the sole Path term by WS children (14.6% of the total terms in TO paths, WS = 5.9). Checking the entire corpus for the Bounded TO Paths, we found that this term was never produced as the sole Path term by either the control children or the adults, who only used the term occasionally in combination with *to* or *towards*, yielding TO Path compound expressions *over to/over towards* (3.9% and 1.1% for adults and controls, respectively). A number of the WS children's uses of *over* were semantically anomalous, for example, describing a tree moving onto the top surface of a block with, "The tree jumped over the block," or a cup moving onto a frog's head as,

TABLE 6
Mean Percentage Production of Five Most Frequent Path Terms for the Three Event Types

	Adults		*Controls*		*Williams Syndrome Group*	
Path Type	*Term*	*%*	*Term*	*%*	*Term*	*%*
Bounded TO[a]	Into	20.5	On	31.9	On	23.3
	On top of	13.4	In	16.5	Over	14.6
	Up to	9.4	To	11.0	To	13.6
	Toward(s)	9.4	Onto	8.8	In	13.6
	On	9.4	Backwards	5.5	Into	12.6
Bounded FROM[b]	Off	63.1	Off	55.9	Off	39.7
	Out	18.2	Out	10.6	Over	17.3
	Away from	9.6	Down	6.4	Down	16.0
	From	4.3	Over	5.3	Out	5.1
	Through	1.1	Away from	3.7	Up	2.6
					Through	2.6
					Backwards	2.6
					Back	2.6
VIA[c]	Through	23.3	Over	26.6	Over	46.7
	Over	22.0	Through	21.9	Around	5.8
	Around	10.7	Past	13.3	Through	5.0
	Past	10.0	Around	7.8	To	4.2
	Backwards	8.7	On	5.5	Past	3.3
					Off	3.3
					Into	3.3
					Back	3.3

[a]n = 12 events. [b]n = 16 events. [c]n = 12 events.

"The cup went over the frog." Such errors may arise from children's use of the term *over* to represent the static final location of the Figure ("over" the block or frog's head), comparable to *above* or *on*.

For Bounded FROM paths, participants in all groups used terms describing motion from a surface (*off*), container (*out*), and point (*away from/from*). There were no violations of the semantic restrictions for these terms (e.g., using *off* for containers or *out* for surfaces). Control children and children with WS also used a simple directional term (*down*) to describe downward motion away from the Ground object. The term *over* was again used frequently by children with WS (17.7% of terms in FROM paths, SE = 5.1) and occasionally by control children (5.3%, SE = 2.5). Children with WS sometimes used it as a general directional term (e.g., "The lady went over") and other times in anomalous fashion (e.g. "The block jumped over the other block" to describe one brick "jumping" down off of another). Several control children also used it in this way.

TABLE 7
Mean Percentages and Standard Errors of Classified Path Expressions for 40 Figure–Ground Events

Path Type	*Participant Group*	*Percent Correct*		*Percent Incorrect*		*Percent Ambiguous Intransitives*		*Percent Omissions*	
		M	*SE*	*M*	*SE*	*M*	*SE*	*M*	*SE*
Bounded TO events	Adults	99.1	0.9	0.9	0.9	0.0	—	0.0	—
	Controls	80.3	3.8	6.9	2.4	5.3	1.9	7.4	2.9
	WS	66.7	8.0	17.2	5.1	4.6	2.9	11.4	4.3
Bounded FROM events	Adults	99.0	0.7	0.5	0.5	0.5	0.5	0.0	—
	Controls	78.0	5.6	11.6	3.3	5.3	2.2	5.1	3.8
	WS	55.7	6.0	16.2	4.0	11.6	2.5	16.6	6.9
VIA events	Adults	97.7	1.2	1.6	1.1	0.7	.7	0.0	—
	Controls	76.9	4.9	9.4	2.7	1.5	1.0	12.3	2.9
	WS	48.0	6.9	19.8	6.2	12.5	3.9	19.7	7.4
All Figure–Ground events	Adults	98.6	1.0	0.4	0.0				
	Controls	78.4	9.3	4.0	8.3				
	WS	56.8	17.7	9.6	15.9				

Note. WS = Williams syndrome.

For VIA paths, participants in all groups used *over, through, around*, and *past* to describe motion with respect to the Ground object. The only obvious difference in distribution of the terms was the very high frequency of use of *over* by children with WS and relatively low use of *through*. Many of the WS children's uses of *over* occurred in contexts in which the control children and adults used *through*, cases where one object threaded itself through a tube like Ground object.

In sum, the top choices of Path terms were organized similarly across the three groups, suggesting generally appropriate choice of terms for different Path types among both controls and children with WS. However, there were also several indications that the children with WS used certain Path terms, in particular, *over*, in contexts that resulted in semantically anomalous encoding of the Path.

These patterns were quantified by coding all descriptions in terms of correct, incorrect, ambiguous intransitives, and omissions. The data are presented in Table 7 by Path type (Bounded TO, FROM, and VIA). A first analysis was conducted on the percentage of correct responses by the children (*M*s = 78% and 56% for the controls and the children with WS, respectively). A 2 (Group) × 3 (Path type) ANOVA revealed reliable main effects of Group, $F(1, 22) = 10.9$, $p < .05$, and Path type, $F(2, 44) = 3.73$, $p < .05$. Control children produced reliably more correct terms than children with WS over all Path types, and across groups, reliably more correct terms were produced for the Bounded TO Paths than for either the Bounded FROM or VIA paths (Tukey's HSD = 10.2). Planned comparisons revealed that the controls did not differ in the proportion of correct terms across the three Path types (all *t*s < 2.0, *df*s = 44, *ns*). However, the children with WS produced reliably more correct terms for Bounded TO paths than for either Bounded FROM or VIA paths (*t*s = 2.4 and 3.17, respectively; *df*s = 44, $p < .05$). Moreover, control children produced reliably more correct terms than children with WS for every Path type (all *t*s > 2.0, *df*s = 44, $p < .05$). A second analysis considered the proportions of these correct terms that also matched the modal term produced by adults for each event, and this revealed the same effects.[2]

The remaining categories include incorrect Path terms, ambiguous intransitives (*over, around, away*, and *back/backwards*), and omissions. Incorrect Path terms by themselves indicate an error in linguistic encoding of the Path type portrayed. A 2 (Group) × 3 (Path type) ANOVA on these data revealed only a marginal effect of Group, $F(1, 22) = 3.6$, $p = .07$; children with WS produced more errors. Both of the remaining categories reflect the child's tendency not to code a specific Path: Omissions are cases where no specific Path has been encoded, and ambiguous intransitives are Path terms that do not clearly express a particular Path. These two categories were collapsed, and the data were entered into a 2 (Group) × 3 (Path type) ANOVA, resulting in a main effect of Group, $F(1, 22) = 4.3$, $p < .05$, and of Path type, $F(2, 44) = 2.99$, $p = .06$, and an interaction of the two, $F(2, 44) = 2.96$, $p = .06$. Children with WS produced more of these responses than control children, and VIA Paths elicited more of this response type than Bounded TO Paths (Tukey's HSD = 8.5). Planned comparisons were used to examine the interaction of Group and Path type. Controls showed no reliable differences in these responses over the three different Path types, whereas children with WS showed reliably more of these responses for Bounded FROM and VIA events than Bounded TO events, *t*s = 2.43, 3.25, *df*s = 44, $p < .05$.

To summarize, the children with WS tended to produce fewer correct terms than control children and more combined omissions and ambiguous intransitives than controls. Both of these patterns interacted with Path type: The children with WS performed better when describing Bounded TO Paths than either Bounded FROM or VIA Paths, whereas the control children showed no such effects. This effect of Path type is reminiscent of the pattern seen for Ground objects: There, children with WS omitted reliably more Ground objects than controls, but their omissions were less frequent for Bounded TO Paths than Bounded FROM Paths, with VIA Paths falling in between the two other Path types.

---

[2]Like the first analysis, there were reliable main effects of Group, $F(1, 22) = 18.14$, $p < .05$, and Path type, $F(2, 44) = 7.48$, $p < .05$. Planned comparisons for these data again showed that the children with WS produced reliably more best matches for Bounded TO Path types than either FROM or VIA Path types (*t*s = 2.2 and 3.76, respectively, *df*s = 44, $p < .05$). In addition, comparisons showed that control children produced reliably more best matches for FROM Path types than VIA path types ($t = 2.17$, $df = 44$, $p < .05$).

DISCUSSION

The evidence shows that children with WS control much of the linguistic structure required for expressing motion events. When considering the rich requirements for producing semantically coherent descriptions of such events, we find it remarkable that such competence can be found in the context of profoundly impaired nonlinguistic spatial cognition. However, the children also show some clear limitations in their linguistic encoding of the motion event. We speculate that these limitations are tied to their nonlinguistic spatial deficit and reflect the difficulty of representing spatial information about motion events over time. This combination of strengths and limitation can shed light on the interaction of spatial language with nonlinguistic spatial cognition: Although the children with WS have semantic and syntactic knowledge of the components of the motion event, they cannot always use this knowledge to describe visually perceived events.

Preservation of spatial–linguistic structure was observed in several domains. First, the encoding of Figure and Ground objects as named object kinds was preserved, as was the representation of their spatial roles, seen through their syntactic encoding as subject and object of the preposition, respectively. Across the 480 descriptions of events involving both Figure and Ground objects, the children produced only three syntactic reversals of Figure and Ground objects. Thus the object kinds represented by the Figure and Ground, the basic spatial roles played by the two objects, and their mapping onto syntactic position all appear to be intact. The accurate naming of the objects by children with WS suggests that their representation of objects for the purposes of naming may not be impaired, consistent with evidence from Wang et al. (1995) and Hoffman and Landau (2000). In addition, the accurate assignment of object names to Figure and Ground roles suggests that the children's understanding of the relative spatial roles of the two objects is preserved. Finally, the correct mapping of these roles into syntactic position suggests preservation of the syntactic–semantic mapping between the spatial representation of the event and the corresponding linguistic structures.

Children also encoded the Figure object's motion properly, including the specific Manner of Motion portrayed. We note again that it would be perfectly possible for children to encode any of the portrayed motions in terms of spatially simpler verbs that indicate only motion, for example, *go, move*, etc. The accurate mapping of the portrayed motion indicates, we believe, intact perception of the different manners of motion as they were portrayed in our stimuli as well as intact ability to encode these with the appropriate verbs.

This conclusion does not necessarily suggest that all aspects of motion perception are intact in children with WS. For example, the results from Atkinson et al. (1997) suggest that children with WS are impaired in some aspects of motion perception. Atkinson et al. asked children with WS (ages 4–14 years) to detect and report the direction of common motion of a set of dots when it was embedded in background noise made up of dots moving in the opposite direction to the target set. Compared to normal participants of roughly the same chronological age, children with WS showed a higher threshold for detection, suggesting more disruption of the ability to perceive directional motion as noise increased. Our stimuli were clearly suprathreshold, and so it would be possible for our WS participants to perceive these stimuli sufficiently well to allow linguistic encoding, even if more subtle aspects of their motion perception are impaired. Key questions are what aspects of motion perception and what degree of sparing are necessary for the accurate linguistic encoding of motion events. One intriguing and relevant finding is from a recent study by Jordan et al. (2002), who found that under a range of conditions, children with WS are unimpaired in detecting and reporting both direction and kind of biological motion (e.g., jumping vs. walking). In that study, children with WS performed better than mental age-matched controls and at a level similar to normal adults. Jordan et al.'s findings suggest that children with WS have intact perception of both the qualitative nature of different kinds of motion and their direction, a conclusion that is consistent with the capacity of children, reported here, to accurately name different manners of motion. Clearly, however, further research is required to fully understand how motion perception operates in children with WS and how it delivers information to the linguistic system for appropriate encoding.

Of all the components of the motion event, the Path exhibited the most fragility: Children with WS both omitted Path altogether and produced vague intransitive Path expressions more often than normally developing children of the same mental age. Yet even this fragility occurred in the context of surprising control over the rich and subtle semantic structure required for the proper use of spatial terms. For example, the three Path types portraye (Bounded TO, FROM, and VIA) each elicited a different, constrained set of terms among children with WS that overlapped considerably with those of control children and even adults. Violations resulting from inappropriate use of a term from one Path type to another were rare, with the exception of the use of *over* to describe Bounded TO Paths, Bounded FROM Paths, and VIA Paths (in the latter, incorrectly expressing "through" Paths). We speculate that the abundant use of *over* stems in part from its high degree of polysemy in the language (Brugman, 1981; Lakoff, 1987) and possibly its relatively high frequency in the language. The result of polysemy could be that the child's representation of *over* is more loosely constrained than that of other terms and therefore it becomes the default term to be retrieved under conditions of uncertainty. Other major violations that crossed Path type were possible but did not occur; for example, *on* was never used instead of *off*, or *in* instead of *out*. Moreover, there were no violations of Ground object selection; for example, *on* and *off* were used in combination with "surface" Ground objects, and *in* and *out* were produced for "container" Ground objects.

The most pronounced and systematic difference between the children with WS and the normal children was not, however, the tendency to produce blatantly incorrect Path terms. Rather, the children with WS tended to either omit mention of the Path at all, to do so in a truncated or highly general fashion by using ambiguous intransitives (largely, *over*), or to omit mention of the Ground object. Each of these patterns suggests a certain fragility in the construction of the Path expression. Importantly, however, these patterns did not occur in blanket fashion across the events. Rather, they were constrained by the type of Path portrayed. Children with WS tended to omit expressions or use vague expressions of Path in contexts where the event portrayed a Figure object moving either away from a Ground object (Bounded FROM) or along a path passing the Ground object (VIA), but not in contexts where the Figure moved to a Ground object (Bounded TO). Their omissions were grammatical; they just failed to express the Path selectively in these contexts, whereas control children tended to include mention of the Path more often and did not show any effects of Path type on their omissions.

We believe that this pattern of selective fragility is best explained as a consequence of the interaction of the children's linguistic representations with their nonlinguistic spatial system, which is impaired. The nonlinguistic spatial deficit characteristic of WS appears most prominently in tasks requiring the retention of visual–spatial information over time (Wang & Bellugi, 1994), for example, the representation of spatial relationships, which then must be reconstructed in an adjacent but separate space. In the auditory domain, Vicari, Brizzolara, Carlesimo, Pezzini, and Volterra (1996) found that children with WS show the normal recency effect in memory for lists, with an advantage for items at the end of a list, but they do not show the normal primacy effect, as they show no advantage for items presented at the beginning of the list (Vicari et al., 1996). Our findings suggest a possibly parallel effect for visual–spatial memory, which could be responsible for selective difficulty encoding the Ground object in Bounded FROM and VIA Paths relative to encoding these in Bounded TO Paths. In the former two path types, the Figure's final resting place does not coincide with the Ground object, perhaps making it more difficult to retain an accurate representation of the Ground object. Similarly, relative difficulty in representing and retaining the Ground object would have an impact on the accurate representation of Path because the nature of the Path depends on the relationship between the Figure and Ground at the beginning of the event compared to their relationship at its conclusion.

We favor this account of Path and Ground object omissions because it closely ties the fragility that we observed in the children's spatial language to the mechanisms by which we can describe what is currently or recently perceived. Put simply, if the child cannot retain a representation of the Ground object or Path over time, he or she will not be able to talk about them. This explanation suggests that the observed fragility resides in spatial cognition, but is reflected in spatial language. Interestingly, this idea is compatible with the fact that languages, by and large, have more resources devoted to expressing TO paths than FROM paths. For example, there are more languages whose case system formally marks the former than the latter Path type. Further, there are a number of prepositions that mark both static locations "at" a Ground object and Paths TO a Ground object (e.g., in, under, between), whereas there are none that double in marking FROM paths and static locations "NOT at" a Ground object (R. Jackendoff, personal communication).

Other possibilities seem less likely to us. For example, the fragility could in principle be due to the status of Path terms as closed class terms. However, the names for Ground objects, which are open class terms, are also selectively omitted under the same circumstances as Path terms, suggesting that the problem cannot be completely explained by the closed class/open class distinction. This possibility could be directly tested, however, by examining the language of children with WS who are learning Path-incorporating languages such as Spanish or French. If the fragility is due to a nonlinguistic spatial deficit, and not to the difficulty of acquiring closed class items, the children should show fragility in the expression of Path (encoded by verbs) and Ground objects when talking about FROM and VIA Paths. Another possibility is that the fragility reflects a deficit in the actual meanings encoded by Path terms; that is, the idea that the meanings of the omitted elements are more difficult, or less richly represented, than those that are preserved. We regard this as unlikely because of the overwhelming evidence for rich spatial structure in the semantics of the Path expressions produced by the children with WS. With very few exceptions, the terms that were produced by the children reflected the appropriate semantic constraints characteristic of each of the components of the motion event, including all Path types. The fragility appeared in highly selective fashion—in just those contexts where it might be difficult to retain spatial information about the event. Thus it seems likely that it is linked to the nonlinguistic representation of the event: In FROM-path events, the Ground object and Path were not represented in a fashion robust enough to receive linguistic encoding.

Although our explanation links the selective deficit in spatial language to a selective nonlinguistic spatial impairment in WS, we cannot rule out the possibility that other kinds of mental retardation would lead to the same selective deficit. Moreover, because our normally developing children had above average IQs, it is possible that the fragility seen among children with WS was accentuated (see Mervis & Robinson, 1999, for discussion of issues pertaining to control groups). However, we view the highly selective deficit in spatial language among our children with WS as strongly compatible with our proposed explanation.

The general pattern of sparing and selective deficit can be used to gain an understanding of how spatial cognition interacts with the acquisition and use of spatial language in children. The strengths displayed by the children with WS in describing motion events reflect, we believe, knowledge of spatial language that has emerged in spite of the children's spatial deficit. Appropriate encoding of the central elements of a motion event in grammatical structures reflects the capacity to represent those aspects of objects, motions, and spatial relationships that are encoded by language. The performance by the children with WS suggests that, despite their profound spatial deficit, they have the capacity to acquire and use rich spatial representations embodied in the semantics of natural languages. Even the most fragile elements—Path terms—are acquired, and hence are part of the children's representations of spatial language.

How, then, can one explain the acquisition of such spatial language, in the face of profound deficit in other arenas of spatial representation? We speculate that spatial language, like many other systems of spatial cognition, has developed evolutionarily as a system which is specialized in the sense of having properties that are not directly and completely mapped from other spatial systems. Because of this specialization, the properties of space that must be represented in order to competently talk about space may be rather different from those properties of space that are required for competence in other spatial domains. The upshot is that it may be possible to acquire most aspects of spatial language even when other aspects of spatial representation are impaired.

This speculation rests on two pieces of evidence. The first is burgeoning evidence from cognitive neuroscience that spatial cognition is not one monolithic system, but rather, multiple systems specialized to represent different kinds of spatial information. One prominent example is provided by Milner and Goodale (1995), who argued that the system guiding action has quite different functional requirements from the system guiding perception; these different requirements are embodied in the computations performed by the two systems. The motor system, for example, must compute precise metric information continuously online as actions are applied to objects in the world. The perceptual system, in contrast, computes a different kind of information, building representations of the enduring qualities of objects. These two spatial systems appear to be represented by different areas of the brain, and perhaps as a consequence are differentially affected by different kinds of brain damage. Although research on brain structure in individuals with WS is in its infancy, evidence is compatible with the idea that there may be differential sparing of areas involved in spatial computations. In particular, there may be disproportionate reduction of volume in parietal and occipital lobes relative to the frontal lobe (Reiss et al., 2000).

The second piece of evidence supporting our speculation concerns the nature of spatial language, which appears to encode properties of objects and spatial relationships that are quite different from, and, in many cases, much coarser than, those required by the action or perception system. The Path types we have considered in this article serve as a good example. To navigate along a specific path, one would need to represent detailed metric information about its contours. However, such detail is not encoded by languages, which tend instead to encode only relatively coarse information, such as the distinction among Bounded TO, Bounded FROM, and VIA Paths. Within these Path types, English further distinguishes among paths on other bases, for example, the distinction between conclusion at an object's surface versus its interior (*on* vs. *in*). Such coarse coding of spatial information has been noted frequently as a characteristic of the incomplete mapping between spatial language and other spatial cognitive systems (e.g., Landau & Jackendoff, 1993; Talmy, 1983). Objects provide another example. Nonlinguistic representations of objects preserve shape and are sensitive to orientation relative to the viewer (Tarr & Bülthoff, 1995); they can also encode the orientation of the object relative to the head, the hand, and other body frames of reference for the purposes of reaching and grasping (Milner & Goodale, 1995). However, names for objects range over sets of similar objects and disregard specific orientation and location.

Thus spatial language would appear to possess properties distinct from other spatial cognitive systems. Given the requirements for rather different kinds of representations, the development of spatial language might not require that all aspects of nonlinguistic spatial cognition be fully intact. That is, it may be possible to acquire representations that encode distinctions pertinent to spatial language while failing to acquire representations pertinent to another spatial system. Recalling our discussion of motion perception, we suggested that it could be possible to normally acquire and use manner-of-motion verbs even if certain aspects of motion perception are impaired. Because language tends to encode spatial properties relatively coarsely, acquiring spatial language may not require that all aspects of spatial representation are intact. We speculate that this is the case in children with WS, who exhibit profound deficits in certain domains of spatial cognition, but show remarkably spared and rich knowledge of the language by which we represent spatial events.

ACKNOWLEDGMENTS

We thank James Hoffman, Helene Intraub, Ray Jackendoff, Michael McCloskey, and Colin Phillips for helpful comments on a draft of this article. We also thank Ted Supalla and Elissa Newport for making available the stimuli from their Verbs of Motion Production task, and Nicole Kurz and Litza Stark for help in transcribing and coding the data reported in this article. We thank the children who participated in these studies, their parents, and the organizations that helped us locate these participants. The latter organizations include the Williams Syndrome Association, the University of Delaware Preschool, and the Mom's Club chapters of Hockessin, Pike Creek, and Newark, Delaware. This research was supported in part by Grant No. 12-FY99-670 from the March of Dimes Birth Defects Foundation and Grant SBR-9808585 from the National Science Foundation.

REFERENCES

Atkinson, J., King, J., Braddick, O., Nokes, L., Anker, S., & Braddick, F. (1997). A specific deficit of dorsal stream function in Williams' syndrome. *NeuroReport, 8,* 1919–1922.

Bellugi, U., Bihrle, A., Neville, H., Doherty, S., & Jernigan, T. L. (1992). Language, cognition, and brain organization in a neurodevelopmental disorder. In M. Gunnar & C. Nelson (Eds.), *Developmental behavioral neuroscience: The Minnesota symposia on child psychology.* Hillsdale, NJ: Lawrence Erlbaum Associates, Inc.

Bellugi, U., Wang, P. P., & Jernigan, T. L. (1994). Williams syndrome: An unusual neuropsychological profile. In S. H. Broman & J. Grafman (Eds.), *Atypical cognitive deficits in developmental disorders* (pp. 23–56). Hillsdale, NJ: Lawrence Erlbaum Associates, Inc.

Bihrle, A. M., Bellugi, U., Delis, D., & Marks, S. (1989). Seeing either the forest or the trees: Dissociation in visuospatial processing. *Brain and Cognition, 11,* 37–49.

Bowerman, M. (1996). Learning how to structure space for language: A crosslinguistic perspective. In P. Bloom, M. A. Peterson, L. Nadel, & M. F. Garrett (Eds.), *Language and space* (pp. 385–436). Cambridge, MA: MIT Press.

Brown, R. (1973). *A first language: The early stages.* Cambridge, MA: Harvard University Press.

Brugman, C. (1981). *Story of over.* Unpublished manuscript, Indiana University Linguistics Club.

Clahsen, H., & Almazan-Hamilton, M. (1999). Syntax and morphology in Williams syndrome. *Cognition, 68,* 167–198.

Clark, H. H. (1973). Space, time, semantics, and the child. In T. E. Moore (Ed.), *Cognitive development and the acquisition of language.* New York: Academic.

Elliot, C. D. (1990). *Differential Abilities Scale.* San Diego, CA: Harcourt Brace.

Fillmore, C. J. (1997). *Lectures on deixis.* Stanford, CA: CSLI.

Gruber, J. (1976). *Lexical strucures in syntax and semantics.* Amsterdam: North-Holland.

Herskovits, A. (1986). *Language and spatial cognition: An interdisciplinary study of the prepositions in English.* Cambridge, England: Cambridge University Press.

Hoffman, J., & Landau, B. (2000). *Preservation of object recognition despite profound spatial deficit: Evidence from children with Williams syndrome.* Poster presented at the Annual Meeting of the Cognitive Neuroscience Society, San Francisco.

Hoffman, J., Landau, B., & Pagani, J. (in press). Spatial breakdown in spatial construction: Evidence from eye fixations in children with Williams syndrome. *Cognitive Psychology.*

Jackendoff, R. (1983). *Semantics and cognition.* Cambridge, MA: MIT Press.

Johnson, S. C., & Carey, S. (1998). Knowledge enrichment and conceptual change in folkbiology: Evidence from Williams syndrome. *Cognitive Psychology, 37*(2), 156–200.

Jordan, H., Reiss, J. E., Hoffman, J. E., & Landau, B. (2002). Preserved perception of biological motion in the fact of severely impaired spatial cognition: Williams syndrome. *Psychological Science, 13*(2), 162–167.

Karmiloff-Smith, A., Grant, J., Berthoud, I., Davies, M., Howlin, P., & Udwin, O. (1997). Language and Williams syndrome: How intact is "intact"? *Child Development, 68*(2), 246–262.

Kaufman, A. S., & Kaufman, N. L. (1990). *Kaufman Brief Intelligence Test.* Circle Pines, MN: American Guidance Service.

Lakoff, G. (1987). *Women, fire, and dangerous things.* Chicago: University of Chicago Press.

Landau, B., & Jackendoff, R. (1993). "What" and "where" in spatial language and spatial cognition. *Behavioral and Brain Sciences, 16,* 217–265.

Langacker, R. W. (1987). *Foundations of cognitive grammar.* Stanford, CA: Stanford University Press.

Mervis, C. B., & Bertrand, J. (1997). Developmental relations between language and cognition: Evidence from Williams syndrome. In L. B. Adamson & M. A. Romski (Eds.), *Communication and language acquisition: Discoveries from atypical language development* (pp. 75–106). Baltimore: Brookes.

Mervis, C. B., & Robinson, B. F. (1999). Methodological issues in cross-syndrome comparisons: Matching procedures, sensitivity (SE) and specificity (SP). In M. Sigman & E. Ruskin (Eds.), *Continuity and change in the social competence of children with autism, Down syndrome, and developmental delays* (pp. 115–130). London: Blackwell.

Mervis, C. B., Morris, C. A., Bertrand, J., & Robinson, B. F. (1999). Williams syndrome: Findings from an integrated program of research. In H. Tager-Flusberg (Ed.), *Neurodevelopmental disorders: Contributions to a new framework from the cognitive neurosciences* (pp. 65–110). Cambridge, MA: MIT Press.

Milner, A., & Goodale, M. (1995). *The visual brain in action.* New York: Oxford University Press.

Newport, E. L. (1990). Maturational constraints on language learning. *Cognitive Science, 14,* 11–28.

Pustejovsky, J. (1991). The syntax of event structure. *Cognition, 41,* 47–81.

Reiss, A. L., Eliez, S., Schmitt, J. E., Straus, E., Lai, Z., Jones, W., et al. (2000). Neuroanatomy of Williams syndrome: A high-resolution MRI study. *Journal of Cognitive Neuroscience, 12*(1), 65–73.

Singleton, J., & Newport, E. L. (in press). When learners surpass their models: The acquisition of American Sign Language from inconsistent input. *Cognitive Psychology.*

Stevens, T., & Karmiloff-Smith, A. (1997). Word learning in a special population: Do individuals with Williams syndrome obey lexical constraints? *Journal of Child Language, 24,* 737–765.

Supalla, T. (1982). *Structure and acquisition of verbs of motion and location in American Sign Language.* Unpublished PhD thesis, University of California, San Diego.

Talmy, L. (1975). Semantics and syntax of motion. In J. Kimball (Ed.), *Syntax and semantics* (Vol. 4, pp. 181–238). New York: Academic.

Talmy, L. (1983). How language structures space. In H. Pick & L. Acredolo (Eds.), *Spatial orientation: Theory, research, and application* (pp. 225–282). New York: Plenum.

Tarr, M. J., & Bülthoff, H. H. (1995). Is human object recognition better described by geon- structural-descriptions or by multiple-views? *Journal of Experimental Psychology: Human Perception and Performance, 21,* 1494–1505.

Vicari, S., Brizzolara, D., Carlesimo, G. A., Pezzini, G., & Volterra, V. (1996). Memory abilities in children with Williams syndrome. *Cortex, 32,* 503–514.

Wang, P. P., & Belllugi, U. (1994). Evidence from two genetic syndromes for a dissociation between verbal and visual–spatial short-term memory. *Journal of Clinical and Experimental Neuropsychology, 16*(2), 317–322.

Wang, P. P., Doherty, S., Rourke, S. B., & Bellugi, U. (1995). Unique profile of visuoperceptual skills in a genetic syndrome. *Brain and Cognition, 29,* 54–65.

APPENDIX
Descriptions of the 80 Events, Taken From Newport (1990)

Figure-Only Events

1. A loop moves diagonally upward
2. A ruler moves across a lawn
5. A baby wanders across the floor
7. A porcupine walks, turns, and walks again
11. An ashtray zigzags across a lawn
12. An airplane moves, turns, and moves
13. An airplane hops in a straight line
15. A barrel hops downhill
19. A man rolls across a lawn

21. A green locomotive moves, turns, and moves
22. A yellow towel zigzags across a lawn
23. An upright wooden bar falls over
27. A broom sweeps slowly and randomly across the floor
28. A toilet moves across the floor
29. A tree hops in a straight line
30. A hen hops uphill
33. A tree moves in a straight line
35. A paper glider flies up and down through the air
39. An upright phonebook falls down
40. A green creature flies through the air in a spiral fashion
42. A cylinder rolls across a lawn
43. A balsa wood glider moves, turns, and moves again
45. A knife moves, turns, and moves
47. A Band-Aid moves, turns, and moves
48. A palm tree flies through the air in a spiral fashion
52. An airplane flies through the air in a spiral fashion
53. A fire hydrant moves, turns, and moves again
54. A thin oil paint brush flies backward in a spiral fashion
56. A fat yellow bee wanders across the floor
57. An upright roll of duct tape falls over
59. A movie reel rolls diagonally upward
61. A rabbit hops slowly downhill
62. A motorcycle moves, turns, and moves
63. A cactus falls over
67. A barrel-half tips over
69. A piece of bone falls over
70. An egg flies up and down through the air
72. A rescue truck zigzags uphill
76. A motorcycle hops slowly downhill
78. A wooden bar spins slowly downhill

Figure-Ground Events

3. A girl jumps into a plumbing nut
4. A cylinder falls off of a swing
6. A white pipe cleaner jumps from a cactus
8. An airplane flies through a plastic T-pipe
9. A Christmas tree jumps up onto a box
10. A wreath falls down from above a fireplace
14. A tractor moves backward and turns toward a book

16. A loop jumps over a tree
17. A chick flies diagonally up to a wooden rod
18. A tricycle moves toward a mail truck and turns to avoid it
20. A dart with a suction cup flies and hits the wall of a building
24. A tail wing falls off of a Lego airplane
25. A duck walks past a thin loop
26. A bed moves around a prone man
31. A cup jumps onto the head of a frog
32. A missile jumps backward on top of another missile
34. A metal washer jumps out of an ashtray
36. A lawnmower moves toward a palm tree and turns to avoid it
37. A roll of paper jumps through a roll of tape
38. A dog jumps backward over a bed
41. A brick jumps down off of another brick
44. A Q-tip flies through a metal washer
46. A VW bug falls off of a thick loop
49. A pickup truck hits a tree
50. A woman walks backward past a dog
51. An airplane takes off from the back of a tugboat
55. A hollow log jumps over a stump
58. A farmer falls from the branch of a tree
60. A soup can falls off of an upright dart
64. A green jeep pulls out of a hollow log
65. A doll jumps down from the head of another doll
66. A doll walks by an airplane and turns to it
68. A floor lamp moves toward a table and turns to avoid it
71. A thick paint brush moves backward into an empty tin can
73. An evergreen falls down off of a red pole
74. A tugboat moves backward from a yellow pole
75. A turtle walks backward and turns toward a tree
77. A robot walks and turns toward a motorcycle
79. A rabbit falls backward from the back of a zebra
80. A pencil moves backward from a yardstick

Neurobiological Models of Visuospatial Cognition in Children With Williams Syndrome: Measures of Dorsal-Stream and Frontal Function

Janette Atkinson, Oliver Braddick, Shirley Anker, Will Curran, Rachel Andrew, John Wattam-Bell, and Fleur Braddick

Visual Development Unit
Department of Psychology
University College London
London, England

We examine hypotheses for the neural basis of the profile of visual cognition in young children with Williams syndrome (WS). These are: (a) that it is a consequence of anomalies in sensory visual processing, (b) that it is a deficit of the dorsal relative to the ventral cortical stream, (c) that it reflects deficit of frontal function, in particular of frontoparietal interaction, and (d) that it is related to impaired function in the right hemisphere relative to the left. The tests reported here are particularly relevant to hypotheses 2 and 3. They form part of a more extensive program of investigating visual, visuospatial, and cognitive function in large group of children with WS children, aged 8 months to 15 years. To compare performance across tests, avoiding floor and ceiling effects, we have measured performance in children with WS in terms of the "age equivalence" for typically developing children. In this article the relation between dorsal and ventral function is tested by motion and form coherence thresholds, respectively. We confirm the presence of a subgroup of children with WS who perform particularly poorly on the motion (dorsal) task. However, such performance is also characteristic of normally developing children up to 5 years; thus the WS performance may reflect an overall persisting immaturity of visuospatial processing that is particularly evident in the dorsal stream. Looking at the performance on the global coherence

Requests for reprints should be sent to Janette Atkinson, Department of Psychology, University College London, Gower Street, London WC1E 6BT, England. E-mail: j.atkinson@ucl.ac.uk

tasks of the entire WS group, we find that there is also a subgroup who have both high form and motion coherence thresholds, relative to the performance of children of the same chronological age and verbal age on the British Picture Vocabulary Scale, suggesting a more general global processing deficit.

Frontal function was tested by a counterpointing task, ability to retrieve a ball from a "detour box," and the Stroop-like "day–night" task, all of which require inhibition of a familiar response. When considered in relation to overall development as indexed by vocabulary, the day–night task shows little specific impairment, the detour box shows a significant delay relative to controls, and the counterpointing task shows a marked and persistent deficit in many children. We conclude that frontal control processes show most impairment in WS when they are associated with spatially directed responses, reflecting a deficit of frontoparietal processing. However, children with WS may successfully reduce the effect of this impairment by verbally mediated strategies. On all these tasks we find a range of difficulties across individual children and a small subset of children with WS who show very good performance, equivalent to chronological age norms of typically developing children. Overall, we conclude that children with WS have specific processing difficulties with tasks involving frontoparietal circuits within the spatial domain. However, some children with WS can achieve similar performance to typically developing children on some tasks involving the dorsal stream, although the strategies and processing may be different in the 2 groups.

It is well known that children with Williams syndrome (WS; or infantile hypercalcemia) typically show a very uneven profile of neuropsychological development, with expressive language abilities being relatively strong combined with unusual semantics, and spatial cognition severely impaired (e.g., Bellugi, Bihrle, Trauner, Jernigan, & Doherty, 1990; Bellugi, Lichtenberger, Mills, Galaburda, & Korenberg, 1999; Bellugi, Sabo, & Vaid, 1988; Bellugi, Wang, & Jernigan, 1994; Karmiloff-Smith, 1998; Klein & Mervis, 1999; Pezzini, Vicari, Volterra, Milani, & Ossella, 1999). This characteristic profile offers the possibility of understanding distinct brain systems underlying different domains of cognitive development.

We have been engaged in an extensive program to test young children with WS on a wide range of functions, starting in 1994. The goal of this program is to relate functional deficits in vision and spatial cognition to possible neurobiological accounts of the disorder, based on our knowledge of normal visual development, primate studies of brain circuitry, and neuropsychological studies of patients with specific brain lesions. We consider the following possible hypotheses for WS visuospatial, visuocognitive, and visuomotor deficits:

1. These are related directly and causally to visual sensory abnormalities. We have found a high incidence of binocular disorders, reduced acuity, and refractive errors in children with WS (Anker & Atkinson, 1997; Atkinson et al., 2001; Braddick & Atkinson, 1995). Binocular deficits, in particular, might be expected

to degrade the quality of spatial information available with consequential effects on development.

2. These are due to a deficit in the parietal lobe, and specifically in the dorsal cortical stream of visual information. There is now a wealth of evidence, from primate and neuropsychological studies, of a dissociation between ventral and dorsal streams of visual cortical processing (Milner & Goodale, 1995; Mishkin, Ungerleider, & Macko, 1983). The ventral stream carries information to the temporal lobe as a basis for object and face recognition, whereas the dorsal stream carries information to the parietal lobe as a basis for processing spatial relationships and for the visual control of spatially directed actions (Rizzolatti, Fogassi, & Gallese, 1997). This distinction appears to map well onto the contrast seen in WS between impaired spatial cognition, particularly on constructional tasks, and spared face recognition. A dorsal stream deficit might be primary, or might be a consequence of abnormal competition in development between the two cortical streams.

3. These are due to a deficit in the prefrontal executive control processes required for spatial processing. Such a deficit might be in prefrontal structures themselves or in the two-way transmission of information between prefrontal areas and the parietal mechanisms involved in spatial representation. Again, such deficits would relate to dorsal rather than ventral stream processing.

4. These problems may be associated with impaired function in the right hemisphere development relative to the left. The linguistic capabilities that are relatively preserved in WS are presumably left hemisphere-based, whereas right hemisphere lesions in children impair spatial performance in ways similar to those seen in WS (Beret, Bellugi, Hickok, & Stiles, 1996; Stiles & Nass, 1991). (It is worth noting, however, that children with focal lesions commonly overcome these spatial problems in a way not seen in WS [Beret et al., 1996].) Right hemisphere deficits might lead to similar problems to those seen in adult patients with right hemisphere parietal lesions who show spatial neglect.

Children with WS show quite diverse levels and patterns of abilities. Thus it cannot be assumed that a single pattern of anomalous brain development is common to all WS individuals. It is also possible that the initial anomaly is not associated with a specific brain system, but becomes expressed in one or more systems as the endpoint of a developmental process (Karmiloff-Smith, 1998).

The first stage of our program (Anker & Atkinson, 1997; Atkinson & Braddick, 1994; Atkinson et al., 2001; Braddick & Atkinson, 1995) concentrated on the relationship between visual measures and a range of visuospatial and cognitive measures on over 100 children with WS under the age of 14 years. Vision tests included orthoptic and refractive examination, stereo and acuity testing, visual field testing, and a range of tests of functional vision constituting the Atkinson Battery of Child Development for Examining Functional Vision (Atkinson, 2000; Atkinson & Van

Hof-van Duin, 1993).Visuospatial cognition was examined with subtests of the Wechsler Preschool and Primary Scale of Intelligence (WPPSI; e.g., object assembly), block construction (Atkinson, Macpherson, Rae, & Hughes, 1994; using the developmental sequence derived from Stiles-Davis, 1988), and Hood's (1995) spatial tubes test. We also measured some aspects of language ability with the British Picture Vocabulary Scale (BPVS), the Test for Reception of Grammar (TROG; Bishop, 1979), or, in children below the level appropriate for these, the MacArthur Inventory of language and communication (Fenson et al., 1993; adapted by us for British English; Atkinson & Knapper, 1993).

In these first studies we also found that certain sensory visual problems were much more common in WS than in the general population of the same age. About half of the children with WS were strabismic or showed stereo deficits, marked refractive errors, or reduced acuity. (Anker & Atkinson, 1997; Atkinson et al., 2001; Braddick & Atkinson, 1995). We also found substantial corelation among the different spatial tasks, and between spatial tasks and the TROG test of grammatical understanding. However, the severity of spatial problems (in terms of delays in age equivalence terms) on tasks such as block construction, errors with invisible displacements in the tubes test, and WPPSI object assembly was not well-correlated with the occurrence of these sensory visual deficits in individual children, and many children with WS with severe spatial deficits did not have marked sensory visual losses (Anker & Atkinson, 1997; Atkinson et al., in press; Braddick & Atkinson, 1995). We conclude that the first hypothesis, of a direct causal relationship between the sensory visual losses and problems of spatial cognition, is implausible.

This part of our study also provided evidence relevant to hypothesis 4 of a lateralized deficit in WS. We saw very little evidence of asymmetries in visual fields, optokinetic responses, or saccadic shifts of fixation of the kind that might be associated with lateralized focal brain lesions (Atkinson & Hood, 1994; Atkinson, Braddick, & Wattam-Bell, 1993; Braddick et al., 1992; Mercuri et al., 1996; Mercuri, Atkinson, Braddick, Anker, et al., 1997) or adult stroke patients with right parietal lesions. We will present some more detailed evidence on this point from fixation shifts. Thus if there are right hemisphere abnormalities in WS, they do not appear to be reflected in asymmetric visual responses on the particular tests we have used. However, stroke patients with right parietal lesions often show constructional apraxia, which can be likened to the problems seen in many children with WS on block construction tasks.

Following this initial part of the study, we have concentrated on tests relevant to parietal, dorsal-stream, and frontal function. We have used two approaches to distinguish dorsal from ventral stream function (Atkinson, Braddick, & Nokes, 1997). Form and motion coherence tasks are based on differences among the types of visual information analyzed in the two pathways. The "postbox" task, based on the work of Milner and Goodale (1995), examines differences between using the same visual information (slot orientation) in the dorsal-based task of controlling a posting action versus the ventral-based task of matching the perceived angle. Both methods found a substantial deficit in dorsal relative to ventral performance in a subset of children with WS. However, more recently, studies on other clinical groups have suggested that the dorsal stream deficiency revealed by motion coherence may not be specific to WS, but may reflect a more general vulnerability of this system (Atkinson et al., 1999). To examine this point, later in this article we present more extensive results with the form and motion coherence tests on both children with WS and controls.

The postbox task requires the transmission of visual spatial information via the parietal lobe to action control systems. We have examined such systems more broadly by using the Movement Assessment Battery for Children (Henderson & Sugden, 1992), which assesses a range of visuomotor skills. We find that 4- to 12-year-old children with WS have at least an average 2-year delay in both fine and coarse visuomotor skill tasks (Atkinson et al., 1996). Of course, a wide variety of brain structures as well as parietofrontal systems are involved in motor control. One such structure is the cerebellum. Morphological differences of the cerebellum and parietal lobe have been found in our study of 2 very young children with WS (Mercuri, Atkinson, Braddick, Rutherford, et al., 1997), suggesting that these differences are present very early in development. Cerebellar changes have also been identified in adult WS in a number of other studies (Galaburda, Wang, Bellugi, & Rossen, 1994; Jernigan & Bellugi, 1990; Jernigan, Bellugi, Sowell, Doherty, & Hesselink, 1993; Rae et al., 1998; Wang, Hesselink, Jernigan, Doherty, & Bellugi, 1992). However, the relationship between cerebellar morphology and the cognitive and visuomotor characteristics of WS is not yet understood.

The function of interactions between parietal and frontal structures is not simply to provide visuospatial input for motor control. Some of the characteristics seen in children with WS, particularly in the control of attention, resemble those described for adult patients with frontal lobe lesions, including distractibility, impulsivity, and difficulty in grasping the global aspects of a complex task or situation and mastering new tasks. The frontal lobes in adults have been considered as a complex of systems involved in the executive control of behavior, including spatial planning, working memory, maintaining attention on the task in hand, cognitive flexibility in switching between tasks when necessary, and inhibiting well-learned responses that are inappropriate to the present situation (e.g., Duncan, Emslie, Williams, Johnson, & Freer, 1996; Goldman-Rakic, 1996, Passingham, 1996; Robbins, 1996; Shallice & Burgess, 1996). It is possible that children with WS show differences from normal development in all these areas, but the ubiquitous spatial deficits in WS point to the possibility that frontal control in the visuospatial domain is more affected than that related to verbal responses.

Here we report results with children with WS on a range of tasks designed to test frontal function, specifically the ability to inhibit a familiar response when it is inappropriate to the task in hand, which has been associated with area 46 of dorsolateral prefrontal cortex (Diamond, 1996). The tasks differ both in being appropriate to different developmental levels and also in the degree to which the stimulus–response relations they involve are spatial versus nonspatial. Some preliminary results from these frontal tests have been reported (Atkinson et al., 1997).

In all these studies, as in our earlier work, we have not adopted the common methodology of comparing performance of the WS group with a group or groups of individuals who are attempted to be matched for chronological or mental age. Because the cognitive profile in WS is so uneven, it is difficult to select and justify a particular measure as the basis for matching. Rather, we have taken a range of tasks on each of which we have data about the age function of typical development. We then examine whether, in terms of equivalences to this typical developmental pattern, there are differences between the age trends of our WS group on different tasks.

Individuals with WS of the same chronological age can vary quite widely in their cognitive performance. Consequently, we have not looked at WS developmental trends solely in terms of chronological age. We also plot data for individuals with WS in terms of an age equivalent derived from their performance on the British Picture Vocabulary Scale (BPVS; Dunn, Whetton, & Burley, 1997), as a broad indicator of general intellectual development. This is not a basis for matching to another group, but rather a way to take into account some of the variance within the WS group. We recognize that this vocabulary measure is in an area where individuals with WS generally show good performance compared to other cognitive tests; we use it because there seems little to be gained by looking at visuospatial cognition as a function of test scores that themselves strongly reflect visuospatial performance.

In the first part of this article, we consider the hypothesis that children with WS have processing difficulties in tasks that depend on the dorsal stream relative to the ventral stream, using an expanded data set measuring form and motion coherence sensitivity on a large group of children with WS. In the second part of the article we look at the evidence for a general frontoparietal deficit in tasks that involve executive control as well as the earlier levels of dorsal stream function.

FORM AND MOTION COHERENCE SENSITIVITY

A key structure in the early parts of the dorsal stream is cortical area V5 (MT). Its large, directionally selective receptive fields are highly sensitive to coherent global motion in the presence of noise (Britten, Shadlen, Newsome, & Movshon, 1992) and the detection of motion coherence is severely impaired by lesions of V5 in macaques (Newsome & Paré, 1988) and humans (Baker, Hess, & Zihl, 1991). Thus we have taken signal/noise thresholds for coherent motion as an index of dorsal stream function. However, a deficit on this task might reflect a more general problem with attention or with extracting a global signal in the presence of noise. We have therefore compared it with a new task designed to place comparable demands on global processing of static form in the presence of noise by the ventral cortical stream. In this task participants must detect the organization of short line segments into concentric circles, with noise introduced by randomizing the orientation of a proportion of the line segments. Neurons responding to concentric organization of this kind have been reported in the ventral stream area V4 in macaques (Gallant, Braun, & Van Essen, 1993).

We have recently identified from functional magnetic resonance imaging studies of normal adults specific areas involved in our form and motion coherence tasks (Braddick et al., 1998; Braddick, O'Brien, Wattam-Bell, Atkinson, & Turner, 2000). This study shows that anatomically distinct circuits are activated in global processing of form and motion, but each circuit involve parts of both the parietal and the temporal lobes, and cannot therefore be said to be strictly dorsal or ventral. However, the activated areas do include dorsal stream areas V5 and V3A for motion and ventral stream area V4 for form.

We have reported results showing that a subgroup of children with WS are impaired on the motion coherence relative to the form coherence task (Atkinson et al., 1997, 1999). Here we report on a larger number and age range of children and relate them to age norms of control children on the same tasks. This study also uses a limited lifetime version of the motion coherence display, which provides a purer test of global motion integration than the earlier version.

METHODS

Motion coherence thresholds were tested with a computer-generated display previously used for preferential looking testing of infants (Wattam-Bell, 1994). A random array of bright dots (density 4 dots/deg^2) was presented on a dark screen (area 33 × 21 deg). Signal dots moved horizontally at 5.3 deg/sec. The trajectory of each signal dot lasted six video frames (120 msec). The direction of movement reversed every 0.33 sec. The remaining noise dots were randomly repositioned on each 50-Hz video frame. Participants had to locate a 13.4 × 6.7-deg target strip, presented either left or right of center, in which the signal dots moved in the opposite direction to those in the surrounding region.

Form coherence thresholds were tested with an array of short line segments, each 0.41 deg long, randomly jittered from positions on a 0.8 × 0.8-deg grid, giving a density of 19 segments/deg over a 33 × 21-deg display. Within a target region of 13 deg diameter, centered 8.3 deg left or right of center, a proportion of line segments was aligned tangentially to concentric circles; this proportion defined the value of form coherence. Remaining segments in this region (noise) and all segments in the rest of the display were randomly oriented. Figure 1 shows a schematic of these displays.

In both form and motion coherence tasks, the child viewed the display from 40 cm and had to indicate whether the target was left or right of center. Usually we asked the child to put his or her hand on the side of the screen containing the global coherence. Each task was initially explained with coherence set to 100%.

Children of mental age 4 years and above can readily understand each task if it is explained with examples and with descriptions such as "the snow is falling, and you have to find the road" (strip of coherent motion in noise running across the center of the screen) and "can you see the ball hidden in the grass" (circular array among random orientations in the form coherence task). The motion and the form coherence tests were run in successive blocks; which test was run first was alternated from one participant to the next. When it was verified that the child had understood the task and could indicate the target reliably at 100% coherence, coherence was progressively reduced until the first error was made and then adjusted by a two-up, one-down staircase rule. The coherence threshold was estimated as the mean of the last four reversal values of the staircase. Motion coherence values reported here take into account the noise created by the disappearance of signal dots at the end of their lifetime as well as the explicitly introduced noise.

(a)

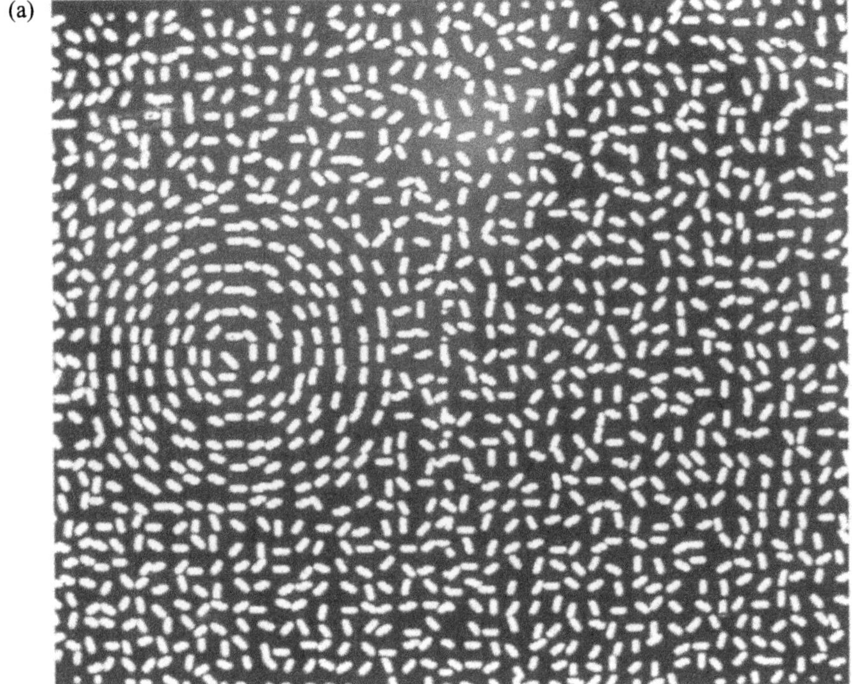

FIGURE 1 Displays used for testing form and motion coherence thresholds. (a) Form coherence display. The case illustrated is 70% coherence, with the concentrically aligned line segments appearing on the right. (b) Motion coherence display. The direction of motion of signal dots at a particular instant is indicated by the arrows. Noise dots (without arrows) appear at new locations on each video frame. The dashed lines were not visible on the display, but are used here to illustrate the boundaries that are visible because of differential motion in the display.

(b)

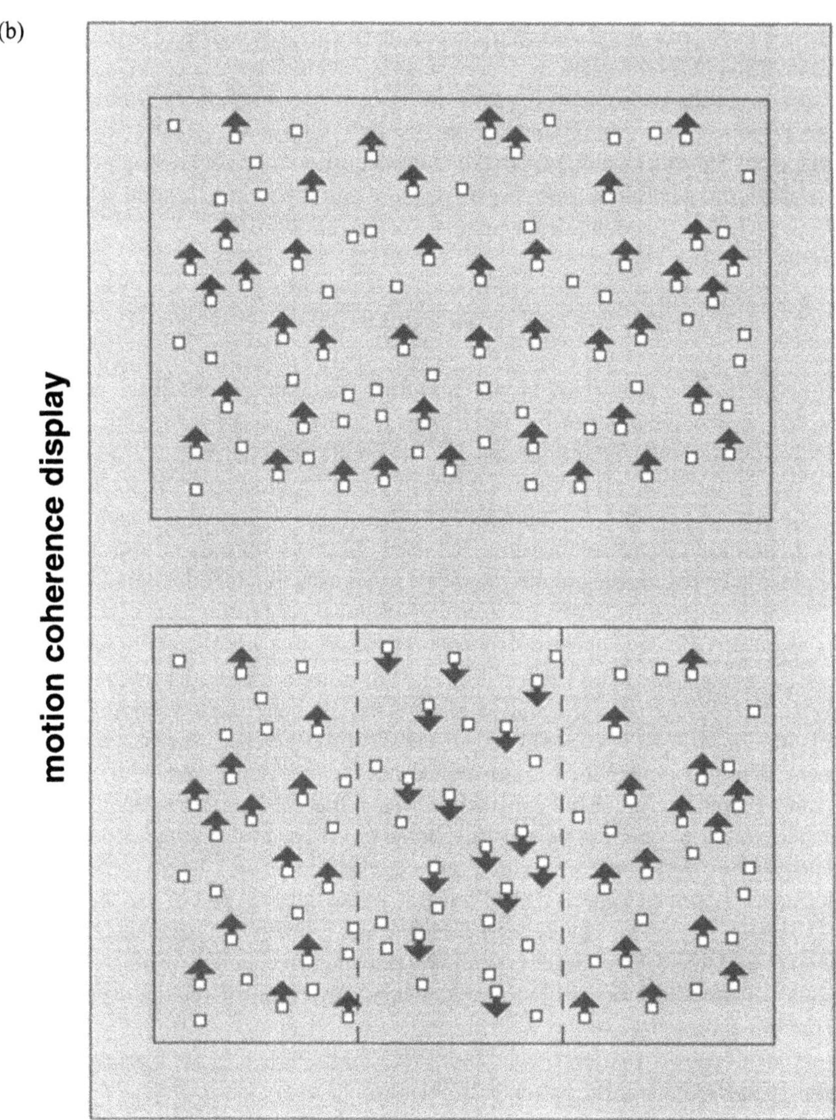

FIGURE 1 *(Continued)*.

Participants

We report here the results on 45 children with WS, who were tested as one component of a wider assessment of their visual and visuocognitive capabilities at the Visual Development Unit. Their ages were in the range 4 years, 8 months (4:8) to

15:4, with a mean of 9:5. All children reached an age equivalent of 4 years or better on the BPVS.

Their results are compared with control data from 76 children from 4-, 5-, 6-, and 7-year-old age groups in a London primary school; 64 visually normal children aged 5:6 to 6 taking part in the follow-up of a vision screening program in Cambridge; 13 children from the 10-year-old age group in a London school; and 35 young adults (students at University College London).

RESULTS

Figure 2 shows a plot of the motion and form coherence thresholds as a function of age for each member of the WS group, together with the 10th, 50th, and 90th percentiles from the control groups. It is apparent that about 40% of the WS group lie beyond the 90th percentile in each plot (19/45 for motion, 18/45 for form), but that there is a tendency for these to be further from the normal results in the case of the motion coherence measure. However, 12 of 45 were on or above the 90th percentile on both form and motion tasks, suggesting that these children had a significant problem on all tasks of detection of global coherence.

However, the developmental pattern for the control groups is different for the two thresholds. The adult values for the two thresholds are similar (median = 14% for form, 16% for motion), but whereas there is a very shallow improvement to this level from 4- to 5-years-old in the case of form coherence, there is a much more marked improvement for motion coherence. In particular, the 90th percentile shows a rapid decline in the early school years, that is, there is a substantial group of the youngest children whose thresholds are high, in the range 35% to 55%. Thus motion performance is much more age-sensitive, and the poor motion performance of some children with WS is not unlike the poor end of the normal 4- to 5-year-old range. This can be seen if BPVS age is taken as a reasonable developmental measure for the children with WS (the uneven cognitive profile of WS implies that no measure will fully reflect their development relative to controls). Figure 3 shows plots of the WS data in this way. The outliers from the 90th percentile of controls are now much fewer (8/45 for motion, 6/45 for form) and do not appear more deviant for motion than for form.

Figure 4 compares form and motion thresholds in individual children and shows the variation which occurs. It is apparent that over the group there is an association between the two thresholds, and in particular that the children who show high form coherence thresholds also show high thresholds for motion. The overall correlation is $r = .324$ ($p < .03$). (Neither the motion nor the form coherence threshold showed significant correlation with age or with BPVS age equivalent in this group, whereas in the control group both thresholds declined significantly with age, $r = -.51$, $p < .001$, for motion; $r = -.356$, $p < .003$, for form.)

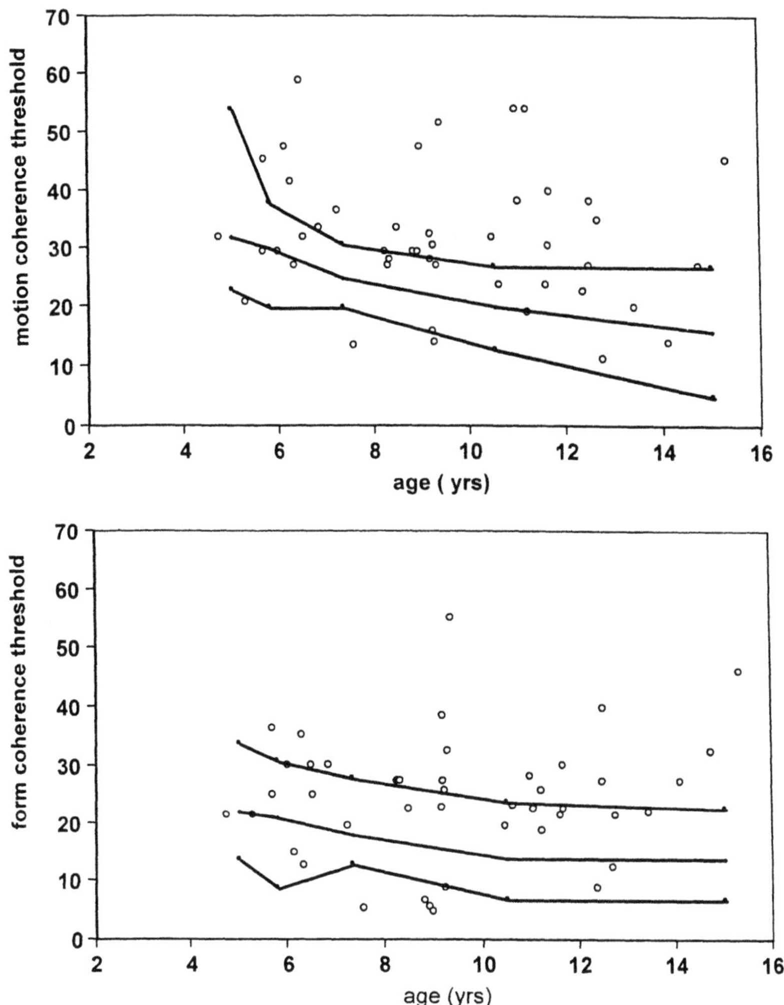

FIGURE 2 Motion (above) and form (below) coherence thresholds for individual children with Williams syndrome as a function of age for each member of the Williams syndrome group. The superimposed lines show the 10th, 50th, and 90th percentiles of results from the control groups aged 4 to 5.5, 5.5 to 6.9, 7 to 8, and 10 to 11 years, and adults.

Overall, if the scores of children with WS are converted into standard scores based on the mean and standard deviation within the same age group of typically developing children, the form and the motion scores do not differ significantly for the WS group as a whole (both average about 0.5 *SD* above the typically developing mean). Any differences are seen in the cases of very high thresholds. There is

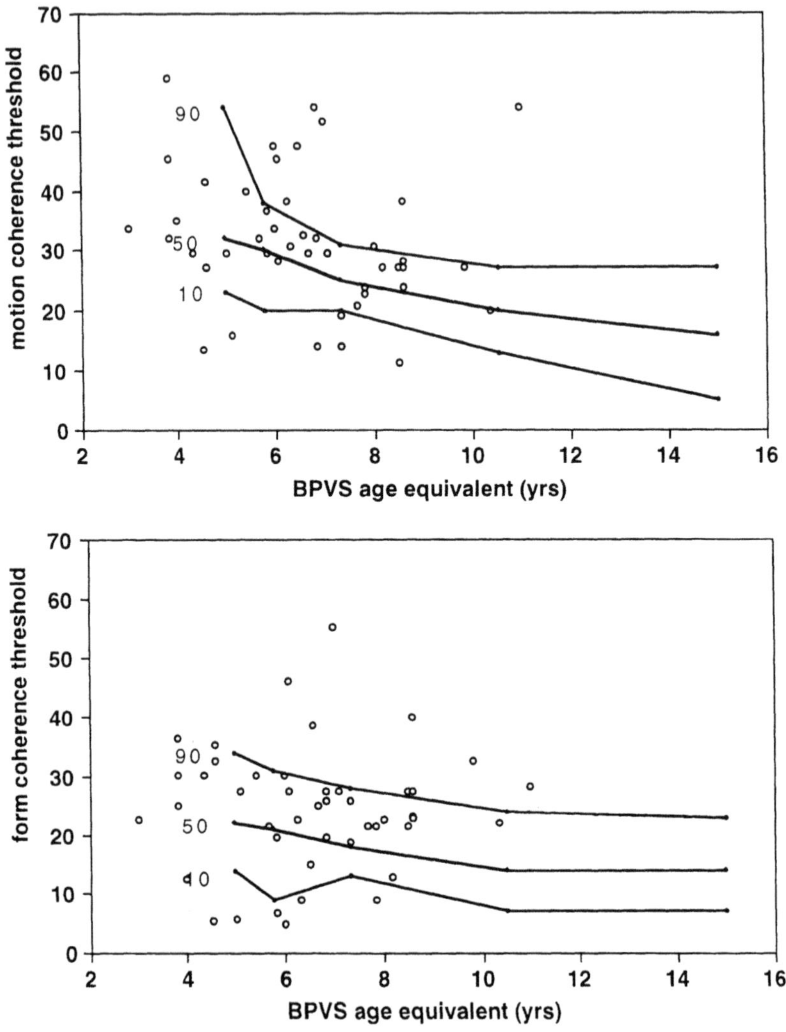

FIGURE 3 Motion and form coherence thresholds as in Figure 2, with children with Williams syndrome plotted against age equivalence on the British Picture Vocabulary Scale. The control data percentiles are plotted as a function of chronological age.

a group in the top left corner of the plot, similar to those highlighted by Atkinson et al., (1997), who perform relatively well on form coherence but have poor motion performance (thresholds over 40%). In contrast, we do not see the converse pattern of good motion with poor form performance, although there are a number of children with poor thresholds (over 40%) on both. Finally, a small subset of the

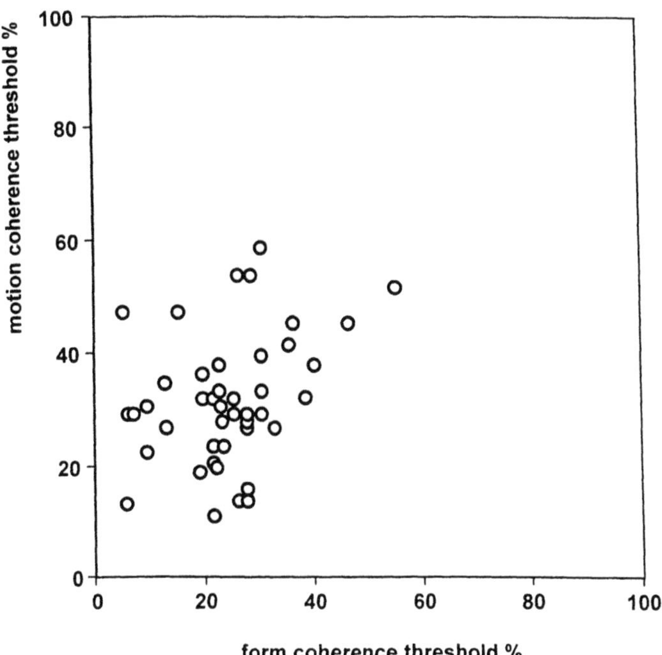

FIGURE 4 Scatter plot of form and motion thresholds for individual children with Williams syndrome.

children achieve high performance (at the 10th percentile or better for their chronological or vocabulary age).

DISCUSSION

Our earlier report (Atkinson et al., 1997) pointed to a group of children with WS who showed poor performance on motion coherence relative to form as evidence for a deficit in global processing in the dorsal relative to the ventral stream. The data presented have show some similar examples, but make it clear (a) that they are a subset of the WS group and (b) that they must be considered in the light of normal development. Dorsal stream function, as indexed by motion coherence thresholds, is relatively immature at 4 to 5 years and shows much more marked development in middle childhood compared to the ventral function tested by form coherence thresholds. Thus the children with WS who show high motion thresholds resemble a group of normal 4- to 5-year-olds in this respect, and indeed, when considered in terms of BPVS age equivalent, resemble them in other cognitive respects also. It is unlikely that this represents a simple delay in development because children who show this performance are scattered through the age range up to 15 years. Children with WS typically show very slow development of spatial tasks beyond the normal 3- to 6-year-old level (e.g., Atkinson et al., 2001; Bellugi et al., 1999; Braddick & Atkinson, 1995; Jarrold, Baddeley, & Hewes, 1998) and this may also be the case for these tasks.

A relatively large group of children with WS find both the motion and the form coherence tasks difficult. This may reflect a general factor such as difficulty in attending to global aspects of the pattern, which has been proposed as a feature of perceptual performance in WS (e.g., Birhle, Bellugi, Delis, & Marks, 1989), but the idea of a general global deficit in WS has been challenged (Bertrand, Mervis, & Eisenberg, 1997; Pani, Mervis, & Robinson, 1999). Normal adults comment that at coherence levels of 40% and above, the task seems effortless and automatic, whereas at lower coherence levels the task requires more explicit effort in spatial integration of information. This skill may be difficult for many children with WS to acquire and some may never acquire it. Those individuals who do perform well often spend a quite extended time scrutinizing the displays, and may be using specific strategies that extract information more locally than in normal performance. Further testing, with modified stimuli, would be necessary to test this hypothesis.

The general conclusion concerning relative dorsal versus ventral stream functioning is that there is both a subgroup of children with WS who have significantly higher thresholds on motion than form and a subgroup who are poor on both tasks (thereby showing a general deficit in global processing).

FIXATION SHIFTS, AND POINTING AND COUNTERPOINTING TESTS

A number of years ago, we developed the fixation shift paradigm for examining the ability of infants to make saccadic shifts of attention from a foveated target to one in the left or the right peripheral field (Atkinson & Braddick, 1985; Atkinson, Hood, Braddick, & Wattam-Bell, 1988; Atkinson, Hood, Wattam-Bell, & Braddick, 1992). This test reveals that normal infants under 3 to 4 months show difficulties of disengaging from the central target under conditions where the central and peripheral targets simultaneously compete for attention. This "sticky fixation" persists in some older children with cortical and basal ganglia lesions (Atkinson et al., 1993; Braddick et al., 1992; Mercuri et al., 1996; Mercuri, Atkinson, Braddick, Anker, et al., 1997). This test provides an indicator of the maturation and asymmetries of cortical mechanisms controlling the disengagement and shift of attention. It is likely to be related to hemianopia often seen alongside neglect in adult stroke patients.

The test of "antisaccades," in which participants are required to make a saccade in the opposite direction to a target, has been widely used to investigate higher levels of cortical control of eye movements in adult pathologies; in particular it is argued that problems with this task result from deficits in frontal mechanisms required to inhibit the prepotent fixation response (e.g., Pierrot-Deseilligny, Rivaud, Gaymard, & Agid, 1991; Pierrot-Deseilligny, Rivaud, Pillon, Fournier, & Agid, 1989). However, this antisaccade task is difficult to explain and to monitor with young children. To test the ability to override a prepotent spatial orienting response in the WS group, we have devised an analogous manual "pointing/counterpointing" task using a fixation shift display in which the child has to point to the target as it appears or to the opposite side to where it appears. Figure 5 shows a schematic illustration of this test.

Methods

For each of these tests (fixation shift, pointing and counterpointing), participants are seated 40 cm in front of a large, computer-controlled monitor, 51 × 38 cm. On each trial they initially fixate a central facelike figure, which alternates between two formats at 3 Hz. When they are fixating, a target appears 13.5 cm either left or right of center. The target consists of adjacent bright and dark stripes, each 2.9 cm wide by 14.7 cm high, reversing in contrast at 3 Hz. In 50%

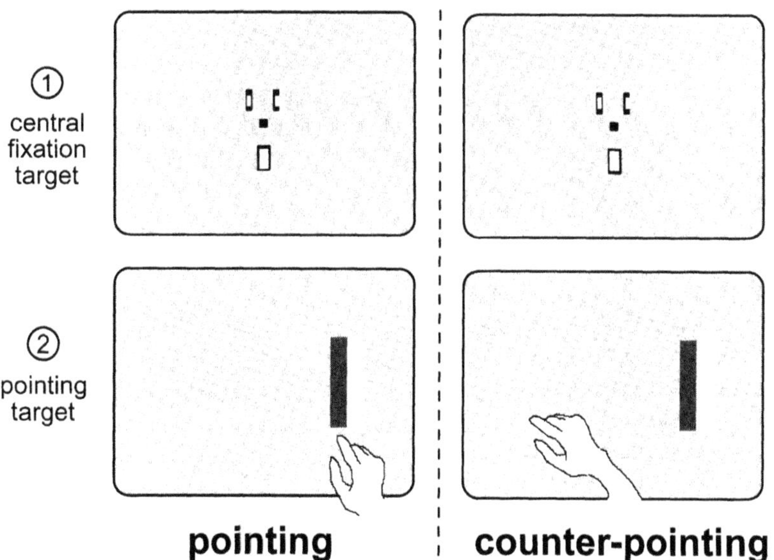

FIGURE 5 Schematic illustration of the pointing and the counterpointing tasks.

of trials (competition condition) the central figure remains; in the other 50% (noncompetition condition) it disappears at the time of target onset.

In the *fixation shift test*, an observer who is blind as to target location or condition presses a button to record the time and direction of the child's first fixation toward one or the other target location. The target then disappears, and the display is ready for the next trial. Twenty trials are run, with the order of locations and conditions randomized.

The pointing/counterpointing test is appropriate for children of a developmental age who can understand instructions to point toward and away from the targets. In the *pointing* condition, the task is to point to the target as quickly as possible after it appears. Most young children found it easier to put their hand on the target, thus making the point explicit. In the *counterpointing* condition, when the target appears the requirement is to point as quickly as possible to the opposite side of the screen from the target. In either case, an observer watches the participant's actions on video and presses a button by which the computer records the latency in touching the screen. The pointing condition is tested first, starting with a demonstration and test that the child understands the task, followed by 20 trials. The counterpointing task is then introduced, if necessary with an explanation that "the computer is trying to catch you out—don't let it trick you, point to the other side from the stripes to make the stripes disappear." When the child has shown that he or she can perform this task by giving three consecutive correct responses, 20 trials are run in the counterpointing condition.

Fixation Shifts

Seventy-two children with WS were tested using the fixation shift task. The older children (over about 5 years) generally responded promptly in both noncompetition and competition conditions and had no difficulty with the tasks (see Atkinson & Braddick [1994] and Braddick and Atkinson [1995] for initial reports of parts of these data). The performance of the younger children with WS was more varied. Here we report results from 19 young children of this larger group of 72, who were all those under 6 years (aged 8 months to 5:10, with a mean of 3:4) in the sample. In comparison with normals, all these children should have had no difficulty with either noncompetition or competition, in that normal infants over 5 months of age show similar mean latencies on both conditions.

Pointing and Counterpointing Task

We report here the results from 25 children with WS aged 4:7 to 14:7, with a mean 9:4, taking part in assessments at the Visual Development Unit. Eleven of these children also participated in the tests of form and motion coherence.

For comparison, we report also results from 13 normal control children, aged 4:1 to 13:5 (*M* = 8:1).

Results: Fixation Shifts

Most of the initial fixations observed in the entire WS group were in the correct direction, with most of the older children (over 6 years) showing similar mean latencies for the noncompetition and the competition conditions. In the 19 children who were under 6 years (*M* age = 35 months) there was a significantly greater number of errors in the competition condition (*M* = 18%) than in the noncompetition condition (*M* = 6%; *p* = .002, Wilcoxon matched-pairs test). The mean measured latencies of the correct responses in the two conditions for each child are shown in Figure 6. There is a clear tendency for longer mean latencies in the competition condition, which is very marked (1–3 sec difference) in a subset of the group. Overall, the difference is significant, with *p* = .006 (Wilcoxon matched-pairs test). For many

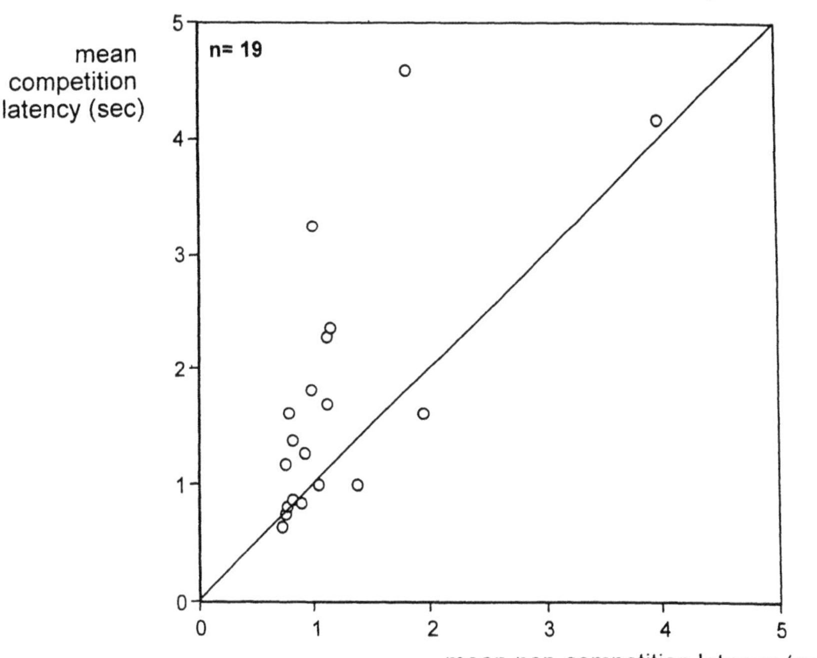

FIGURE 6 Mean latencies of the correct responses in the two conditions (noncompetition and competition) of the fixation shift test for each child with Williams syndrome tested under 6 years of age.

of these young children with WS, the latency varied across trials, with occasional very long latencies in the competition condition when the child appeared to get fixed on the central stimulus and was unable to unlock his or her attention from it. They seemed to have difficulty disengaging similar to problems seen in very young normally developing infants. Specifically, 7 of the 19 children (*M* age = 38 months) showed some latencies over 4 sec, on a median 18% of competition trials.

Figure 7 shows a plot of the latencies for left-field versus right-field targets for each child. It is clear that there is no general advantage for one or other half-field in this group.

Discussion: Fixation Shifts

A penalty for fixation shifts from a competing central target in terms of latency and correct responses is a feature of very young normal infants (Atkinson et al.,

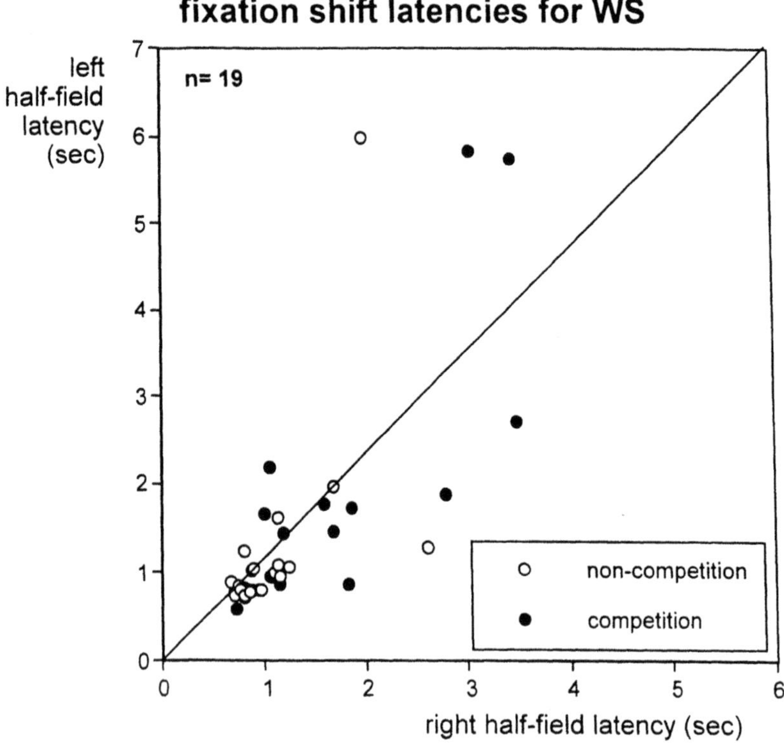

FIGURE 7 Mean latencies for left-field versus right-field fixation shifts (correct responses) for each child with Williams syndrome whose data appear in Figure 6. Noncompetition and competition trials are averaged separately.

1988; Atkinson & Hood, 1992). However, by about 6 months of age, this penalty has become very small, with recorded times for both conditions below 1 sec. Many of the children with WS, across the entire age range, show this pattern. However, about one third of the WS group under 6 years of age show substantial effects of competition (latency penalty of 0.8 sec or above), which is very marked in a few children. This phenomenon of "sticky fixation," in which the child finds it difficult to disengage his or her gaze from the current object of fixation, is a characteristic of Balint's syndrome resulting from bilateral parietal damage. However, the selection and implementation of saccade targets involves a wider neural circuit, in particular with connections between parietal structures, the frontal eye fields, and subcortical structures (Schiller, 1985) and the problems manifested in the performance of some children with WS might reflect parietal processing, frontal processing, or the connections between the two.

There is no difference between performance in the two half-fields. Thus these results, like the results of our visual field testing (Atkinson et al., 2001; Braddick & Atkinson, 1995), give no support to the view that children with WS might show a lateralized hemispheric deficit on these particular tasks. This also does not support the hypothesis that the problems seen in children with WS are similar to those seen in adult patients with right parietal lesions, who show attentional deficits in the left visual field.

Results: Pointing and Counterpointing

In the pointing condition, both children with WS and control children pointed to the correct side on every trial. In the counterpointing condition, all control children were correct on 100% of trials. Many children with WS made a number of errors: For the group as a whole, responses were to the correct side on an average of 88% of counterpointing trials, with most children scoring above 75%, but one child gave only 10% correct responses (with this child excluded, the group M = 92%).

Figure 8 plots for each child the mean latency of correct responses, with counterpointing latencies plotted against pointing latencies. Figure 9 shows the mean latency in each condition for the two groups.

It is apparent from Figure 8 that there is much overlap between the WS and control groups. However, Figure 9 illustrates that the WS group, although slower overall, is worse affected on the counterpointing than on the pointing task: Analysis of variance showed both a significant main effect of group, $F(1, 36) = 18.58$, $p = .0001$ and a significant Group × Task interaction, $F(1, 36) = 6.041$, $p = .019$. The requirement to override the spatially compatible response of pointing to the target causes special difficulty to many of the children with WS. This was apparent from the error rates as well from latency data. In a number of cases the long latencies on counterpointing were associated with overt difficulty in inhibiting the compatible response, for example, false starts of pointing toward the target, with

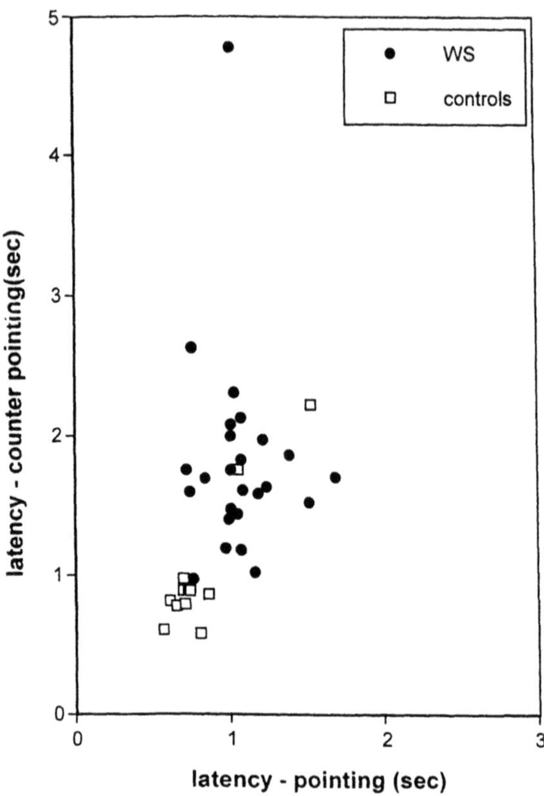

FIGURE 8 Mean latency of correct responses on pointing and counterpointing tasks for each child with Williams syndrome and control child.

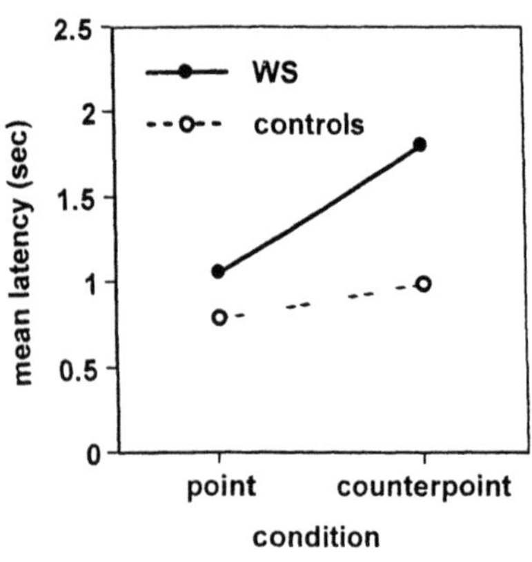

FIGURE 9 Mean latency of pointing and counterpointing responses (data from Figure 8) for the Williams syndrome group and the control group.

late correction of the hand or verbal strategies to maintain focus on the task (such as saying "opposite, opposite"). The counterpointing task, therefore, appears sensitive to the difficulties of children with WS in maintaining executive control of spatially directed actions and in particular inhibiting a prepotent response.

DETOUR BOX AND "DAY–NIGHT" FRONTAL TESTS

Methods

Detour Box

This apparatus, originally devised by Hughes and Russell (1993) as a test of executive function in young and autistic children, consists of a box with an aperture at the front through which the child can see a brightly colored ball on a platform. The tester explains to the child that this is a "magic box" and demonstrates that, if he or she reaches through the aperture to pick up the ball, the ball falls through a trapdoor in the platform and disappears from view. (This is achieved by the hand interrupting an invisible photocell beam, which controls an electrically operated latch.) The tester then demonstrates that the ball can be obtained by a less direct method. In the *lever task*, a lever mounted on a shaft coming through the side of the box rotates a visible paddle, which pushes the ball off the platform; the ball rolls down a chute into a tray where the child can pick it out. In the *switch task*, the paddle is locked so that the lever method does not work, but a switch on the other side of the box can be operated to inactivate the photocell and allow the ball to be retrieved directly by reaching out with the hand. In this condition, the activation of the photocell is signaled to the child by red lights on either side of the aperture. Because there is no visible connection between operating the switch and physical access to the ball in the switch task, young children find it harder than the lever task; normative data (Biro & Russell, 2001; Drake, Lee, & Russell, 1993) indicate that it is typically mastered by age 3.5 years compared to 2.5 years for the lever task.

The lever task is tested first. The child is allowed to reach directly and sees the effect of interrupting the beam; the tester then reaches directly and shows that he or she gets the same effect. The tester then demonstrates three times how the ball can be retrieved successfully by operating the lever. The child is then encouraged to retrieve the ball. Each trial is scored as a correct response or as an error (direct reach, or no response until prompted). After an error, a child is reminded of the correct method. Trials continue until three successive correct responses are made (to a maximum of 15 trials). Performance is measured by the number of errors before this criterion is reached.

The switch task is then tested by a similar procedure. In this case, attempting to operate the level counts as an error.

Day and Night Task

This is a variant of the Stroop test, devised by Gerstadt, Hong, and Diamond (1994) to examine frontal control processes in normal children aged 3.5 to 7 years. The task requires children to overcome a familiar verbal response by saying "day" to a card with a cartoon picture of the moon in a starry dark sky and saying "night" to a cartoon picture of the sun among clouds in a bright sky. The results are compared with a control task in which the responses day and night are arbitrarily assigned to patterns with no preexisting associations (one card showing a red–green checkerboard and another with a wavy stripe across each diagonal of the card). The sun–moon test is run first, with the tester demonstrating the correct responses and then giving the child two practice trials, one with each card. Practice continues until the child produces a correct response to each card at least once. Sixteen trials with the sun/moon cards in random order are then given, without feedback. The control task is then run with a similar procedure.

Participants

We report here the results of 36 children with WS who performed the detour box task, aged 2:7 to 13:5 (M = 7:8) and of 45 who performed the day–night task, aged 4:8 to 15:3 years (M = 10:0). All children in the latter group had a vocabulary age, on the BPVS, of at least 3 years. Twenty-six of the children participated in both tests. Norms on these tests are derived from published data (Biro & Russell, 2001; Drake et al., 1993; Gerstadt et al., 1994).

Results

Detour Box

Figure 10 shows a plot of the number of errors to criterion for the lever and the switch tasks. The large majority of children, throughout the age range, could perform error-free on the lever task; the mean error rate was 1.58. In contrast, in the more demanding switch task, the mean error rate was 7.86, and 11 children, over a wide range of ages, never learned the task. The dotted lines indicate the percentiles found for normal children aged 2 to 3.5 years by Drake et al. (1993), showing that almost half the children with WS (15/36) did not attain the performance of normal 3.5-year-olds.

In Figure 11 we replot the switch task data as a function of the children's age equivalents on the BPVS vocabulary test. Two features are apparent: Children with WS show as sharp an increase of performance with age as do normal

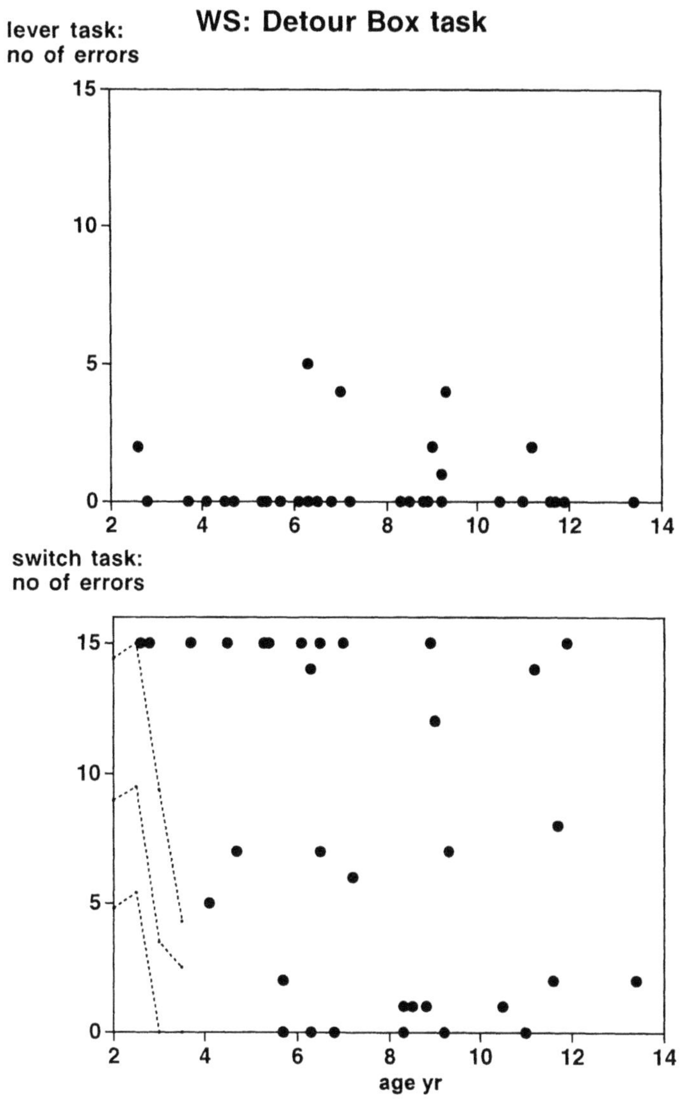

FIGURE 10 Plots of the number of errors to criterion for the lever and the switch tasks on the detour box against chronological age for each child with Williams syndrome. The dashed lines indicate the 10th, 50th, and 90th percentiles of normal performance from the data reported by Drake et al. (1993).

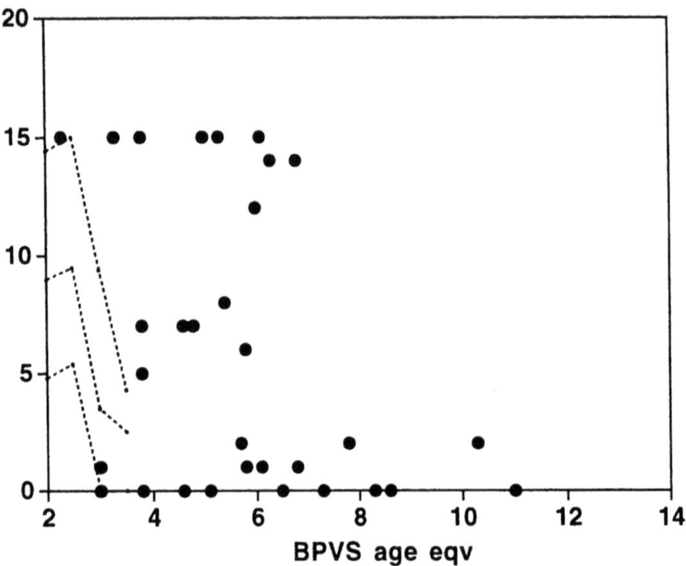

FIGURE 11 Detour-box switch task data from Figure 10, replotted as a function of the Williams syndrome's children age equivalents on the British Picture Vocabulary Scale vocabulary test. The 10th, 50th, and 90th percentiles of normal performance (dashed lines) are plotted as in Figure 10 in terms of chronological age.

children, but this improvement is seen around a mental age (in vocabulary terms) of 7 years in WS, whereas it occurs around 3 years of age in normal development.

Day and Night Task

Figure 12 shows the percentage of correct trials achieved by children with WS on the control task (M = 86%). Thirteen of the 45 children gave more than two errors (dashed line) and so their performance on the day–night test may reflect an inability to learn a new association rather than inability to overcome the established association. Figure 13 shows the percentage of correct trials on the test as a function of age (M = 76% for all children; 83% for those who made two errors or less on the control task). The results can be compared with the norms for 3- to 7-year-old children. The great majority of children with WS who can do the control task perform at or above the 5-year-old level.

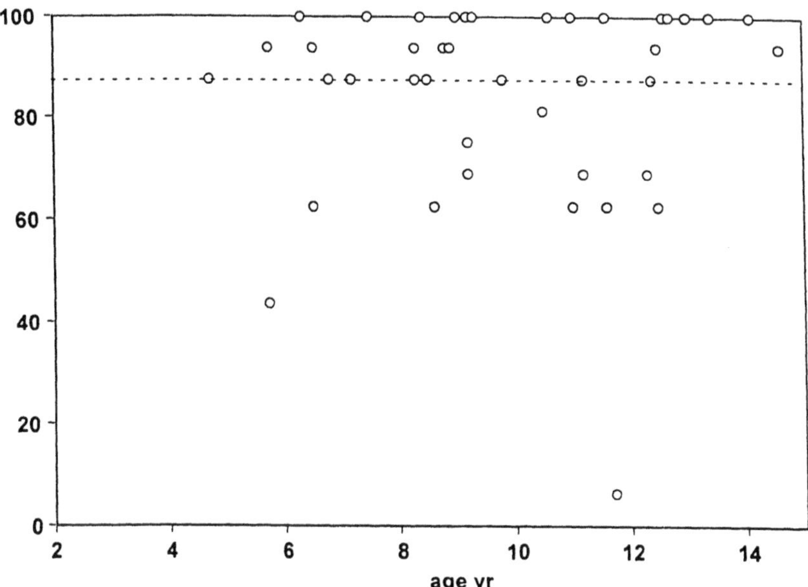

FIGURE 12 Percentage of correct trials achieved by children with Williams syndrome on the control task of the day–night test as a function of chronological age. The dashed line indicates the cutoff used to divide the data in Figures 13 and 14.

When the data are plotted in terms of the vocabulary age equivalent (Figure 14), most of the children with WS perform around or above their verbal age-equivalent level. Again, there is a special group of children with WS who perform very well on this task, in the upper percentiles for their chronological age.

Relation Among Frontal Tasks

Tables 1 and 2 present intercorrelations among scores on the frontal tests (day–night, detour box switch task, and counterpointing). Table 1 includes the correlation of each score with the children's BPVS age equivalence, and Table 2 shows the intercorrelations when the effect of BPVS has been partialed out. It should be noted that, because the different tests were appropriate for different levels of developmental age, the numbers of children for whom we have data on both of a particular pair of tests is in some cases quite small. Nonetheless, we can say (a) that there does appear to be a general "frontal factor," in the sense

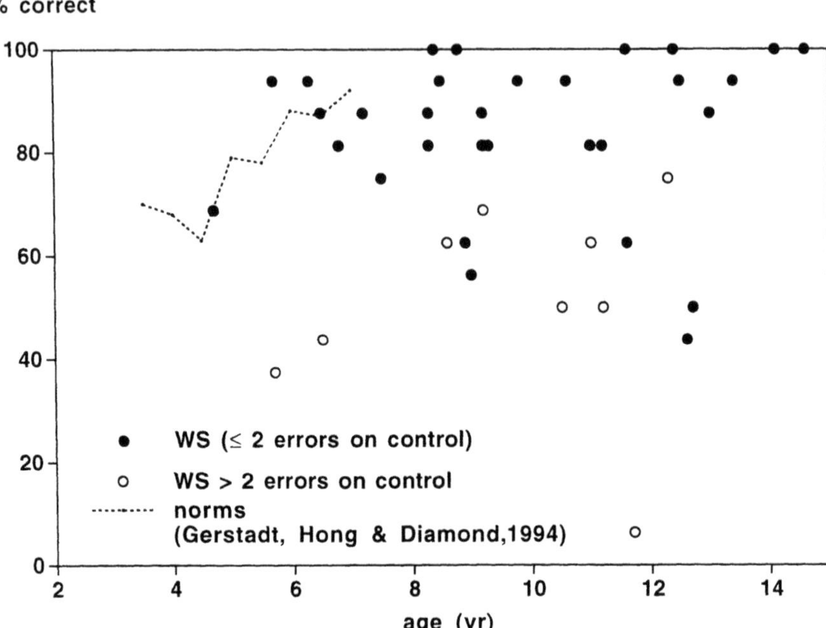

FIGURE 13 Percentage of correct trials on the day–night Stroop test as a function of chronological age for each child with Williams syndrome. Children who succeeded (two errors or less) on the control task are plotted separately from those who failed. The dashed line shows the age-group means from the normative data of Gerstadt et al. (1994).

that detour box and day–night performance are markedly correlated, even when the association with vocabulary age indexed by the BPVS is taken out, (b) that the correlation of counterpointing with detour box performance appears substantially higher than that with day–night performance, although this must be tentative given the numbers involved, and (c) that the detour box test shows the clearest relationship to BPVS age, a statement which is reinforced by our earlier discussion of the data shown in Figure 11.

Discussion

The comparison of these two frontal tasks makes it clear that, as well as considerable variation among individuals, which is not closely tied to their chronological age, the performance of children with WS on frontal tasks is highly task-dependent. A number of them did not show sufficiently secure associative learning on the control task (showing many errors) for the day–night results to be

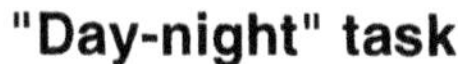

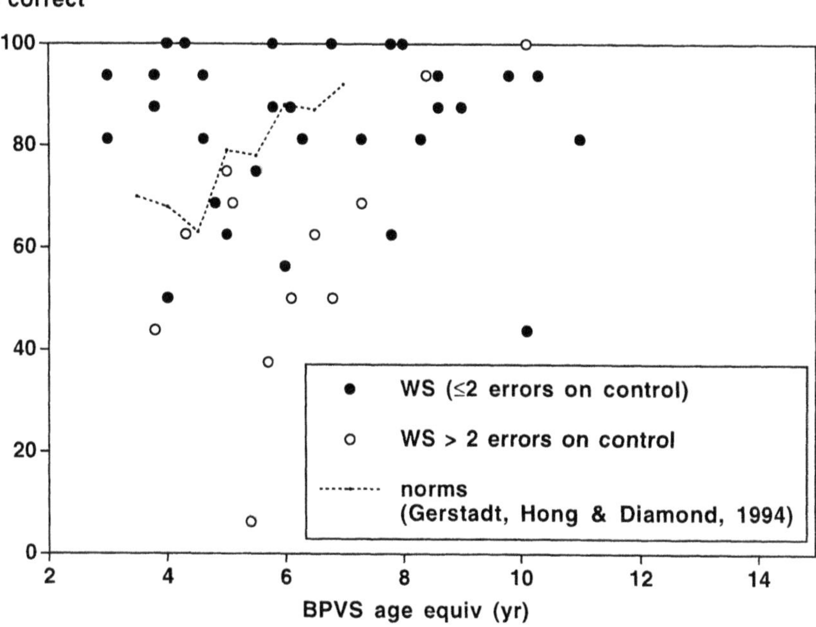

FIGURE 14 Results of the day–night Stroop test from Figure 13 replotted as a function of British Picture Vocabulary Scale equivalent verbal age for each child with Williams syndrome. The normative data (dashed line) are plotted in terms of chronological age.

TABLE 1
Intercorrelations Among Frontal Tasks

	BPVS Age	*Day–Night Errors*	*Detour-Box Switch Errors*
Day–night errors	−0.27*[a]	—	—
Detour-box switch errors	−0.44**[a]	0.47***[c]	—
Counterpoint–point latency	−0.55*[b]	0.29****[b]	0.43*****[d]

Note. BPVS = British Picture Vocabulary Scale.
[a]n = 34. [b]n = 10. [c]n = 25. [d]n = 8.
*p = .10. **p = .008. ***p = .02. ****p = .24. *****p = .29.

revealing. However, the remainder performed the task at a level that was broadly in line with their verbal ability as reflected in vocabulary. In contrast, performance on the detour box showed a considerably greater deficit relative to controls across the majority of the group, but again there is a small group who perform well for their chronological age.

TABLE 2
Intercorrelations Among Frontal Tasks, With BPVS Age Equivalence Partialed Out

	Day–Night Errors	*Detour-Box Switch Errors*
Detour-box switch errors	0.51*,[a]	—
Counterpoint–point latency	0.21**,[b]	0.37***,[c]

Note. BPVS = British Picture Vocabulary Scale.
[a]$n = 25$. [b]$n = 10$. [c]$n = 8$.
*$p = .01$. **$p = .56$. ***$p = .37$.

GENERAL DISCUSSION

We have looked at a large group of children with WS in early life with detailed assessment of their visual and spatial abilities. All our tests show considerable diversity in the performance of individuals with WS, and any account in neurobiological terms must allow for this variation in the degree of deficit and possibly variations in the structures and neural processes affected.

The general pattern of WS performance, in particular the difficulties with visuospatial constructive tasks, is consistent with the involvement of the parietal lobe, the destination of the dorsal stream of visual processing. Our visual coherence measures designed to compare dorsal and ventral function do show that some children with WS find global processing based on the dorsal stream especially difficult. However, our control data show that motion coherence performance, relative to form, matures more slowly in middle childhood, and we have also found that it is more vulnerable to perinatal brain damage as indexed by hemiplegia (Atkinson et al., 1999; Gunn et al., 2001). Thus it may be most appropriate to characterize the deficit seen in WS as a persisting immaturity of global visual processing, which shows a similar balance of dorsal and ventral function to that seen in other impaired or immature systems. It remains an interesting question whether the high performance of WS in the ventral stream function of face recognition (Bellugi et al., 1999; Wang, Doherty, Rourke, & Bellugi, 1995) is a special case or reflects a more general aspects of ventral stream recognition function. Our coherence threshold data emphasize a methodological point, that in evaluating developmental deficits in WS it is important to consider the age sensitivity of the measures used.

The age sensitivity of the test is also important in considering our fixation shift results. The ability to disengage in the competition condition is normally found in this particular stimulus paradigm from around 3 to 5 months of age. In general, children in our WS group aged over 5 to 6 years had no difficulties disengaging attention from the central stimulus to make an immediate saccadic shift to a newly appearing target, but a number of them, generally younger than 6 years but over 6 months of age, show "sticky fixation" when competing targets are presented. This suggests that the disengage mechanism, involving both cortical (parietal and frontal) and subcortical circuits (see Atkinson, 2000 for details of this circuitry) can be late to mature in WS and may not operate faultlessly even at an older age. The saccadic system is the first cortical action system to develop and mature normally in early infancy, and it is possible that poor development in this domain could have a cascade of effects on other, more complex action systems based on spatial representations which interlink with these eye movement systems.

The tasks that children with WS find particularly difficult (e.g., block constructions, drawing, complex visually controlled actions) require that visual spatial information should not simply be analyzed, but that it should be transmitted to action systems and that it should be subject to control processes. Both these processes require communication between parietal spatial information and frontal lobes, so that the spatial problems of WS may reflect frontal involvement. We have taken several different approaches to frontal function in these studies, and the differences between them are of interest.

The three tests discussed here—counterpointing, detour box, and day–night—all involve the requirement to inhibit a prepotent response. Of the three, the day–night task showed the least evidence of a consistent deficit, with some children performing at age norms and many more performing in line with or better than their vocabulary age. For the detour-box switch task, the data in Figure 11 suggest that children with WS will generally master the task requirement, at least if they achieve a vocabulary age of 7 years. For the counterpointing task, the majority seem to show a persisting deficit. Thus response inhibition does not create a uniform problem, but one that is to some degree domain-dependent. The day–night task requires suppression of a pictorial–verbal association, without any spatial component. Both the detour box and the counterpointing tasks, in contrast, require suppression of a spatially directed response. In the case of counterpointing the stimulus–response relation to be suppressed is a particularly simple and direct one, whereas the required response has the difficulty that it has to be directed to a featureless region of the display. The results suggest that frontal response inhibition is particularly problematic for individuals with WS when it is associated with spatially directed and spatially organized actions.

There is some evidence that, within dorsolateral prefrontal cortex, there are segregated subsystems involved in the control of spatial and nonspatial behavors (Goldman-Rakic, 1996). It is possible, therefore, that WS is associated with a deficit in a specific frontal subsystem. Alternatively, the connectivity between frontal and parietal systems may be abnormal. This possibility would be consistent with findings of white-matter abnormalities in the developing brain of young children with WS (Mercuri, Atkinson, Braddick, Rutherford, et al., 1997).

In terms of the hypotheses in the Introduction, evidence for both parietal and (nonuniform) frontal or frontoparietal deficits may be found in WS. Of course, this analysis leaves open the question of the neurodevelopmental sequence that leads to such deficits. Even by 3 to 4 years, there would ample opportunity for an initial anomaly in one cerebral system to affect the development of others, by providing deficient or anomalous input, abnormal regulation, or competition in the course of plastic reorganization.

It should be noted that the pattern of frontal deficit in WS we have described here is in relation to norms from typically developing children. We do not have corresponding data on other groups with mental retardation. Consequently, we cannot say how far this pattern is specific to WS and how far it might be shared with other atypically developing groups.

In all the tasks reported here, we find a subset of children with WS who can perform in line with their chronological age norms and others who show no deficit greater than would be expected from their development in terms of vocabulary (which would usually be the cognitive area in which they are closest to normal). However, the fact that a child with WS and a normally developing child attain the same score does not mean that their performance is identical. We have already noted that children with WS with good coherence thresholds sometimes appear to achieve these by close local scrutiny of the display and that they may succeed at the counterpointing task by employing verbal mediation. Similar, verbally based strategies were apparent in some cases in the other frontal tasks. Levine et al. (1996) also commented on the use of verbal mediation in some WS cases who show unusually high function in cognitive tasks. It is important to remember these possible processing or strategy differences in comparing identical numerical scores (for example, in error rate) in children with WS and typically developing children.

The performance of this small subset raises the question of whether these children continue to show superior performance during development, and how far their use of explicit verbal strategies to overcome difficulties in the learning and automatic execution of novel spatial rules is helpful in everyday spatial tasks, such as putting on shoes and socks or making a sandwich. If so, would those who do not spontaneously use such strategies find them useful if guided toward them? One hope for the future is that from observing the very varied approaches taken by children with WS in overcoming their severe spatial difficulties we may be able to plan and test out remedial strategies appropriate for a wide range of children with WS, given their uniquely developing brains.

ACKNOWLEDGMENTS

We thank all members of the Visual Development Unit for their help in running these studies. We thank Ursula Bellugi, Joan Stiles, Liz Bates, Larry Fenson, Orlee Udwin, Annette Karmiloff-Smith, Dorothy Bishop, Sheila Henderson, Adele Diamond, and Jim Russell for helpful discussions and advice on specific testing methods. We thank the Williams Syndrome Foundation of Great Britain for their help, and, most of all, the children and their families for their cooperation and enthusiasm. This work is supported by program Grant G7908507 from the Medical Research Council (UK).

REFERENCES

Anker, S., & Atkinson, J. (1997). Visual acuity measures in a sample of Williams syndrome. *Perception, 26,* 763.

Atkinson, J. (2000). *The developing visual brain.* Oxford, England: Oxford University Press.

Atkinson, J., & Braddick, O. J. (1985). Early development of the control of visual attention, *Perception, 14,* A25.

Atkinson, J., & Braddick, O J. (1994). *Comparison of visual, visuo-spatial and cognitive development in young Williams syndrome children (1–12 years).* Poster at the Sixth National/International Conference of the Williams Syndrome Association, San Diego,CA.

Atkinson, J., & Hood, B. (1994). Deficits of selective visual attention in children with focal lesions. *Infant Behaviour and Development, 17,* 423.

Atkinson, J., & Knapper, S. (1993). *Communicative development in 16–30 month toddlers.* Undergraduate dissertation, Department of Experimental Psychology, University of Cambridge.

Atkinson, J., & Van Hof-van-Duin, J. (1993). Assessment of normal and abnormal vision during the first years of life. In A. Fielder & M. Bax (Eds.), *Management of visual handicap in childhood.* (pp. 9–29). London: MacKeith.

Atkinson, J., Anker, S., Macpherson, F., Nokes, L., Andrew, R., & Braddick, O. (2001). Visual and visuo-spatial development in young children with Williams syndrome. *Developmental Medicine and Child Neurology, 43,* 330–337.

Atkinson, J., Braddick, F., & Nokes, L. (1997). Frontal control processes in Williams syndrome children. *Perception, 26,* 763.

Atkinson, J., Braddick, O., Anker, S., Ehrlich, D., Macpherson, F., Rae, S., et al. (1996). *Development of sensory, perceptual, and cognitive vision and visual attention in young Williams syndrome children.* Presentation and poster at the Seventh International Professional Conference on Williams Syndrome, King of Prussia, PA.

Atkinson, J., Braddick, O. J., Lin, M. H., Curran, W., Guzzetta, A., & Cioni, G. (1999). Form and motion coherence: Is there dorsal stream vulnerability in development? *Investigative Ophthalmology and Visual Science, 40,* S2079.

Atkinson, J., Braddick, O. J., & Wattam-Bell, J. (1993). Infant cortical mechanisms controlling OKN, saccadic shifts, and motion processing. *Investigative Ophthalmology and Visual Science, 34,* S1357.

Atkinson, J., Hood, B., Braddick, O. J., & Wattam-Bell, J. (1988). Infants' control of fixation shifts with single and competing targets: Mechanisms of shifting attention. *Perception, 17,* 367–368.

Atkinson, J., Hood, B. Wattam-Bell, J., & Braddick, O. J. (1992). Changes in infants' ability to switch visual attention in the first three months of life. *Perception, 21,* 643–653.

Atkinson, J., King, J., Braddick, O., Nokes, L., Anker, S., & Braddick, F. (1997). A specific deficit of dorsal visual stream function in Williams syndrome. *NeuroReport, 8,* 1919–1922.

Atkinson, J., Macpherson, F., Rae, S., & Hughes, C. (1994). Block constructions in young children's development of spatial grouping ability. *Strabismus, 2,* 41.

Baker, C. L., Hess, R. F., & Zihl, J. (1991). Residual motion perception in a "motion-blind" patient, assessed with limited-lifetime random dot stimuli. *Journal of Neuroscience, 11,* 454–461.

Bellugi, U., Bihrle A., Trauner, D., Jernigan, T., & Doherty, S. (1990). Neuropsychological, neurological, and neuroanatomical profile of Williams syndrome children. *American Journal of Medical Genetics, 6*(Suppl.), 115–125.

Bellugi, U., Lichtenberger, L., Mills, D., Galaburda, A., & Korenberg, J. R. (1999). Bridging cognition, the brain, and molecular genetics: Evidence from Williams syndrome. *Trends in Neurosciences, 22,* 197–207.

Bellugi, U., Sabo, H., & Vaid, J. (1988). Spatial deficits in children with Williams syndrome. In J. Stiles-Davis, M. Kritchevsky, & U. Bellugi (Eds.) *Spatial cognition: Brain bases and development* (pp. 273–298). Hillsdale, NJ: Lawrence Erlbaum Associates, Inc.

Bellugi, U., Wang, P. P., & Jernigan, T. L. (1994). Williams syndrome: An unusual neuropsychological profile. In S. H. Broman & J. Grafman (Eds.), *Atypical cognitive deficits in developmental disorders: Implications for brain function* (pp. 23–56). Hillsdale, NJ: Lawrence Erlbaum Associates, Inc.

Beret, N., Bellugi, U., Hickok, G., & Stiles, J. (1996). *Integrative spatial deficits in children with Williams syndrome and children with focal brain lesions: A comparison.* Presentation at the Seventh International Professional Conference on Williams Syndrome, King of Prussia, PA.

Bertrand, J., Mervis, C. B., & Eisenberg, J. D. (1997). Drawing by children with Williams syndrome: A developmental perspective. *Developmental Neuropsychology, 13,* 41–67.

Birhle A. M., Bellugi, U., Delis, D., & Marks, S. (1989). Seeing either the forest or the trees: Dissociation in visuospatial processing. *Brain and Cognition, 11,* 37–49.

Biro, S., & Russell, J. (2001). The execution of arbitrary procedures by children with autism. *Development and Psychopathology, 13,* 97–110.

Bishop, D. V. M. (1979). Comprehension in developmental language disorders. *Developmental Medicine and Child Neurology, 21,* 225–238.

Braddick, O. J., & Atkinson, J. (1995). Visual and visuo-spatial development in young Williams syndrome children. *Investigative Ophthalmology and Visual Science, 36*(Suppl.), S954.

Braddick, O., Atkinson, J., Hood, B., Harkness, W., Jackson, G., & Vargha-Khadem, F. (1992). Possible blindsight in babies lacking one cerebral hemisphere. *Nature, 360,* 461–463.

Braddick, O. J., Hartley, T., O'Brien, J., Atkinson, J., Wattam-Bell, J., & Turner, R. (1998). Brain areas differentially activated by coherent visual motion and dynamic noise. *NeuroImage, 7,* S322.

Braddick, O. J., O'Brien, J. M. D., Wattam-Bell, J., Atkinson J., & Turner, R. (2000). Form and motion coherence activate independent, but not dorsal/ventral segregated, networks in the human brain. *Current Biology, 10,* 731–734.

Britten, K. H., Shadlen, M. N., Newsome, W. T., & Movshon, J. A. (1992). The analysis of visual motion: A comparison of neuronal and psychophysical performance. *Journal of Neuroscience, 12,* 4745–4765.

Diamond, A. (1996). Evidence for the importance of dopamine for prefrontal cortex early in life. *Philosophical Transactions of the Royal Society of London B, 351,* 1483–1494.

Drake J., Lee, S., & Russell, J. (1993). *The development of detour-reaching ability in toddlers.* Undergraduate dissertation, Department of Experimental Psychology, Cambridge University.

Duncan, J., Emslie, H., Williams, P., Johnson, R., & Freer, C. (1996). Intelligence and the frontal lobe: The organization of goal-directed behavior. *Cognitive Psychology, 30,* 257–303.

Dunn, L., Whetton, C., & Burley, J. (1997). *British Picture Vocabulary Scale.* Windsor, England: NFER-Nelson.

Fenson, L., Dale, P., Reznick, J. S., Thal, D., Bates, E., Hartung, J., et al.(1993). *The MacArthur Communicative Development Inventories: User's guide and technical manual.* San Diego, CA: Singular.

Gallant, J. L., Braun, J., & Van Essen, D.C. (1993). Selectivity for polar, hyperbolic, and Cartesian gratings in macaque visual cortex. *Science, 259,* 100–103.

Galaburda, A. M., Wang, P. P., Bellugi, U., & Rossen, M. (1994). Cytoarchitectonic anomalies in a genetically based disorder. *NeuroReport, 5,* 753–757.

Gerstadt, C. L., Hong, Y. J., & Diamond, A. (1994). The relationship between cognition and action: Performance of children 3 ½–7 years old on a Stroop-like day–night test. *Cognition, 53,* 129–153.

Goldman-Rakic, P. S. (1996) The prefrontal landscape: Implications of functional architecture for understanding human mentation and the central executive. *Philosophical Transactions of the Royal Society of London B, 351,* 1445–1453.

Henderson, S. E., & Sugden, D. A. (1992). *The Movement ABC manual.* London: Psychological Corporation.

Hood, B. (1995). Gravity rules for 2–4 year olds. *Cognitive Development, 10,* 577–598.

Hughes, C., & Russell, J. (1993). Autistic children's difficulty with mental disengagement from an object: Its implications for theories of autism. *Developmental Psychology, 29,* 498–510.

Jarrold, C., Baddeley, A. D., & Hewes, A. K. (1998). Verbal and nonverbal abilities in the Williams syndrome phenotype: Evidence for diverging development trajectories. *Journal of Child Psychiatry and Psychology, 39,* 511–523.

Jernigan, T., & Bellugi, U. (1990). Anomalous brain morphology on magnetic resonance images in Williams syndrome and Down syndrome. *Archives of Neurology. 47,* 529–533.

Jernigan, T. L., Bellugi, U., Sowell, E., Doherty, S., & Hesselink, J. R. (1993). Cerebral morphologic distinctions between Williams and Down syndromes. *Archives of Neurology, 50,* 186–191.

Karmiloff-Smith, A. (1998). Development itself is the key to understanding developmental disorders. *Trends in Cognitive Sciences 2,* 389–398.

Klein B. P., & Mervis C. B. (1999). Contrasting patterns of cognitive abilities of 9 and 10-year- olds with Williams syndrome or Down syndrome. *Developmental Neuropsychology, 16,* 177–196.

Levine, K., Castro, R., Kelley, K., Correia, A., Shea, A., Pober, B., et al. (1996). *Above average intellectual ability in two individuals with Williams syndrome.* Presentation at the Seventh International Professional Conference on Williams syndrome, King of Prussia, PA.

Mercuri, E., Atkinson, J., Braddick, O., Anker, S., Nokes, L. Cowan, F., et al. (1996). Visual function and perinatal focal cerebral infarction. *Archives of Disease in Childhood, 75,* F76–F81.

Mercuri, E., Atkinson, J., Braddick, O., Anker, S., Nokes, L. Cowan, F., et al. (1997). Basal ganglia damage in the newborn infant as a predictor of impaired visual function. *Archives of Disease in Childhood, 77,* F111–F114.

Mercuri, E., Atkinson, J., Braddick, O., Rutherford, M., Cowan, F., Counsell, S., et al. (1997). Chiari I malformation and white matter changes in asymptomatic young children with Williams syndrome: Clinical and MRI study. *European Journal of Paediatric Neurology, 5/6,* 177–181.

Milner A. D., & Goodale, M. A. (1995). *The visual brain in action.* Oxford, England: Oxford University Press.

Mishkin, M., Ungerleider, L., & Macko, K. A. (1983). Object vision and spatial vision: Two cortical pathways. *Trends in Neuroscience, 6,* 414–417.

Newsome, W. T., & Paré, E. B. (1988). A selective impairment of motion processing following lesions of the middle temporal area (MT). *Journal of Neuroscience, 8,* 2201–2211.

Passingham, R. (1996). Attention to action. *Philosophical Transactions of the Royal Society of London B, 351,* 1473–1479.

Pani, J. R., Mervis, C. B., & Robinson, B. F. (1999). Global spatial organization by individuals with Williams syndrome. *Psychological Science, 10,* 453–458.

Pezzini, G., Vicari, S., Volterra, V., Milani, L., & Ossella, M. T. (1999). Children with Williams syndrome: Is there a single neuropsychological profile? *Developmental Neuropsychology, 15,* 141–155.

Pierrot-Deseilligny, C., Rivaud, S., Gaymard, B., & Agid, Y. (1991). Cortical control of reflexive visually-guided saccades. *Brain, 114,* 1473–1485.

Pierrot-Deseilligny, C., Rivaud, S., Pillon, B., Fournier E., & Agid, Y. (1989). Lateral visually-guided saccades in progressive supranuclear palsy. *Brain, 112,* 471–487.

Rae, C., Karmiloff-Smith, A., Lee, M. A., Dixon, R. M., Grant, J., Blamire, A. M., et al. (1998). Brain biochemistry in Williams syndrome—Evidence for a role of the cerebellum in cognition? *Neurology 51,* 33–40.

Rizzolatti, G., Fogassi, L., & Gallese, V. (1997). Parietal cortex: From sight to action. *Current Opinion in Neurobiology, 7,* 562–567.

Robbins, T. W. (1996). Dissociating executive functions of the prefrontal cortex. *Philosophical Transactions of the Royal Society of London B, 351,* 1463–1471.

Schiller. P. H. (1985). A model for the generation of visually guided saccadic eye movements. In D. Rose & V. G. Dobson (Eds.), *Models of the visual cortex* (pp. 62–70). Chichester, England: Wiley.

Shallice, T., & Burgess, P. (1996). The domain of supervisory processes and temporal organization of behaviour. *Philosophical Transactions of the Royal Society of London B, 351,* 1405–1412.

Stiles, J., & Nass, R. (1991). Spatial grouping activity in young children with congenital right and left hemisphere brain injury. *Brain & Cognition, 15,* 201–222.

Stiles-Davis, J. (1988). Developmental change in young children's grouping ability. *Developmental Psychology, 24,* 522–531.

Wang, P. P., Doherty, S., Rourke, S. B., & Bellugi, U. (1995). Unique profile of visuo-perceptive skills in a genetic syndrome. *Brain and Cognition, 29,* 54–65.

Wang, P. P., Hesselink, J. R., Jernigan, T. L., Doherty, S., & Bellugi, U. (1992). Specific neurobehavioral profile of Williams syndrome is associated with neocerebellar hemispheric preservation. *Neurology, 42,* 1999–2002.

Wattam-Bell, J. (1994). Coherence thresholds for discrimination of motion direction in infants. *Vision Research, 34,* 877–883.

Visuospatial Cognition in Williams Syndrome: Reviewing and Accounting for the Strengths and Weaknesses in Performance

Emily K. Farran and Christopher Jarrold
Department of Experimental Psychology
University of Bristol
Bristol, United Kingdom

Individuals with Williams syndrome typically show relatively poor visuospatial abilities in comparison to stronger verbal skills. However, individuals' level of performance is not consistent across all visuospatial tasks. The studies assessing visuospatial functioning in Williams syndrome are critically reviewed, to provide a clear pattern of the relative difficulty of these tasks. This prompts a possible explanation of the variability in performance seen, which focuses on the processing demands of some of these tasks. Individuals with Williams syndrome show an atypical processing style on tests of construction, which does not affect tests of perception.

Ever since the pioneering work of Bellugi, Sabo, and Vaid (1988) it has been clear that a fundamental aspect of the psychological profile of individuals with Williams syndrome (WS) is their relatively poor performance on tests of visuospatial cognition (Karmiloff-Smith, Klima, Bellugi, Grant, & Baron-Cohen, 1995; Mervis, 1999). Many researchers describe the cognitive profile of WS by detailing the marked contrast that is seen between these individuals' verbal and visuospatial abilities. For example, Bellugi, Wang, and Jernigan (1994) described a "Pattern of linguistic preservation and marked spatial cognitive deficit" (p. 44), whereas Udwin and Yule (1991) suggested that "overall their

---

Emily K. Farran is now at the Department of Psychology, University of Reading, Reading, United Kingdom.

Requests for reprints should be sent to Emily K. Farran, Department of Psychology, University of Reading, Earley Gate, Reading, RG6 6AL, United Kingdom. E-mail: E.k.farran@reading.ac.uk

verbal abilities are markedly superior to their visuo-spatial and motor skills" (p. 233). In general it is the case that the verbal abilities of individuals with WS are superior to their nonverbal abilities (Grant et al., 1997; Howlin, Davies, & Udwin, 1998). However, Jarrold, Baddeley, and Hewes (1998) and Jarrold, Baddeley, Hewes, and Phillips (2001) claimed from cross-sectional and longitudinal data, respectively, that in WS, verbal ability improves at a faster rate than nonverbal ability, so that as individuals develop, an increasing discrepancy between these two domains emerges. This is supported by Atkinson et al. (2001), who reported steeper slopes in improvement with age in vocabulary and grammar ability than the comparatively slow rate of improvement in ability with age on three visuospatial tasks. Although the discrepancy between verbal and nonverbal ability is, broadly speaking, characteristic of WS, the situation is complicated by the considerable variance between the composite measures of any IQ score. These composite scores often hide an interesting pattern of differences in abilities shown on tests that measure particular aspects of cognition within the verbal or visuospatial domains. Karmiloff-Smith et al. (1997) showed, for example, that performance is not uniform on a range of tasks measuring different aspects of verbal ability. The purpose of this article is to critically review the research carried out to date in the area of *visuospatial* cognition in WS, with the aim of explaining the reasons for the varying levels of performance between different visuospatial tasks. As this is arguably the weakest of all aspects of cognition in WS, it is particularly important to provide potential explanations for the difficulties these individuals encounter on visual and spatial tests.

METHODOLOGICAL ISSUES

Methodological issues need to be taken into account when evaluating the findings of any study; however, particular methodological problems arise when working with special populations in general, and with individuals with Williams syndrome (WS) specifically. Consequently, before reviewing the studies of visuospatial cognition in WS we provide a brief outline of these methodological concerns and their potential effects on these studies.

Floor and ceiling effects can be a major problem when testing atypical populations. Clearly, when either effect occurs, the test used may be artificially constraining the possible range of performance. Floor effects are particularly prevalent when testing visuospatial processing in WS because this is such a weak area of cognition. This is evident in studies employing the Benton Lines Orientation test to assess individuals with WS (Benton, Varney, & Hamsher, 1978; see Bellugi et al., 1988; Rossen, Klima, Bellugi, Bihrle, & Jones, 1996; Wang, Doherty, Rourke, & Bellugi, 1995). Such results can only tell us that a group's abilities are at or below the lowest level that the test purports to measure, and thus that the group's scores may not be truly representative of their actual skills. In this context, ceiling effects are commonly seen in comparison or control groups. When WS participants are matched to a control group for chronological age (CA), it is difficult to find a test that encompasses the range of abilities seen across the two groups. If the test is too easy for the control group, they will score at ceiling, and as a consequence the performance of the WS group may erroneously appear to be close to that of controls. This possibility will be discussed in relation to much of the research that addresses face recognition in WS, where CA-matched control groups are often employed (e.g., Karmiloff-Smith, 1997).

The problem of floor and ceiling effects can be overcome somewhat by matching individuals with WS to typically developing (TD) groups for mental age (MA). This approach has been adopted by Bertrand, Mervis, and Eisenberg (1997), for example, who, in addition to typically developing CA matched controls, also employed a typically developing control group matched for MA. This reduces the problem of differing levels of ability, but creates a new concern due to the discrepancy that will necessarily arise between the CAs of each group. The higher CA of the WS group will equate to them also having more experience, more practice in using their skills, and more strategic coping styles (although this may also be linked to MA), which can introduce confounds into the experiment. This can be overcome by employing groups of individuals with learning difficulties as controls (Crisco, Dobbs, & Mulhern, 1988), or in addition to TD controls (Jarrold, Baddeley, & Hewes, 1999), because these individuals can potentially be matched to WS groups for both CA and MA.

However, an additional issue that arises whenever a control group is employed concerns the criteria used to match groups. This follows from the uneven profile of abilities of individuals with WS in contrast to the flat profile seen in typical development. A CA-matched control group is likely to differ from a WS group in all areas of intelligence, but more so in the visuospatial domain and less so in the verbal domain. When matching groups by general MA, a control group will have higher visuospatial skills and lower verbal skills than the WS group. Any discrepancies in results that then emerge among groups could be primarily due to these differences in levels of ability, rather than in performance on the task in question. Visuospatial cognition in WS is particularly susceptible to the problems of matching by general MA because level of ability in this area is so low.

A related problem occurs when test batteries such as the Wechsler scales (Wechsler, 1974, 1981) or the Differential Ability Scales (DAS; Elliot, 1990) are employed. These batteries use a large number of tests to determine an individual's Full-Scale IQ (FSIQ) or level of development (MA). The uneven profile of abilities in WS means that performance will not be equivalent across all of the individual subtests of a test battery. It is therefore important to consider the number and the type of subtests used to determine which specific abilities are contributing to the composite measure of FSIQ. The Wechsler scales contain five nonverbal and five verbal subtests, whereas the DAS contains six subtests in total. Shortened versions of the Wechsler Intelligence Scale for Children (WISC) are also used (e.g., Grant et al., 1997). Speculatively, the more subtests employed, the more likely will the average score encompass the full range of abilities, thus producing a more reliable measure of general ability. However, although FSIQ can reliably assess general ability, due to the imbalance in skill in individuals with WS, an IQ score is not necessarily a particularly valid measure. It merely represents an averaged score of many differing levels of ability, and is therefore unlikely to be a powerful predictor of functioning on other tests of interest (as in typical development). In the case of WS, the individual subtests arguably provide more informative details of cognition than a composite IQ score.

These problems of matching are exacerbated when individuals with learning difficulties are used as controls because the cognitive profile of these controls may also be less uniform than that seen in typical development. For example, individuals with Down syndrome (DS) are often used as controls for individuals with WS (e.g., Bellugi, Bihrle, Neville, Doherty, & Jernigan, 1992; Bellugi et al., 1988; Rossen et al., 1996; Wang et al., 1995). The choice of DS controls is based on the assumption that these individuals exhibit a flat profile of abilities. However, Klein and Mervis (1999) presented evidence against this assumption. They suggested that individuals with DS have a relative strength in the area of visuospatial construction and a relative weakness in verbal ability (see also Chapman, 1995; Fowler, 1990; Jarrold & Baddeley, 1997; Miller, 1987). In light of this, where studies have used individuals with DS as controls, any observed differences in scores could be due to strengths or weaknesses in the DS control group as much as in the WS group.

To overcome these difficulties, control groups can be matched by their performance on a single measure. For matching to be appropriate, the measure used must be drawn from the same area of cognition as the area under investigation. This ensures that the scores of the control group are predictive of the expected level of performance of the WS group in the test condition, although none of the studies reviewed here adopt this approach. A further problem can arise if the predictive MA measure and the testing measure are too closely related. In this case the experimenter might just be testing the same abilities twice in both groups, and any interesting results that might indicate a deviation from typical development will be wiped out (Bishop, 1997). Bishop (1997) claimed that even when a difference is noted in these cases, one cannot be sure that this is not simply due to differences in the relative reliability of the two tasks.

In summary, every method has some weaknesses, and research with individuals with WS is particularly susceptible to the problems of floor and ceiling effects and of matching controls appropriately. This emphasizes the importance of employing a number of methodological techniques in a single study, with the intention of counteracting the weaknesses of one methodology with the strengths of another, for example, matching by both MA and by CA as in Bertrand et al. (1997), or employing both TD controls and controls with moderate learning difficulties (see Jarrold et al., 1999). In the following two sections we review the main body of research in the area of visuospatial cognition in WS, discussing first studies that used test batteries such as the Wechsler scales, and second those that employed tests of specific aspects of visuospatial ability. Clearly, all of these studies need to be interpreted in the light of the methodological concerns raised here.

STUDIES EMPLOYING STANDARDIZED TEST BATTERIES

Nonverbal Subtests of the Wechsler Adult Intelligence Scale and Wechsler Intelligence Scale for Children

The WS cognitive profile has been primarily documented using standardized test batteries such as the Wechsler Intelligence Scale for Children–Revised (WISC–R) and the Wechsler Adult Intelligence Scale–Revised (WAIS–R; Wechsler, 1974, 1981). Five studies provided information on the individual scores of each subtest of the battery (Arnold, Yule, & Martin, 1985; Dall'oglio & Milani, 1995; Howlin et al., 1998; Udwin & Yule, 1991; Udwin, Yule, & Martin, 1987), although the sample employed by Udwin and Yule (1991) was a subset of that employed by Udwin et al. (1987). Mean subtest scores where provided (two studies: Howlin et al., 1998; Udwin et al., 1987) are given in Table 1. The five nonverbal subtests of the WISC–R and the WAIS–R provide a measure of Performance IQ (PIQ). These are: Picture Completion, where a picture is presented and the participant has to indicate what is missing; Picture Arrangement, which involves placing a series of pictures into a sequential order of events; Block Design, where the participant is instructed to use colored blocks to model an example pattern; Object Assembly, which is a jigsaw-type task; and Coding, which is a timed task where the participant uses a key to draw specified symbols below a set of numbers.

Dall'oglio and Milani (1995) assessed 16 individuals with WS aged 4 years, 10 months (4:10) to 15:4 (no mean age given) using the WISC–R. Their participants showed poor performance on the Block Design, Coding, and Picture Arrangement subtests, in contrast to better performance on the Picture Completion and Object Assembly subtests. Arnold et al. (1985) measured the performance of 23 participants (*M* age = 10:4, range = 7:2–13:1). They reported that Coding was significantly poorer than Picture Completion, Block Design, and Object Assembly. In addition, performance on Picture Completion was higher than Picture Arrangement performance, a result consistent with the data presented by Dall'oglio and Milani (1995).

Howlin et al. (1998) studied 62 individuals with WS who were of mean age 26.5 years (range = 19–39 years). In contrast to the other studies just described,

TABLE 1
Mean Scaled Scores and Standard Deviations on the Subtests of the WISC–R[a] and WAIS–R[b] Across Different Studies

Study	M age (years months)	n	Picture Completion		Picture Arrangement		Block Design		Object Assembly		Coding	
			M	SD	M	SD	M	SD	M	SD	M	SD
Udwin et al. (1987)	11:1	44	3.25	2.18	2.84	2.53	2.14	1.76	3.18	1.82	1.55	1.21
Howlin et al. (1998)	26:6	62	3.39	1.19	3.73	1.77	3.10	1.38	3.30	1.70	2.85	1.11

Note. WISC–R = Wechsler Intelligence Scale for Children–Revised; WAIS–R = Wechsler Adult Intelligence Scale–Revised.
[a]Udwin et al. (1987). [b]Howlin et al. (1998).

they found that scores on the Picture Arrangement task were the highest among the PIQ subtests and was significantly higher than scores on the Coding subtest (referred to as Digit Symbol), where the lowest scores were achieved (see Table 1).

Udwin et al. (1987) originally tested 44 participants with a mean age of 11:1 (range = 6:0–15:9). They did not find highest scores on the Picture Arrangement task, but a subsequent study of 20 of these individuals, who had a mean age of 10:4 (range = 6:5–14:5) did achieve their highest mean score on the Picture Arrangement subtest (Udwin & Yule, 1991). In both studies individuals showed significantly poorer ability in Coding than a combined mean of the scores achieved on the other four Performance subtests (see Table 1).

Although the profile of scores on the five nonverbal subtests of the WISC and WAIS is not entirely consistent across these studies, it is clear that scores on the Block Design and Coding subtests tended to be among the lowest obtained, whereas the Picture Completion and Object Assembly tasks produced consistently higher scores. The ranked position of the Picture Arrangement task was less consistent, with performance varying from a central to a higher position in comparison to other subtests.

A related study (Atkinson et al., 2001) employed three tasks, two of which were an Object Assembly subtest (taken from the Wechsler Preschool and Primary Scale of Intelligence–Revised [WPPSI–R]; Wechsler, 1989) and a block construction task (Atkinson, Macpherson, Rae, & Hues, 1994). The performance of 73 children with WS (*M* age = 7:3, range = 8 months–13:7) was compared against a set of norms obtained in a previous study (Atkinson et al., 1994). Graphical information clearly indicates that the performance of individuals was poor on these tasks with respect to age norms. Thus, the performance of the large sample employed in this study concurs with those of the other studies just reported.

Nonverbal Subtests of the DAS

The DAS consists of two alternative batteries: a Preschool battery (ages = 3:6–6:11) and a School-age battery (ages = 5:0–17:11). The Preschool version has six subtests, three of which are used to derive nonverbal mental age. These are: Picture Similarities, which requires the participant to match a sample card to one of four pictures based on perceptual similarity or semantic association; Pattern Construction, a task similar to the Block Design subtest of the Wechsler scales; and Copying, where the individual copies line drawings. Four school-age measures, two labeled as nonverbal and two labeled as spatial, are employed to ascertain nonverbal ability. The nonverbal tasks are Matrices, where the correct design has to be selected to complete a matrix pattern; and Sequential and Quantitative Reasoning, in which items such as a shape have to be selected to complete a sequence of items. The spatial tasks are Pattern Construction, as just described, and Recall of Designs, in which the individual is shown an abstract design for a period of 5 sec, after which it is removed and the child is requested to draw it from memory.

Jarrold et al. (1998) compared selected subtest scores of the DAS battery in their sample of 16 individuals with WS (*M* age = 16:9, range = 6:11–28:0). Among those individuals functioning at the PreSchool level of the DAS the level of performance on the nonverbal tasks employed, ranked in descending order, were as follows: Copying, Picture Similarities, and Pattern Construction. The corresponding order on the three subtests employed for individuals at the School-Age level was Matrices, Sequential and Quantitative Reasoning, and Pattern Construction. The relatively low performance on the Pattern Construction subtest in both DAS batteries is consistent with the results of Block Design performance in the Wechsler studies described earlier.

Summary: The WS Cognitive Profile

The uniformly poor performance seen on the Pattern Construction and Block Design tasks in the DAS and Wechsler test batteries suggests that the skills needed for this kind of task are particularly weak in WS. This has led to the test being investigated as a single measure rather than as part of a composite of subtest scores. Mervis, Morris, Bertrand, and Robinson (1999) assessed performance on the Pattern Construction subtest of the DAS in 80 WS participants (age range 4–47 years). Eighty percent of the sample had a score that corresponded to the 1st percentile or lower for typical performance. Fifty-eight percent of participants were at floor on the task, which may be masking even poorer abilities. Only 10% scored within the normal range. Other studies (e.g., Bellugi et al., 1988, 1992; Frangiskakis et al., 1996) also reported similarly low scores on block construction tasks.

Mervis (1999) used the consistent weakness in Pattern Construction, along with other characteristics of WS, as a basis for a set of psychological criteria for diagnosing WS. These are a "definite strength in auditory short term memory, relative strength in language, and extreme weakness in visuo-spatial construction" (Mervis, 1999, p. 197). The Pattern Construction test was used as the measure of visuospatial construction ability and was involved in two of the criteria. Performance on this test must be below the general MA measure and also below Digit recall score (a measure of verbal short-term memory). A number of studies found high levels of sensitivity and specificity using these criteria to identify individuals who do and do not have WS (Frangiskakis et al., 1996; Jarrold et al., 1998; Mervis, 1999; Mervis et al., 1999; Mervis et al., 2000).

STUDIES EMPLOYING SPECIFIC VISUOSPATIAL TESTS

Tests of Spatial Organization

Bellugi and colleagues (e.g., Bellugi et al., 1988; Bellugi et al., 1992; Bellugi et al., 1994) have suggested that individuals with WS process information at the local level, that is, they focus on the parts of an image rather than its whole. The basis for this claim is the pattern of errors shown by some individuals with WS on the Block Design task. Rather than recreating the overall spatial organization of the pattern, that is, four blocks in a 2×2 square arrangement, individuals with WS may select the appropriate individual blocks, but place them in an unorganized manner that fails to maintain the relationships among blocks. There are a number of factors to take into account when considering this suggestion of a local processing bias. First, young children also produce solutions where the configuration are broken (e.g., Akshoomoff & Stiles, 1996), which suggests that the errors made by individuals with WS might not be due to a deviant processing style. Second, other authors have suggested that a local processing approach should actually be beneficial to performance on the Block Design test (Happé, 1994, 1999; Shah & Frith, 1993). This is because to succeed on this task the individual needs to resist the gestalt form of the overall pattern and analyze the stimulus in terms of its component parts. In support of this, Shah and Frith (1993) showed that typically developing individuals complete test items more rapidly when the stimulus is presegmented into its constituent blocks rather than presented as a whole. In addition, individuals with autism, who are known to show a local visual processing bias on many tasks (Happé, 1999), show particularly strong levels of performance on the Block Design test precisely because the task benefits from a local analysis (Happé, 1994; Shah & Frith, 1993).

If individuals with WS do process information at a relatively local level, then this form of segmentation should not cause response time to decrease. Mervis et al. (1999) investigated the performance of a group of 21 individuals with WS of mean age 29.5 years, using both a standard and a segmented version of the DAS Block Design task. Response times were generally reduced when blocks were segmented. This facilitation suggests that individuals with WS do not rely exclusively on local processing in the standard Block Design task as advocated by Bellugi. Consequently, the authors put forward the suggestion that "individuals with Williams syndrome have difficulty segmenting the whole into its component parts" (p. 94).

Farran, Jarrold, and Gathercole (2001) were interested in the magnitude of this facilitation effect, that is, whether the effect of segmentation observed in WS on this type of task occurs to a greater, equal, or lesser extent than in the typical population. The authors employed a novel task, the Squares task, which is a two-dimensional version of the Block Design task. Individuals were presented with either a segmented or a nonsegmented version of a model image, which could be copied by placing four squares in the correct 2 × 2 formation. Each square was divided centrally into two colors either across the diagonal (oblique squares) or vertically/horizontally (nonoblique squares). The performance of 21 individuals with WS of mean age 19:11 (range = 9:6–38:5) was compared to that of 21 TD controls matched individually by score on the Ravens Coloured Progressive Matrices (RCPM; Raven, 1993). Results showed that both groups were equally facilitated by segmentation. This implies not only that individuals with WS do not show a local processing bias, but that their processing preferences appear to be entirely typical.

Hoffman, Landau, and Pagani (in press) were interested in the process of construction in WS. Hence, they investigated the pattern of eye fixations while participants were completing a computerized block construction task. They reported that, in complex puzzles, 8 individuals with WS (*M* age = 9:5, range = 7:0–13:11) were just as able to detect an error in their solution as a group of 8 TD controls matched for IQ on the Kaufman Brief Intelligence Test (Kaufman & Kaufman, 1990) of mean age 5:3 (range = 5:1–6:4). However, individuals in the WS group were less accurate at choosing the correct puzzle piece, checked their partial solutions less often, and were less likely to change their solution when they detected an error. The authors suggest that these factors account for the significantly lower accuracy overall in the WS group than the control group. This suggests that it is the process of block construction, rather than the perception of the model image, that effects WS performance.

Pani, Mervis, and Robinson (1999) administered a visual search task to test whether individuals with WS are influenced by global information. They employed a task, taken from Banks and Prinzmetal (1976), in which the participant is asked to indicate whether a T or an F is present among the stimuli in a visual array. These targets are presented alongside distracters, which were described as halfway between a T and an F. This task affects the efficiency of global and local processing approaches, depending on how the stimuli are manipulated. Stimulus grouping particularly affects individuals who adopt a relatively global processing approach to the task. In contrast, individuals employing a relatively local approach are more likely to be affected by the number of distracters in the array. Banks and Prinzmetal (1976) found that response times were significantly faster when targets were isolated and the distracters were grouped by proximity than when there were fewer, more evenly spread stimuli. In other words, the effect of gestalt grouping was stronger than the effect of display size, implying a predominance of global over local processing in TD adults. Pani et al. (1999) presented this task to 12 individuals with WS, with a mean age of 30:11 (range = 19:3–47:6), who were matched to 12 TD individuals by gender and CA. Both groups were more influenced by gestalt grouping than by display size, which suggests that individuals with WS have a global processing precedence as seen in typical development. The WS group was less influenced by the number of distracters than the controls. The authors argue that this implies that individuals with WS are less able to disengage from global processing than the controls. The suggestion made by Bellugi and colleagues that individuals with WS have a global processing deficit is therefore not supported by this study.

Farran and Jarrold (2001a) investigated the comprehension of spatial relations in WS. Global accuracy is dependent on reproducing the spatial relations among the parts of the image, and therefore spatial relations are particularly important in tasks in which an image must be reproduced. Twenty-one individuals with WS of mean age 21:2 and 21 TD controls of mean age 6:3 were matched individually by level of performance on the RCPM. Three tasks were administered: Two tasks measured categorical spatial relations and coordinate spatial relations, respectively, and a third task measured the comprehension of visual relations. Categorical spatial relations refer to linguistic categories such as "next to," "to the left of," and "above" and are used to describe the spatial layout of a scene. Coordinate spatial relations refer to distances, and are useful for spatial navigation. In both of the spatial relations tasks, participants were shown an image of a man holding a bat. Following the appearance of a ball, participants were asked whether the ball was above or below the bat (categorical relations), or whether the ball was in or out (coordinate relations). In the visual relations task, the individual was presented with three colored squares. The two outer squares were blue and green, respectively, and the middle square varied in hue between blue and green. Participants were asked to judge whether the middle square was more like the green square or more like the blue square. In all three tasks, experimental trials followed a set of 12 practice/training trials. Results showed that the WS group, although showing a similar pattern of performance to the TD controls, was significantly poorer than the TD controls in completing both the spatial relations and the visual relations tasks. This suggests that individuals with WS find it difficult to comprehend both the spatial relationship among elements of an image and also variations in color hue, which are also important indicators of spatial organization. It is possible that this apparent deficit in spatial relational understanding has a negative affect on the ability of individuals with WS to reproduce images accurately.

Tests of Drawing

Bellugi et al. (1988) employed a subtest of the Boston Diagnostic Aphasia Examination (BDAE; Goodglass & Kaplan, 1972) to assess drawing skills in WS. In this task the individual is asked to draw a set of common objects, first from memory and then using a model. The objects become increasingly complex (i.e., cross, cube, flower, house) as the task progresses. Bellugi et al. (1988) observed that 3 individuals with WS, aged 11, 15, and 16 years, drew parts without integrating the drawings into functional objects; drawings also lacked representation of depth and perspective. These authors also administered the Developmental Test of Visual–Motor Integration (VMI; Beery & Buktenica, 1967), which consists of a set of 24 geometric figures of varying complexity, which have to be copied. These are divided into four categories, which are, in order of increasing difficulty, single lines, simple shapes, intersection of lines, and items involving integration of two or more shapes. The 3 individuals with WS in this study again lacked the ability to organize their drawings. Of the 24 figures, only the first 8, belonging to the single lines and simple shapes categories, were completed by all 3 children. This is the level that a child aged 4:11 would be expected to reach and was considerably below these participants' CA. Bellugi et al. (1988) interpreted these results as an "inability to maintain two hierarchically organised levels in their drawings" (p. 295).

Wang et al. (1995) employed the VMI in a study with 10 participants with WS (*M* age = 15.7 years, range 11–18 years, and FSIQ of 48.9) and a control group of individuals with DS matched for CA and FSIQ. The WS participants successfully completed a mean of 7.5 figures, a level significantly below that obtained by the DS group, although this may be due to elevated performance among the DS group, as their visuospatial construction abilities are stronger than their verbal abilities (Klein & Mervis, 1999). The authors suggested that the individual drawings of the participants with WS indicate that qualitatively there is "an impairment in global coherence" (p. 58) and that "local features were not oriented correctly with respect to each other" (p. 59).

Bertrand et al. (1997) also employed the object drawing subtest of the BDAE and a reduced version of the VMI (Beery, 1989). In study one, 18 children with WS of mean CA 9:11 (range = 9:2–10:7) and mean MA 5:6 (range = 3:0–7:0) participated and were compared to two control groups of TD individuals. One control group was matched by MA (*M* CA = 5:6, range = 3:5–6:11) and the other by CA (*M* CA = 9:11, range = 9:2–10:8). The performance level of the WS group on the VMI was equivalent to that of typical children of age 4:10 and was significantly lower than that observed in both control groups. On the BDAE, individuals with

WS produced significantly fewer recognizable drawings, fewer major parts, and more disorganized drawings than CA-matched controls. Recognizability and disorganization of WS drawings was not significantly different from that of the MA-matched controls' drawings, although significantly fewer major parts were produced by the WS group. In a second study, Bertrand et al. (1997) investigated the developmental progression of typically developing individuals aged 4 to 7 years on the two tests just described. Results from the VMI revealed that copying geometric forms that require the integration of component parts is a skill that is not fully acquired until 6 years. The drawings of 4-year-old children and many of the 5-year-olds were unintegrated, resembling those of the WS group in the first study. The drawings from the BDAE of older children were significantly more recognizable, included more major parts, and were more organized than those of younger children. Again, the level of disorganization at 4 years resembled that of the individuals with WS in the first study. Bertrand and Mervis (1996) reported developmental improvements in the drawings of six adolescents with WS between two testing points, one at age 9 and 10 years and the second at 12 to 14 years, which followed the same path as typically developing individuals.

The Delis Hierarchical processing task, also known as the Navon task (Navon, 1977), is another task that can involve drawing. This test focuses more directly on the issue of global and local levels of processing. A figure is presented, which consists of local features such as small L's, which, when seen as a whole, make up a larger shape or letter such as a D. The individual is invited to draw the figure from memory or to copy it. In each case both local and global processing are required if both the parts and the whole are to be drawn accurately.

Bihrle, Bellugi, Delis, and Marks (1989) compared the performance on this task of 14 individuals with WS, of mean age 13.12 years (range = 9–18 years) and mean IQ 57.42 (range = 49–77), with that of a group of 10 CA-matched TD controls and 9 children with DS matched for CA and IQ. In the memory condition, the TD group performed significantly better than both children with WS and children with DS. However, of particular interest is a significant interaction between group and hierarchical level that emerged from the analysis. Individuals with WS were significantly more accurate at drawing local features relative to global figures, whereas individuals with DS showed the opposite pattern. Participants with DS omitted significantly more global forms than both DS and TD groups. In the copy condition the same group-by-hierarchical level interaction emerged. Individuals in the TD group were equally competent at copying both global and local forms, although this may be because they performed at ceiling on the test. Because of this, it is possible that the significant interactions reported in this study are driven by atypical performance in the DS group, rather than the WS group. Entirely similar results were reported on this task by Rossen et al. (1996), who compared the performance of 6 individuals with WS (*M* age = 14:2; *M* IQ = 50.8) to that of 6 individuals with DS matched for CA and IQ. No statistical analysis was given and comparison with a TD control group was not made, so once again it is difficult to establish whether the performance of the WS group is atypical. However, these two studies point toward a possible preference for local processing in WS in drawing.

The Delis task was also employed by Stevens (1997), who asked 13 individuals with WS, of mean CA 18:10 and mean MA 5:3, to both draw the stimuli themselves and give verbal instructions to another person as to how to draw each figure. Stevens did not find that the WS group as a whole showed a local bias in their drawings, although this was seen among the drawings of 5 of the 13 individuals with WS. When participants were asked to give instructions to someone else there was much less evidence of any local bias. In this case only 1 individual showed a consistent local preference, and that individual's responses contained some global elements. As a result Stevens suggests that any local bias seen on the Delis task is unlikely to be due to an abnormality of visuospatial perception, but that it could emerge during the planning or execution of a motor response.

Farran, Jarrold, and Gathercole (in press) compared the drawing ability of the Navon figures to perception of the same figures in WS. Twenty-one individuals with WS of mean age 20:9 (range = 10:2–39:2) and 21 TD participants of mean age 6:7 years (range = 5:9–7:9) were matched individually by performance on the RCPM. Performance on the drawing task showed significantly better local accuracy than global accuracy in the WS group, whereas the performance of the control group was comparable in local and global accuracy, thus replicating the results of previous studies (Bihrle et al., 1989; Rossen et al., 1996). Two perceptual versions of the Navon task, measuring divided and selective attention, respectively, were adapted from Plaisted, Swettenham, and Rees (1999). In the divided attention task, the individual was required to indicate whether the large letter (global level) or the small letter (local level) was a letter A, and hence was required to switch attention across the hierarchical levels. In the selective attention task, attention was focused on one hierarchical level at a time. In one condition, participants were required to focus at the global level and had to indicate whether the large letter was an H or an S. In the other condition, attention was directed to the local level and participants indicated whether the small letter was an S or an H. In contrast to the results from the drawing task, Farran, Jarrold, et al. (in press) found that at the perceptual level, individuals with WS showed the same pattern of performance as the TD controls, with no evidence of either a global or a local processing preference. This suggests that the local preference seen in the drawing abilities of individuals with WS does not reflect a local perceptual processing bias.

Tests of Visual Closure

Perceptual closure is the ability to use fragmented information to obtain a configural percept. This is essential in cases of object recognition when information about the object's global configuration is incomplete. In these instances the individual needs to construct a global percept from the available information, rather than focusing on the local, fragmented elements of the stimulus. A well-known example of a test of visual closure is the Mooney Faces Test (Mooney, 1957), in which the participant must discriminate between faces and nonfaces that have highly exaggerated shadows and highlights. Bellugi et al. (1988) presented this test to their 3 individuals with WS and observed higher performance levels than would be expected for these individuals' CA. They took this to indicate "intact abilities to perceive and differentiate shape and form" (p. 293). Wang et al. (1995) also gave the Mooney Faces Test (Mooney, 1957) to their 10 individuals with WS. In contrast to Bellugi et al.'s results, they found that performance on this and other tests of visual closure was not significantly different from that of a comparison group of 9 individuals with DS matched for CA and IQ. The performance of both groups fell within the range expected for preschool and young school-aged children, which was consistent with these individuals' MA levels. Although both of these studies employed relatively small samples and lacked a control group other than individuals with DS, their results suggest that individuals with WS may be able to perceive the global aspects of an image.

Tests of Face Recognition

Face recognition is viewed as an area of relative strength within the domain of visuospatial cognition in WS (e.g., Bellugi et al., 1988; Rossen et al., 1996). The Benton Test of Facial Recognition (Benton, Hamsher, Varney, & Spreen, 1983) has been administered in a number of studies (Bellugi et al., 1988; Bellugi et al., 1992; Karmiloff-Smith, 1997; Rossen et al., 1996; Wang et al., 1995). In this test the participant is initially shown a front-view photograph of a face and is then asked to identify this target from among distracters. In a subsequent section of the task, the target and the distracters are presented in three-quarter view, and in the final section the target appears among faces that are photographed under different lighting conditions.

Three studies have compared the performance on the Benton Faces Test of individuals with WS against that of individuals with DS matched for CA and FSIQ (Bellugi et al., 1992; Rossen et al., 1996; Wang et al., 1995). In each case the WS groups outperformed their controls. However, as already noted, this discrepancy may be primarily due to reduced performance in the DS group, rather than to particularly unusual performance among individuals with WS. If this is the case, then this alone does not necessarily indicate preserved face recognition in WS. Nevertheless, in these studies the levels of performance shown by individuals with WS fell within the normal range. Similar results were reported by Bellugi et al. (1988), who found average performance levels across the whole test of 74%, 87%

and 80% correct, respectively, of their 3 individuals with WS. A score of below 70% is considered to indicate defective processing on the Benton Faces Test; thus these individuals appear to be performing at a normal level. However, it is important to note that the Benton faces test is designed primarily for use with individuals with neuropsychological deficits. The narrow range of normal performance on the task, between 70% and 100% suggests that it is relatively easy for the general population. This raises the possibility that ceiling effects might be present in the standardization data.

Karmiloff-Smith (1997) assessed 10 individuals with WS with a mean CA of 22:8, a mean verbal MA of 10:5, and a mean performance MA of 6:8. In contrast to the studies reviewed thus far, these individuals were matched individually by CA to a control group of 10 TD individuals. Seven members of the WS group scored within the normal range on the Benton Test, 2 were borderline normal, and 1 individual showed impairment. All of the control group scored within the normal range. However, because detailed scores are not given, there remains the possibility that ceiling effects are present in this control group.

An interview following the task revealed that individuals with WS recognized the faces by specific features such as a cheek bone or the shape of the nostrils, whereas the control group talked about the face as a whole. Karmiloff-Smith therefore suggested that the apparently normal levels of performance of the WS participants may be reached by a different means than that of TD controls (see also Wang et al., 1995). Karmiloff-Smith (1997) assessed the same participants in a second face recognition experiment, which employed a computerized discrimination task taken from Campbell, Bruce, Import, and Wright (1995). This task requires the individual to discriminate among different faces that vary by a number of different facial elements. These are facial speech (lip reading), emotional expression, eye gaze direction, and the identity of the faces (all features visible, or hairline or eyes masked; Djabri, 1995). Stimuli were presented full face or oriented to the right or to the left; some of the faces were very similar to each other, whereas others were very dissimilar. Individuals with WS and controls performed at seemingly comparable levels (over 90% for the TD controls and over 80% for the WS participants) with the exception of conditions where "configural processing" was necessary (similar identities, sideways facial orientation, and the masked-features conditions). In these conditions, the performance level of the WS group dropped to chance, whereas the control group continued to perform at a high level. Karmiloff-Smith (1997) attributed this contrast among groups to the type of processing used, suggesting that for individuals with WS to exhibit their characteristically strong face processing skills they need to be able to use facial features rather than processing the global configuration as in typical development. However, Karmiloff-Smith conceded that this is a preliminary study, and hence no statistical analysis was provided. Also, given that the interpretations made are based on data where controls are performing at or near ceiling, one cannot be entirely certain that typically developing individuals would not find certain conditions particularly difficult if the task was made somewhat harder.

Deruelle, Mancini, Livet, Casse-Perrot, and Schonen (1999) employed a similar face matching task to test 12 individuals with WS of mean CA 11.9 years and mean MA of 5.9 years, matched to two TD control groups, one by CA and one by MA. The WS group performed at the same level as MA controls (accuracy: WS = 87.7%, MA = 89.3%) and significantly below the CA controls (95.2% accurate) when matching faces by gender, age, gaze direction, emotional expression, and identity across different angles, but at the same level as the CA controls in the lip reading condition. The authors argue that this reflects that matching by lip reading requires featural processing, in contrast to configural processing in the other conditions. However, as just noted (Karmiloff-Smith, 1997), the results could reflect the fact that ceiling effects are masking a pattern of results in the CA controls that would otherwise be similar to that of the WS group.

Tests of Object Recognition

The Canonical–Noncanonical Views Test (Carey & Diamond, 1990) measures the recognition of familiar objects. The ability to name objects from noncanonical or atypical views (such as a teapot viewed from above) is determined from an individual's performance on two subtests, each containing 25 pictures. The first subtest shows objects from noncanonical views. These same 25 objects are then shown from canonical views (e.g., a teapot viewed from the side) to ensure that the individual is familiar with them. A noncanonical views score is calculated as the number of items that were correctly named on the noncanonical subtest as a percentage of those items correctly named on the canonical subtest.

Wang et al. (1995) used this test to compare the performance of their groups of individuals with WS and DS. Similar numbers of canonical views were recognized in both groups (WS 23.3 and DS 22.7 of 25); however, the groups differed significantly in their ability to recognize noncanonical views, with the WS group obtaining higher percentage scores (M = 75.9%) than the DS group (M = 66.4%). The authors viewed this as a "relative strength" in the WS profile, which raises the interesting question of whether the studies reviewed that purport to show normal abilities in face recognition do so because of a specific or more general strength in recognition memory. However, again the difference in the performance of these groups could equally reflect particularly poor abilities in the DS group.

Hoffman and Landau (2000) reported the results of a similar canonical views task. In their study, the performance of 12 children with WS of mean age 11:1 (range = 7:5–15:3) was compared to that of 12 adult controls and 12 TD children who were matched for MA by both verbal and nonverbal ability level on the

K–BIT and had a mean age of 5:10 (range = 4:1–7:1). Participants were presented with a computerized task with four conditions (canonical view, clear image; canonical view, blurred image; noncanonical view, clear image; and noncanonical view, blurred image) and were required to name 80 objects, 20 from each condition, taken randomly from a pool of 320 images. Results demonstrated that adults performed better than the two groups of children, and that the WS children performed at the same level as the mental-age-matched controls. The authors suggested that this indicates that "object recognition may be selectively spared" (Hoffman & Landau, 2000). However, the WS group was matched to the controls by both verbal and nonverbal mental age, hence the similarities in the groups' performance indicates that object recognition in WS is at a similar level to their other nonverbal abilities, rather than a spared area of ability.

Tests of Orientation Coding

Atkinson et al. (1997) employed two "post-box" tasks to assess the abilities of 11 children with WS (from a group of 15 WS participants of *M* age = 9.7 years, range = 4–14 years) and a group of 20 TD controls (a subset from a group of 30 TD controls of *M* age = 8.1 years ranging from 4–20 years). The tasks were taken from the neuropsychological literature and are designed to assess the functioning of the two visual systems, the ventral and the dorsal visual streams, responsible for perception and action, respectively (Milner & Goodale, 1995). In both tasks, a cylindrical drum is presented. A slot at the front of the drum can be orientated at 0, 45, 90, or 135 deg. The matching task tests ventral stream functioning: A card is held by a rotatable wooden hand and the individual is asked to rotate the hand so that the card is in the correct position ready to be posted. In the posting task, a test that taps the functions of the dorsal stream, the individual is asked to post the card into the slot. Results indicated that in the matching task the performance of 6 of the individuals with WS was similar to the TD controls, whereas the remaining WS children showed modest deficits. Performance on the posting task was somewhat weaker: 2 individuals with WS displayed errors of a similar magnitude to TD older children and adults, 4 showed errors similar to TD 4-year-old controls, and 5 made errors that were larger than the control group. The results of this study suggest that individuals with WS are able to match orientations, but experience difficulty if an additional motor action is required.

Orientation matching has also been assessed in WS using the Benton Lines Orientation test (Benton et al., 1978; see Bellugi et al., 1988; Rossen et al., 1996; Wang et al., 1995). In this task the participant is presented with a display of 11 lines oriented 18 deg apart and is asked to decide which of these lines matches the orientation of two target lines. Two of Bellugi et al.'s (1988) 3 children with WS scored at or below 35% correct and the third child failed the pretest (which requires passing 2 of 5 practice trials). Wang et al. (1995) reported that only 2 of their 10 individuals with WS passed this pretest. Similarly, Rossen et al. (1996) found that the majority of their 6 participants with WS could not pass the pretest. These obvious floor effects contrast to the results of Atkinson et al. (1997), and tell us only that individuals with WS perform predominantly at a level below that of a "severely deficient" adult, the lowest classification of the test.

Stiers, Willekens, Borghgraef, Fryns, and Vandenbussche (2000) designed a line orientation task, the Preschool Judgement of Line Orientation task, which was set at a more appropriate level for individuals with WS. The task was similar to the Benton Lines Task, that is, the individual had to match target lines to a number of choice alternatives. In this task, however, in blocks 1 to 3, one rather than two target lines was presented. Additionally, the number of choice alternatives varied from 2 in block 1, to 4 in block 2, to 11 in block 3. Block 4 used items from the original Benton Lines Task described previously, with two target lines and 11 response choices. Twenty individuals with WS of ages ranging from 5 to 25 years (no mean given) performed at a level that was slightly below their verbal ability and at the same level as their nonverbal ability as measured by the WPPSI–R. This highlights the importance of employing tasks that measure the correct range of ability and appears to suggest, in contrast to the evidence from the standard Benton Lines Task, and in line with results of Atkinson et al.'s study, that individuals with WS are able to encode differences in line orientations.

Summary

The visuospatial skills of individuals with WS appear to vary considerably among tests. Face recognition is typically seen as a major strength in WS, although the actual evidence for this claim is undermined by the presence of clear ceiling effects among controls or in normative comparison data. Although visuospatial abilities are generally impaired in WS, relatively higher levels of performance are seen on some tests, notably the segmented version of the Block Design task, visual search tasks, and the Canonical–Noncanonical Views Test. This appears to suggest that individuals with WS are able to process visual information at a global level. Relatively weaker performance is seen on the standard Block Design task, in tests of drawing, and in completing drawing versions of the Delis Hierarchical processing task. These difficulties have previously been explained in terms of a local processing bias in WS. This raises a clear contrast: How can individuals with WS show little impairment on such tasks as visual search tasks that require global organization, given the suggestion (e.g., Bellugi et al., 1988) that they have a preference for processing information at a local level? The following section attempts to provide an explanation for this apparent contradiction, as well as for some of the differences seen in performance levels across visuospatial tasks.

THEORETICAL IMPLICATIONS

Having reviewed the available information regarding visuospatial functioning in WS and considered methodological issues in the process, we are now in the position to propose explanations of the results obtained. We have drawn together the whole body of research in the visuospatial domain in an effort to draw conclusions as to what factors might be constraining performance in WS. The uneven profile of performance of individuals with WS on visuospatial tasks may be related to the processing preferences of individuals with WS, such as local or global processing, but additionally it may reflect the specific demands of each task, such as perceptual and constructional requirements.

There is considerable discussion as to whether individuals with WS rely on local methods of processing on visuospatial tasks or use a predominantly global method of processing as in typical development (e.g., Bellugi et al., 1988; Farran, Jarrold, et al., in press; Karmiloff-Smith et al., 1997; Mervis, 1999; Stevens, 1997; Wang et al., 1995). Bellugi and colleagues argued that individuals with WS show a local processing precedence. Mervis and colleagues proposed that they do not have a local bias, but predominantly process information at a global level as in typical development. Pani and colleagues suggested that individuals with WS experience problems in switching from one hierarchical level of processing to another.

Our proposal takes a novel angle by relating the level of performance in WS to the perceptual and constructional demands of the task. We suggest that individuals with WS can perceive information at both global and local levels, as in typical development (as shown by Mervis et al., 1999, and Pani et al., 1999), but that they struggle to use this information to complete visuospatial construction at a global level. This constructional process encompasses the abilities needed to perform an overt motor action, the abilities required to perform the internal manipulations of spatial representations necessary for successful motor planning, and the ability to maintain the correct spatial relationships between the parts of an image when reproducing it. Thus, in reference to local and global levels of processing, we suggest that individuals with WS will only show evidence of a local processing bias in tasks with a constructional component. In addition they will not show any particular evidence of a local bias on tasks that are largely perceptual. This account has the potential to reconcile the apparently contradictory evidence that exists in this area.

As already discussed, the poor performance of individuals with WS on the Block Design task has been seen as evidence for a local processing bias (e.g., Bellugi et al., 1988). However, evidence from autism and other areas (e.g., Shah & Frith, 1993) shows that a local processing bias is actually advantageous on this test. A possible solution to this apparent contradiction is provided by Kohs (1923), who designed the Block Design task. Kohs suggested that the task requires "first the breaking up of each design presented into logical units, and second a reasoned manipulation of blocks to reconstruct the original design from separate parts." Notice that there are two processes involved here. The first—the breaking up of the design—is a perceptual component, and the second—the reconstruction of the design—is constructional. In these terms the evidence suggests that the local processing bias in autism is perceptual (Happé, 1996; Jarrold & Russell, 1997; Shah & Frith, 1993), whereas the local processing bias in WS is constructional (Bellugi et al., 1988).

Other evidence supports the view that perceptual processing in WS is not particularly driven by a local preference. Individuals with WS show a beneficial effect of segmentation on the Block Design task (Mervis et al., 1999), which would be reduced if stimuli were perceived at the local level. They are also predominantly influenced by the global characteristics of stimuli within visual search tasks (Pani et al., 1999). Performance on the Canonical–Noncanonical Views task appears to represent a peak in the WS nonverbal profile, and recognition of the noncanonical views is thought to reflect the ability to use local features of an object to recognize the whole form (Carey & Diamond, 1990). This task therefore requires both local and global perceptual processing styles. However, the claim that face processing in WS is influenced by featural analysis (e.g., Karmiloff-Smith, 1997) seems to contradict this proposal. There may be two explanations for this. First, the evidence of a local bias in face processing in WS comes from studies that employed tasks that may be insensitive to differences in performance levels among controls. Second, even if it is shown that face processing in WS is "particularly local," this could reflect the fact that face processing in typical development is seen by some as a domain-specific process, which is separate from other areas of visuospatial cognition (Farah, 1996). If so, then face processing tendencies may be independent of any general visuospatial processing style. This would accommodate both the claim for a local perceptual bias when processing faces and a relatively global bias for perceiving other visuospatial information.

A local bias in construction in WS is seen not only on block construction tasks, but also in tests of drawing ability (Bellugi et al., 1988; Bertrand & Mervis, 1996, Bertrand et al., 1997; Wang et al., 1995). Wang et al. (1995) explicitly noted evidence of this local approach in WS, and observed that their participants with WS were only able to concentrate on the parts of an image one at a time and did not integrate these to form the global whole. Similarly, Bihrle et al. (1989) and Rossen et al. (1996) concluded from performance on the Delis Hierarchical processing task that individuals with WS approached this task at the local level. However, they reached this conclusion by analyzing the quality of an individual's output, that is, how they had constructed the image, rather than the quality of the input, that is, how the image had been perceived. Farran, Jarrold, et al. (in press) and Stevens (1997) demonstrated that these two levels are dissociable in WS by examining both perception and construction of hierarchical figures. In contrast to previous drawing studies, Stevens (1997) only found evidence of a predominantly local approach in 5 of his 13 individuals with WS. Nevertheless, when asked to describe the same hierarchical letter stimuli, none of his WS participants showed any evidence of a local processing bias. Similarly, Farran, Jarrold, et al. (in press) reported significantly better local than global accuracy in the drawing abilities of their group of WS individuals, which contrasts sharply to the group's perception of these hierarchical figures where no local processing preference was observed.

Atkinson et al. (2001) looked at the occurrence of sensory visual problems, such as strabismus, reduced stereopsis, or visual acuity loss, in WS. They reported that their group of individuals with WS showed no reliable correlation between sensory visual problems and performance on the three visuospatial cognition tasks described earlier. This supports our proposal that visuospatial problems in WS are not perceptual.

Pani et al. (1999) suggested that individuals with WS can process at both local and global levels but experience difficulty in switching between these levels of organization. This differs from our suggestion that the local processing preference in WS is expressed in constructional, but not in perceptual tasks, and is difficult to support for two reasons. First, in the divided attention version of the Delis task, which requires the participant to switch between hierarchical levels, individuals with WS performed at the same level as TD controls (Farran, Jarrold, et al., in press). Second, in the Block Design task, a switch is required at the perceptual stage from global perception of the image to the local perception of the individual blocks. This task demand can be eliminated by presegmenting the image into its constituent parts (e.g., Mervis et al., 1999). The facilitation effect elicited by presegmenting the blocks is equal in WS to that seen in typical development (Farran, Jarrold, et al., 2001), suggesting that the switch is equally demanding for both groups. We suggest that faced with the requirements of constructional tasks, individuals with WS experience the normal levels of difficulty at perception, but at construction adopt a piecemeal approach resulting in relative success in reduplicating the local elements of an image in comparison to the global image. This appears to result from a poor comprehension of spatial relations in WS (Farran & Jarrold, 2001a).

The evidence from Atkinson et al. (1997) indicates a specific problem in performing a motor action in WS. The authors suggested from these results that dorsal stream functioning in WS may be impaired. However, they conceded that this deficit cannot be the only contributing factor to the pattern of visuospatial abilities in WS. Hoffman et al. (in press) indicated, from studying eye movements, that the actual process of construction differed in WS from TD controls. Taken together, the findings of Atkinson et al., Farran and Jarrold (2001a), and Hoffman et al. (in press), support our argument that construction is poor in WS, that is, that the internal manipulation of the individual elements (measured by Hoffman et al., in press), the maintenance of the spatial representation in reproduction (measured by Farran & Jarrold, 2001a), and the overt motor action required to place each element in the correct position (measured by Atkinson et al.) are problematic processes for the WS population to complete.

The poor ability of individuals with WS to complete the global configuration in block construction tasks is similar to that seen in young children (Akshoomoff & Stiles, 1996; Kramer, Kaplan, Share, & Huckeba, 1999). Kramer et al. (1999) reported more broken configurations (defined as any occasion in which the child placed a block outside of the square matrix) produced by children aged 6 to 7 years in comparison to older age groups (8–9, 10–11, 12–13 years). Anecdotal reports suggest that there is a large proportion of broken configurations in WS solutions (e.g., Bellugi et al., 1988). This claim was investigated systematically by Mervis et al. (1999), who found that in 76% of solutions, the overall shape was reproduced correctly in WS. The authors stated that this is equivalent to the proportion of correct global configurations produced by TD children aged 6 to 8 years as reported by Akshoomoff and Stiles (1996). This implies that the presence of broken configurations in WS solutions on this task could indicate that their level of ability is delayed, rather than deviant. This is supported by the evidence that individuals with WS demonstrate a poor level of ability, but a typical pattern of performance in tasks measuring spatial relations (Farran & Jarrold, 2001a), that is, delayed rather than deviant abilities.

The development of drawing abilities in children progresses through a local processing stage. At 4.5 years, typically developing individuals produce unintegrated drawings much like those produced by 9.5-year-old individuals with WS (Bertrand & Mervis, 1996). In addition, the developmental pathway followed by individuals with WS in drawing resembles that seen in typical development (Bertrand et al., 1997). By 13.5 years, the drawings of Bertrand and Mervis's (1996) WS group had become more organized and were now equivalent to the drawings of a child of 5.5 years. Block construction ability in WS also improves during childhood, and by adulthood, level of ability in WS reaches the level of a typically developing 6-year-old child (Mervis et al., 1999). As just noted (Mervis et al., 1999), these results suggest that the local processing bias seen in the drawings and constructional abilities of individuals with WS (e.g., Bellugi et al., 1988; Wang et al., 1995) reflect delayed development. If one were to accept that visuospatial output by construction and drawing in WS is at the level of a typically developing child of approximately 6 years, whereas other skills such as aspects of language are closer to an adolescent's level of performance, can we label these abilities as delayed or deviant? Individuals with WS are aware of their errors, yet still are unable to correct them (Hoffman et al., in press). This contrasts to the performance of young typically developing children, who may fail because they are not sophisticated enough to be aware of their errors; thus errors persist until the children simultaneously develop the ability to see and correct their inaccuracies. Given the huge discrepancy between levels of performance in WS, such a large delay in construction and drawing may in fact be deviant.

The examples just given indicate that an individual with WS has problems not so much in the perception of an image as in its reconstruction. Stevens (1997) argued that this problem occurs in the planning and execution of a motor action, whereas Pani et al. (1999) suggested that having processed information at one level, individuals with WS then experience difficulty when a change in the spatial organization of the image is required. We propose that to produce an image through drawing or construction, the individual with WS is forced to rely on a piecemeal method of approaching the task, hence the appearance of a local processing bias at the expense of maintaining the spatial organization and consequently the loss of the global configuration of the image. The resulting level of output in WS develops until it is at the level of a 6-year-old child, at which point individuals with WS reach a ceiling in ability and these abilities cease to develop further.

This piecemeal approach appears to result from difficulty in encoding the spatial relations among the individual elements (Farran & Jarrold, 2001a). As described earlier, spatial relations refer to the relative position of one object to another such as above or next to (categorical spatial relations), or to the precise distance from one object to another (coordinate spatial relations; Kosslyn & Koenig, 1992). Success in construction tasks, that is, mentally deconstructing and manipulating the parts of a model image and physically reconstructing the image to provide a correct solution, is dependent on accurately preserving the spatial relations between the local elements throughout the construction process. Without this skill or with poor levels of ability, individuals may recreate the local details of the image, but not place these local elements in the correct relationship to one another; thus the global spatial representation may be incorrect. This appears to be what is observed in the solutions of individuals with WS. In contrast to constructional tasks, the spatial relations among elements are always kept constant in perceptual tasks, and so the ability to understand spatial relations is not a crucial factor for successful task completion. This could explain why perceptual but not constructional abilities might be affected in WS by a lack of comprehension of spatial relations, resulting in a local bias on construction.

CONCLUSIONS

A general conclusion that emerges from the review of these studies is that visuospatial abilities in WS are collectively poor, but that the relative level of difficulty of tasks is not consistent across the visuospatial domain. We suggest that this variability is partly due to the methodological problems associated with studying WS, but that there are reliable underlying differences in the levels of performance of individuals with WS across a variety of visuospatial tests. The evidence from methodologically sound studies has led us to argue that many of the strengths and weaknesses in WS performance are the result of the perceptual or the constructional demands associated with a particular task. Other authors have suggested that individuals with WS might adopt a relatively local approach for all visuospatial processing (e.g., Bellugi et al., 1988), yet perceptual ability in WS does not support this hypothesis (e.g., Mervis et al., 1999; Pani et al., 1999). We argue that these accounts highlight that the type of processing preference seen depends on the way in which performance is measured. It appears that individuals with WS show an entirely typical global processing style on tests of perception (Farran, Jarrold, et al., in press; Mervis et al., 1999; Pani et al., 1999), but rely on a local processing approach on tests of construction. Given the need for integration of information (through an accurate comprehension of spatial relations) in constructional tasks, this leads to particular difficulties on these tests and to a loss of global information.

The methodological difficulties inherent in investigating visuospatial abilities in WS emphasize the need for further studies to confirm whether individuals with WS do have particular problems on tasks that require the construction of a global image. This might be done by undertaking further investigations that employ tasks where perceptual and constructional components are dissociable and assessing the particular strategies used by individuals with WS to complete these tests. Other areas clearly need further investigation. The area of face processing in WS would be better understood if harder tasks were employed to reduce the occurrence of ceiling effects. The effects of different facial manipulations in tasks such as those used by Karmiloff-Smith (1997) and Deruelle et al. (1999) could then be compared more reliably with results with typically developing individuals. This would indicate whether the apparent local processing preference in the WS group differs from control groups or the difference among groups in previous studies was simply the result of ceiling effects in the controls.

Mental imagery is one area that deserves more attention in WS investigation (Farran, Jarrold, et al., 2001, in press). This includes the ability to pan, translate, rotate, and scan mental images (Kosslyn, 1994). The processes involved in these transformations and their impact on perception and construction might indicate at which point between apparently intact perceptual abilities and impaired constructional skill individuals with WS begin to experience difficulty. This could range from storing the image, to planning the action at a premotor stage, to making comparisons during construction between the image being constructed and the to-be-constructed image, to the motor act itself. Greater understanding of these processes would be highly beneficial to the theories being developed regarding WS processing.

In summary, our understanding of the unusual pattern of strengths and weaknesses within visuospatial cognition in WS has given rise to a number of interpretations. In order to evaluate these theories, further investigations that both employ methodologically sound techniques in the areas already tapped and examine other, as-yet-untouched areas of visuospatial ability are essential.

ACKNOWLEDGMENT

The work of E. K. F. was supported by a research studentship from the Williams Syndrome Foundation of the United Kingdom.

REFERENCES

Akshoomoff, N., & Stiles, J. (1996). The influence of pattern type on children's block design performance. *Journal of the International Neuropsychological Society, 2,* 392–402.

Arnold, R., Yule, W., & Martin, N. (1985). The psychological characteristics of infantile hypercalcaemia: A preliminary investigation. *Developmental Medicine and Child Neurology, 27,* 49–59.

Atkinson, J., & Braddick, O. (1995, April). *Comparison of visual, visuo-spatial and cognitive development in young Williams syndrome children* (1–12 years). Paper presented at the National Parents Meeting of the IHC Foundation, London.

Atkinson, J., Anker, S., Braddick, O., Nokes, L., Mason, A., & Braddick, F. (2001). Visual and visuospatial development in young Williams syndrome children. *Developmental Medicine and Child Neurology, 43,* 330–337.

Atkinson, J., King, J., Braddick, O., Nokes, L., Anker, S., & Braddick, F. (1997). A specific deficit of dorsal stream function in Williams syndrome. *Neuroreport: Cognitive Neuroscience and Neuropsychology, 8,* 1919–1922.

Atkinson, J., Macpherson, F., Rae, S., & Hughes, C. (1994). Block constructions in young children: Development of spatial grouping ability. *Strabismus, 2,* 41.

Banks, W. P., & Prinzmetal, W. (1976). Configurational effects in visual information processing. *Perception and Psychophysics, 19,* 361–367.

Beery, K. E. (1989). *Developmental test of visual–motor integration* (3rd ed.). Cleveland, OH: Modern Curriculum Press.

Beery, K. E., & Buktenica, N. A. (1967). *Developmental test of visual–motor integration.* Cleveland, OH: Modern Curriculum Press.

Bellugi, U., Bihrle, A., Neville, H., Doherty, S., & Jernigan, T. (1992). Language, cognition and brain organization in a neurodevelopmental disorder. In M. R. Gunnar & C. A. Nelson (Eds.), *Developmental behavioral neuroscience. The Minnesota Symposia on Child Psychology* (Vol. 24, pp. 201–232). Hillsdale, NJ: Lawrence Erlbaum Associates, Inc.

Bellugi, U., Sabo, H., & Vaid, J. (1988). Spatial deficits in children with Williams syndrome. In J. Stiles-Davis, U. Kritchevshy, & U. Bellugi (Eds.), *Spatial cognition: Brain bases and development* (pp. 273–297). Hillsdale, NJ: Lawrence Erlbaum Associates, Inc.

Bellugi, U., Wang, P. P., & Jernigan, T. L. (1994). Williams syndrome: An unusual neuropsychological profile. In S. H. Brodman & J. Grafman (Eds.), *Atypical cognitive deficits in developmental disorders: Implications for brain function* (pp. 23–56). Hillsdale, NJ: Lawrence Erlbaum Associates, Inc.

Benton, A. L., Hamsher, K. deS., Varney, N. R., & Spreen, O. (1983). *Contributions to neuropsychological assessment.* New York: Oxford University Press.

Benton, A. L., Varney, N. R., & Hamsher, K. deS. (1978). Visuospatial judgement: A clinical test. *Archives of Neurology, 35,* 364–367.

Bertrand, J., & Mervis, C. B. (1996). Longitudinal analysis of drawings by children with Williams syndrome: Preliminary results. *Visual Arts Research, 22,* 19–34.

Bertrand, J., Mervis, C. B., & Eisenberg, J. D. (1997). Drawing by children with Williams syndrome: A developmental perspective. *Developmental Neuropsychology, 73,* 41–67.

Bihrle, A., Bellugi, U., Delis, D., & Marks, S. (1989). Seeing either the forest or the trees: Dissociation in visuospatial processing. *Brain and Cognition, 11,* 37–49.

Bishop, D. V. M. (1997). Cognitive neuropsychology and developmental disorders: Uncomfortable bedfellows. *Quarterly Journal of Experimental Psychology, 50A,* 899–923.

Campbell, R. N., Bruce, V., Import, A., & Wright, R. (1995). *Testing face processing skills in children.* Manuscript submitted for publication.

Carey, S., & Diamond, R. (1990). *Canonical–noncanonical views test.* Unpublished manuscript.

Chapman, R. S. (1995). Language development in children and adolescents with Down syndrome. In P. Fletcher & B. MacWhinney (Eds.), *Handbook of child language* (pp. 641–663). Oxford, England: Blackwell.

Crisco, J. J., Dobbs, J. M., & Mulhern, R. K. (1988). Cognitive processing of children with Williams syndrome. *Developmental Medicine and Child Neurology, 30,* 650–656.

Dall'oglio, A. M., & Milani, L. (1995). Analysis of the cognitive development in Italian children with Williams syndrome. *Genetic Counselling, 6,* 175–176.

Deruelle, C., Mancini, J., Livet, M. O., Casse-Perrot, C., & de Schonen, S. (1999). Configural and local processing in Williams syndrome. *Brain and Cognition, 41,* 276–298.

Djabri, W. F. (1995). *Face processing in Williams syndrome: A further case of within-domain dissociations.* Unpublished manuscript, University College London.

Elliot, C. D. (1990). *Differential Ability Scales.* New York: Psychological Corporation.

Farah, M. J. (1996). Is face recognition "special"? Evidence from neuropsychology. *Behavioural Brain Research, 76,* 181–189.

Farran, E. K., & Jarrold, C. (2001a). *The encoding of categorical and co-ordinate spatial relations in Williams syndrome.* Manuscript submitted for publication.

Farran, E. K., & Jarrold, C. (2001b). *Interpreting atypical performance patterns on visuo-spatial tasks: Evidence from Williams syndrome.* Manuscript submitted for publication.

Farran, E. K., Jarrold, C., & Gathercole, S. E. (2001). Block design performance in the Williams syndrome phenotype: A problem with mental imagery? *Journal of Child Psychology and Psychiatry, 42,* 719–728.

Farran, E. K., Jarrold, C., & Gathercole, S. E. (in press). Divided attention, selective attention and drawing: Processing preferences in Williams syndrome are dependent on the task administered. *Neuropsychologia.*

Fowler, A. E. (1990). Language abilities in children with Down syndrome: Evidence for a specific syntactic delay. In D. Cicchetti & M. Beeghly (Eds.), *Children with Down syndrome: A developmental perspective* (pp. 302–328). Cambridge, England: Cambridge University Press.

Frangiskakis, J. M., Ewart, A. K., Morris, C. A., Mervis, C. B., Bertrand, J., Robinson, B. F., et al. (1996). LIM-kinase1 hemizygosity implicated in impaired visuospatial constructive cognition. *Cell, 86,* 59–69.

Goodglass, H., & Kaplan, E. (1972). *Assessment of aphasia and related disorders.* Philadelphia: Lea and Febiger.

Grant, J., Karmiloff-Smith, A., Gathercole, S. E., Paterson, S., Howlin, P., Davies, M., et al. (1997). Phonological short-term memory and its relationship to language in Williams syndrome. *Cognitive Neuropsychiatry, 2,* 81–99.

Happé, F. G. E. (1994). Wechsler I.Q. profile and theory of mind in autism: A research note. *Journal of Child Psychology and Psychiatry, 35,* 1461–1471.

Happé, F. G. E. (1996). Studying weak central coherence at low levels: Children with autism do not succumb to visual illusions. A research note. *Journal of Child Psychology and Psychiatry, 37,* 873–877.

Happé, F. (1999). Autism: Cognitive deficit or cognitive style? *Trends in Cognitive Sciences, 3,* 216–222.

Hoffman, J. E., & Landau, B. (2000). *Spared object recognition with profound spatial deficits: Evidence from children with Williams syndrome.* Paper presented at the 7th Annual Meeting of the Cognitive Neuroscience Society, San Francisco.

Hoffman, J. E., Landau, B., & Pagani, B. (in press). Spatial breakdown in spatial construction: Evidence from eye fixation in children with Williams syndrome. *Cognitive Psychology.*

Howlin, P., Davies, M., & Udwin, O. (1998). Cognitive functioning in adults with Williams syndrome. *Journal of Child Psychology and Psychiatry, 39,* 183–189.

Jarrold, C., & Baddeley, A. D. (1997). Short-term memory for verbal and visuo-spatial information in Down's syndrome. *Cognitive Neuropsychiatry, 2,* 101–122.

Jarrold, C., Baddeley, A. D., & Hewes, A. K. (1998). Verbal and non-verbal abilities in the Williams syndrome phenotype: Evidence for diverging development trajectories. *Journal of Child Psychology and Psychiatry, 39,* 511–523.

Jarrold, C., Baddeley, A. D., & Hewes, A. K. (1999). Genetically dissociated components of working memory: Evidence from Down's and Williams syndrome. *Neuropsychologia, 37,* 637–651.

Jarrold, C., Baddeley, A. D., Hewes, A. K., & Phillips, C. (2001). A longitudinal assessment of diverging verbal and non-verbal abilities in the Williams syndrome phenotype. *Cortex, 37,* 423–431.

Jarrold, C., & Russell, J. (1997). Counting abilities in autism: Possible implications for central coherence theory. *Journal of Autism and Developmental Disorders, 27,* 25–37.

Karmiloff-Smith, A. (1997). Crucial differences between developmental cognitive neuroscience and adult neuropsychology. *Developmental Neuropsychology, 13,* 513–524..

Karmiloff-Smith, A., Grant, J., Berthoud, I., Davies, M., Howlin, P., & Udwin, O. (1997). Language and Williams syndrome: How intact is "intact"? *Child Development, 68,* 274–290.

Karmiloff-Smith, A., Klima, E., Bellugi, U., Grant, J., & Baron-Cohen, S. (1995). Is there a social module? Language, face processing and theory of mind in individuals with Williams syndrome. *Journal of Cognitive Neuroscience, 7,* 196–208.

Kaufman, A. S., & Kaufman, N. L. (1990). *Kaufman Brief Intelligence Test.* Circle Pines, MN: American Guidance Service.

Klein, B. P., & Mervis, C. B. (1999). Cognitive strengths and weaknesses of 9- and 10-year-olds with Williams syndrome or Down syndrome. *Developmental Neuropsychology, 16,* 177–196.

Kohs, S. C. (1923). *Intelligence measurement.* New York: Macmillan.

Kosslyn, S. M. (1994). *Images and brain; The resolution of the imagery debate.* Cambridge, MA: MIT Press.

Kosslyn, S. M., & Koenig, O. (1992). *Wet mind: The new cognitive neuroscience.* Cambridge, MA: MIT Press.

Kramer, J. H., Kaplan, E., Share, L., & Huckeba, W. (1999). Configural errors on the WISC–III block design. *Journal of the International Neuropsychological Society, 5,* 518–524.

Mervis, C. B. (1999). The Williams syndrome cognitive profile: Strengths, weaknesses, and interrelations among auditory short term memory, language, and visuospatial constructive cognition. In R. Fivush, W. Hirst, & E. Winograd (Eds.), *Essays in honor of Ulric Neisser* (pp. 193–227). Mahwah, NJ: Lawrence Erlbaum Associates, Inc.

Mervis, C. B., Morris, C. A., Bertrand, J., & Robinson, B. F. (1999). Williams syndrome: Findings from an integrated program of research. In H. Tager-Flusberg (Ed.), *Neurodevelopmental disorders: Contributions to a new framework from the cognitive neurosciences* (pp. 65–110). Cambridge, MA: MIT Press.

Mervis, C. B., Robinson, B. F., Bertrand, J., Morris, C. A., Klein-Tasman, B. P., & Armstrong, S. C. (2000). The Williams Syndrome Cognitive Profile. *Brain and Cognition, 44,* 604–628.

Miller, J. F. (1987). Language and communication characteristics of children with Down syndrome. In S. M. Pueschel, C. Tingey, J. E. Rynders, A. C. Crocker, & D. M. Crutcher (Eds.), *New perspectives on Down syndrome* (pp. 233–262). Baltimore: Brookes.

Milner, A. D., & Goodale, M. A. (1995). *The visual brain in action.* Oxford, England: Psychological Press.

Mooney, C. M. (1957). Age in the development of closure ability in children. *Canadian Journal of Psychology, 11,* 219–310.

Navon, D. (1977). Forest before trees: The precedence of global features in visual perception. *Cognitive Psychology, 9,* 353–383.

Pani, J. R., Mervis, C. B., & Robinson, B. F. (1999). Global spatial organization by individuals with Williams syndrome. *Psychological Science, 10,* 453–458.

Plaisted, K., Swettenham, J., & Rees, L. (1999). Children with autism show local precedence in a divided attention task and global precedence in a selective attention task. *Journal of Child Psychology and Psychiatry, 40,* 733–742.

Raven, J. C. (1993). *Coloured progressive matrices.* Oxford, England: Information Press.

Rossen, R., Klima, E. S., Bellugi, U., Bihrle, A., & Jones, W. (1996). Interaction between language and cognition: Evidence from Williams syndrome. In J. Beitchman, N. Cohen, M. Konstantareas, & R. Tannock (Eds.), *Language, learning and behaviour disorders: Developmental, behavioural and clinical Perspectives* (pp. 367–392). New York: Cambridge University Press.

Shah, A., & Frith, U. (1993). Why do autistic individuals show superior performance on the block design task? *Journal of Child Psychology and Psychiatry, 34,* 1351–1364.

Stevens, T. (1997). *Language acquisition in Williams syndrome: Lexical constraints and semantic organisation.* Unpublished PhD thesis, University College London and MRC Cognitive Development Unit, London.

Stiers, P., Willekens, D., Borghgraef, M., Fryns, J. P., & Vandenbussche, E. (2000). *Visuo-perceptual and visuo-constructive ability in persons with Williams syndrome.* Paper presented at the 8th International Professional Conference on Williams Syndrome, Dearborn, Michigan.

Udwin, O., & Yule, W. (1991). A cognitive and behavioural phenotype in Williams syndrome. *Journal of Clinical and Experimental Neuropsychology, 13,* 232–244.

Udwin, O., Yule, W., & Martin, N. (1987). Cognitive abilities and behavioural characteristics of children with idiopathic infantile hypercalcaemia. *Journal of Child Psychology and Psychiatry, 28,* 297–309.

Wang, P. P., Doherty, S., Rourke, S. B., & Bellugi, U. (1995). Unique profile of visuo-perceptual skills in a genetic syndrome. *Brain and Cognition, 29,* 54–65.

Wechsler, D. (1974). *Wechsler Intelligence Scale for Children–Revised.* New York: Psychological Corporation.

Wechsler, D. (1981). *Wechsler Adult Intelligence Scale–Revised.* San Antonio, TX: Psychological Corporation.

Wechsler, D. (1989). *Wechsler Pre-school and Primary Scale of Intelligence–Revised.* New York: Psychological Corporation.

Implicit Learning in Children and Adults With Williams Syndrome

Audrey J. Don
Children's Seashore House

E. Glenn Schellenberg
University of Toronto

Arthur S. Reber
Brooklyn College of City University of New York

Kristen M. DiGirolamo
Children's Seashore House

Paul P. Wang
Children's Seashore House and University of Pennsylvania School of Medicine

In comparison to explicit learning, implicit learning is hypothesized to be a phylogenetically older form of learning that is important in early developmental processes (e.g., natural language acquisition, socialization) and relatively impervious to individual differences in age and IQ. We examined implicit learning in a group of children and adults (9–49 years of age) with Williams syndrome (WS) and in a comparison group of typically developing individuals matched for chronological age. Participants were tested in an artificial-grammar learning paradigm and in a rotor-pursuit task. For both groups, implicit learning was largely independent of age. Both groups showed evidence of implicit learning but the comparison group outperformed the WS group on both tasks. Performance advantages for the comparison group were no longer significant when group differences in working memory or nonverbal intelligence were held constant.

Requests for reprints should be sent to Paul P. Wang, Pfizer Global Research and Development, 50 Pequot Avenue, 6025-B2138, New London, CT 06320. E-mail: wangp@mail.med.upenn.edu

Williams syndrome (WS) is a genetic disorder caused by a submicroscopic deletion on chromosome 7 (Ewart et al., 1993). WS is typically manifest in mild to moderate retardation with an unusual cognitive profile, which includes relatively preserved language and music skills, which contrast markedly with extremely weak visuospatial and visuomotor skills (Bellugi, Wang, & Jernigan, 1994; Dilts, Morris, & Leonard, 1990; Don, Schellenberg, & Rourke, 1999; Mervis, Morris, Bertrand, & Robinson, 1999; Udwin & Yule, 1990, 1991). Individuals with WS also tend to be extremely sociable and outgoing (Udwin & Yule, 1990).

Researchers have suggested that implicit learning plays a crucial role in the acquisition of linguistic, social, and motor skills, and possibly other skills as well (Gomez & Gerkin, 1999; A. S. Reber, 1992, 1993). In contrast to explicit learning, implicit learning occurs without conscious awareness and is thought to be a phylogenetically older form of learning, which predates consciousness (A. S. Reber, 1992; P. J. Reber & Squire, 1994). Based on this line of reasoning, A. S. Reber (1992; Abrams & Reber, 1988) proposed that implicit learning should show relatively small variations as a function of individual differences in age and maturity and be relatively unaffected by neurological or psychological disorder. Moreover, in contrast to explicit learning, implicit learning should be relatively independent of measures of higher cognitive functioning (i.e., IQ; A. S. Reber, Walkenfeld, & Hernstadt, 1991). If implicit-learning processes are indeed largely invariant to individual differences in age and IQ, then such processes may be relatively preserved in individuals with WS and underlie their relative strengths in language and social skills.

In this study, we assessed implicit learning in individuals with WS and in a comparison group of typically developing individuals matched for chronological age. Our measures were a language-based artificial grammar learning (AGL) task and a visuomotor rotor pursuit (RP) task. The contrast between relatively strong language abilities and weak visuomotor skills in WS invited comparison among the abstract, nonmotor skills assessed by the AGL task, and the visuomotor skills measured in the RP task.

IMPLICIT-LEARNING PARADIGMS

A large variety of testing paradigms, including AGL and RP, have been used to study implicit learning (A. S. Reber, 1993). The ability of individuals with amnesia to perform successfully on these tasks is often considered evidence of their implicit nature (Abrams & Reber, 1988; Corkin, 1968; Sagar, Gabrielli, Sullivan, & Corkin, 1990). Nonetheless, a few tasks thought to assess implicit learning in normal individuals, such as the Hebb supraspan digits tasks, cannot be learned by patients with amnesia (Charness, Milberg, & Alexander, 1988).

Additional discrepancies among tasks suggest that the processes assessed in the various implicit-learning paradigms may be related but dissociable (Kosslyn & Koenig, 1992; Seger, 1994; Squire, Knowlton, & Mussen, 1993).

The AGL task is one of the most widely used measures of implicit learning (for a descriptive summary, see A. S. Reber, 1993). In the typical paradigm, individuals are presented with strings of letters generated from a finite-state grammar such as the one illustrated in Figure 1. In an initial learning phase, participants are familiarized with a set of strings generated from the grammar. In a subsequent testing phase, participants are asked to distinguish between novel strings that follow the rules of the grammar and those that violate the rules. Ability to distinguish grammatical from ungrammatical strings is taken as evidence that participants have learned the rules of the grammar.

Early studies of AGL focused primarily on participants' ability to distinguish grammatical from ungrammatical strings, whereas recent research has focused more on the nature of the learning and the representational form of the information learned (e.g., Altmann, Dienes, & Goode, 1995; Knowlton & Squire, 1994; Manza & Reber, 1997; Servan-Schreiber & Anderson, 1990; Vokey & Brooks, 1992). Some investigators argue that participants' success on AGL tasks does not reflect an implicit abstraction of the underlying grammatical rules, but, rather, explicit knowledge of permissible bigrams and trigrams (referred to as *chunks*) in

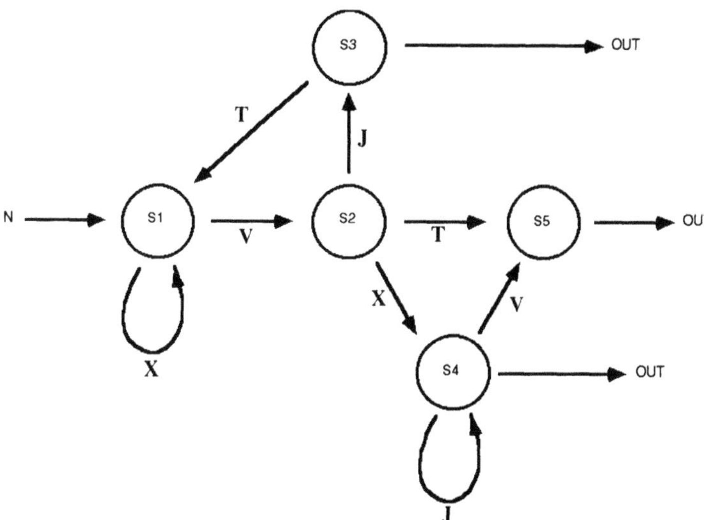

FIGURE 1 Finite-state grammar used by Abrams and Reber (1988). Strings were generated for this experiment by following the arrows from one node to another. Thus, XXVJ and XVTVJ are grammatical strings; XVTJ is ungrammatical.

the test stimuli (Perruchet & Pacteau, 1990). Such knowledge of permissible chunks would be stimulus-specific rather than abstract. Nonetheless, patients with amnesia who were studied by Knowlton, Ramus, and Squire (1992) performed as well as controls on AGL tasks. Because the amnesics had impaired declarative memory for the chunks, explicit knowledge of chunking patterns is unlikely to account for their performance. Moreover, the same patients showed positive transfer to a second AGL task that used an identical grammar instantiated in a new letter set. Again, these findings indicate that the participants' knowledge was not stimulus-specific (Knowlton & Squire, 1994). Normal controls can also transfer a learned artificial grammar across modalities (Altmann et al., 1995) and from one letter set to additional sets (Matthews et al., 1989). This combination of findings provides rather strong support for the proposal that abstract structures (i.e., grammars) are learned implicitly in AGL paradigms.

As with AGL tasks, the RP task has a long history as an implicit-learning paradigm (e.g., Heindel, Butters, & Salmon, 1988). This task requires fine motor and visuomotor skills. Participants are asked to maintain contact between a stylus (a metal pointer) and a target, which is placed near the edge of a horizontally rotating disk. An electric current is established when the stylus is in contact with the rotating target and accumulated contact time is recorded. Over time, performance improves, indicating that learning has occurred. Patients with amnesia demonstrate normal learning on the RP task, which is retained over a delay (e.g., Brooks & Baddeley, 1976; Milner, Corkin, & Teuber, 1968). By contrast, patients with damage to the basal ganglia, such as individuals with Huntington's disease, show impaired learning even after controlling for their baseline motor dysfunction (Heindel et al., 1988). Patients with Parkinson's disease also have basal ganglia pathology and exhibit similar impairment on the RP task (Harrington, Haaland, Yeo, & Marder, 1990), but patients with multiple sclerosis—who have motor impairments not attributable to the basal ganglia—perform normally (Beatty, Goodkin, Monson, & Beatty, 1990). A single neuroimaging study using positron emission tomography also suggests that skilled performance on the RP task depends on the integrity of the basal ganglia (Grafton et al., 1992).

Findings of relatively intact AGL abilities in patients with Parkinson's disease raise the possibility that AGL and RP performance may be dissociable. For example, Meulemans and Van der Linden (1998) reported that immediately after the training phase of their AGL procedure, patients with Parkinson's disease performed as well as controls, although their performance deteriorated to chance levels during the second half of the testing phase. P. J. Reber and Squire (1997) reported more compelling evidence for preserved AGL skills in Parkinson's disease. In their study, participants with Parkinson's disease performed similarly to controls and demonstrated positive transfer to a novel letter set (a new instantiation of the same grammar).

IMPLICIT LEARNING ACROSS DEVELOPMENT AND IN INDIVIDUALS WITH MENTAL RETARDATION

Most studies of implicit learning have been conducted with adults. Although a slight decline in performance is noted in very old adults, implicit learning appears to be remarkably stable across most of adulthood (Curran, 1997; Howard & Howard, 1997; for a review, see A. S. Reber & Allen, 2000). Studies of implicit learning in younger participants indicate that children can learn artificial grammars, but it is uncertain whether their performance matches that of adults. In one study, good AGL performance was evident in children 9 to 11 years of age (Fischer, 1997). In another study, Gomez and Gerkin (1999) used a head-turn preference procedure to assess whether 1-year-old infants could distinguish strings that conformed to an artificial grammar from strings that violated the grammar. Testing was conducted after less than 2 min of exposure to examples of grammatical auditory strings (sequences of nonsense syllables). Infants successfully distinguished between grammatical and ungrammatical strings, and they also transferred their knowledge to a second task in which the same grammar was instantiated in a new vocabulary. Performance could have been influenced, however, by explicit as well as implicit strategies, and the authors did not make any claim about the cognitive strategy used by their infant participants. Nonetheless, other studies with younger infants provide converging evidence of implicit learning in infancy. For example, when presented with structured sequences of nonsense syllables for brief periods of time, 7- and 8-month-old infants subsequently exhibit knowledge of the transitional probabilities between consecutive syllables (Saffran, Aslin, & Newport, 1996) and the grammatical rules that were used to construct the stimulus sequences (Marcus, Vijayan, Rao, & Vishton, 1999). Presumably, such learning in young infants is implicit rather than explicit.

Other studies provide additional support for the idea that implicit-learning abilities are well developed in early childhood and do not vary significantly with increased age. For example, Mecklenbraeuker, Wippich, and Schulz (1998) assessed memory for picture puzzles and found no difference in performance between younger (6–7 years of age) and older (9–10 years of age) children. Meulemans and Van der Linden (1998) found that sequence learning on a serial reaction-time task was equivalent for children (age 6–10) and young adults (age 18–27) and remained equivalent at follow-up 1 week later.

By contrast, Maybery, Taylor, and O'Brien-Malone (1995) observed that performance on an implicit contextual-learning task varied with age but not with IQ. Participants were children from two age groups (5–7 years and 10–12 years) subdivided into three IQ subgroups ranging from the borderline to the superior range. The older children performed at above-chance levels regardless of IQ, whereas the younger groups performed at chance. Another study from the same laboratory examined implicit-learning abilities across an even wider range of IQ (Fletcher, Maybery, & Bennett, 2000). Participants who were diagnosed with mental retardation performed less well on the contextual learning task than did participants with IQ scores in the normal range.

Other studies of individuals with mental retardation have used visual-priming paradigms to assess implicit memory rather than implicit learning. In priming tasks, participants are exposed to stimuli without explicit instructions to memorize the stimuli. Priming is inferred if subsequent identification of the same stimuli (often degraded) is facilitated. Priming can result from a single prior presentation, whereas implicit-learning paradigms involve multiple presentations of the information that is to be learned.

Results from priming studies of individuals with mental retardation are equivocal. In a large-sample study, Wyatt and Connors (1998) found that 6- to 17-year-olds with mental retardation performed similarly to a control group (matched for age) on a visual priming task (picture-fragment completion). In other words, performance on this task appeared to be independent of IQ. Nonetheless, age-related increases in performance were observed for both groups. Similarly, Vicari, Bellucci, and Carlesimo (2000) reported that repetition priming was preserved in 14 individuals with Down syndrome (*M* age = 21 years), who were compared to a control group matched for mental age (*M* chronological age = 5 years). These investigators also administered a simplified version of Nissen's serial reaction-time test (Nissen, Willingham, & Hartman, 1989) and found preserved performance on that task as well. By contrast, Mattson and Reilly (1999) found that mentally retarded children with Down syndrome showed significantly less priming than two control groups (both with higher mean IQ scores), who performed equivalently.

In sum, the existing literature leads to competing hypotheses about the implicit-learning abilities of individuals with WS. On the one hand, A. S. Reber (1992) contended that implicit learning should be robust in the face of neurological disorder. The findings of some investigators that implicit learning is preserved in populations with mental retardation are consistent with this proposal. On the other hand, the basal ganglia appear to subserve some forms of implicit learning, and MRI findings indicate that basal ganglia volumes are diminished in WS (Jernigan, Bellugi, Sowell, Doherty, & Hesselink, 1993). Moreover, other investigations have reported implicit-learning and priming deficits in samples of mentally retarded individuals. In other words, predictions about implicit learning in WS were unclear. Nonetheless, because explicit learning is impaired in WS, we predicted that the comparison group would attend more than the WS group to the chunk strength of the stimuli in the AGL task. Moreover, marked visuospatial and motor impairments in WS led us to expect that implicit learning would be better preserved in the AGL task than in the RP task.

METHOD

Participants

The WS group consisted of 27 individuals (14 male, 13 female) between 9 and 49 years of age (*M* = 23 years, 7 months; *SD* = 13 years, 6 months). The age-matched comparison group consisted of 27 normally developing adolescents and adults (11 male, 16 female), who ranged in age from 9 to 50 years (*M* = 23 years, 7 months; *SD* = 13 years, 4 months). Matching was within 6 months for participants 9 to 13 years of age, within 1 year for 14- to 29-year-olds, and within 2 years for those 30 years and over. Participants with WS were recruited through the local chapter of the Williams Syndrome Association and through national and regional meetings of the same organization. The comparison group consisted of siblings of the WS participants, employees of the institution where the research was conducted, and others recruited by word of mouth. All participants spoke English as their primary language and were without significant sensory or physical handicaps.

Measures

Implicit learning was assessed with an AGL task and an RP task. Short-term memory, working memory, receptive vocabulary, and nonverbal reasoning were also assessed to investigate the relationship between these variables and the implicit-learning measures.

Implicit-learning tasks. For the AGL test, we generated 36 letter strings from the finite-state grammar shown in Figure 1 (Abrams & Reber, 1988). This grammar was used to create 16 training strings and 20 test strings, each of which was two to five letters in length. In addition, 20 ungrammatical letter strings of two to five letters were created. Each ungrammatical string violated the rules of the grammar at only one position in the string, and such violations occurred at all positions. The 20 grammatical and ungrammatical strings were paired by length. Grammatical strings and foils were also paired on the basis of *chunk strength*, a term that refers to the presence of potentially familiar fragments within the strings.

Chunk strength was calculated in the manner of Knowlton and Squire (1996). The 16 training stimuli were examined to determine the frequency with which each possible bigram and trigram appeared across the training set. This frequency parameter has been termed the associative strength of each chunk. Each test stimulus was then examined to determine the number of bigrams and trigrams that appeared in each stimulus. For example, in the stimulus string XXVJ, the bigrams

XX, XV, and VJ appear, as do the trigrams XXV and XVJ. The chunk strength of each stimulus was calculated by averaging the associative strength of all the bigrams and trigrams that it contained. Half of the targets and half of the foil strings were created as high-chunk-strength strings. The other half had low chunk strength. The grammatical high-chunk-strength stimuli had a mean chunk strength of 6.81 (SD = 1.13); the low-chunk-strength stimuli averaged 3.60 (SD = 0.74). The ungrammatical, high-chunk-strength strength stimuli averaged 6.14 (SD = 1.26); the ungrammatical, low-chunk-strength strength stimuli averaged 3.42 (SD = .58).

Five pairs of each possible combination of high-chunk-strength and low-chunk-strength targets and foils were included in the set of 20 grammatical/ungrammatical test pairs (i.e., five sets each of high/high, low/low, high/low, or low/high target-foil combinations). The number of letters per string was matched in each pair.

The 16 training strings were printed in large bold letters on 3 × 5-in. cards and decorated with dinosaur stickers to create interest. Participants were shown the complete deck of training stimuli three times (48 training trials in total) in standard order and asked to spell the stimuli (called "dinosaur words") out loud each time. Testing immediately followed training. Test items consisted of 20 pairs of target–foil strings printed the same size as the training stimuli and placed one pair per page. One string was placed at the top of the page; the other was placed at the bottom. The placement of the target and the foil on the page was pseudorandom, with the target never appearing more than four times consecutively in one position. Participants were shown the new words, in pairs, and asked to spell both words out loud. They were then asked to identify the dinosaur word in each pair. This "forced-choice" design is a departure from the more typical classification task that has been used in other AGL studies. The method was modified to minimize yes or no response biases that might occur for individually presented stimuli. The entire block of 20 pairs was repeated immediately after the first block with string placement reversed and page sequence randomized. Thus, participants identified dinosaur words in a total of 40 string pairs. The outcome measure was the number of items answered correctly.

The motor-learning task was a standard RP task. Participants were asked to maintain contact between a stylus and a target on a rotating disk. On each trial, the disk rotated at 30 RPM for 20 sec. Trials were presented in blocks of four, with a rest period of 20 sec between trials. Duration of contact was recorded for each block. Six blocks were completed in a single testing session with a rest of approximately 1 min after blocks 1, 3, and 5 and a rest of about 3 min after blocks 2 and 4. The primary outcome measure was duration-of-contact on the sixth (final) block. We also examined participants' improvement in performance across the six blocks.

Supplementary measures. The Peabody Picture Vocabulary Test–Revised (PPVT–R; Dunn & Dunn, 1981) was used to assess receptive vocabulary. The

Matrices subtest of the Kaufman Brief Intelligence Test (K–BIT; Kaufman & Kaufman, 1990) was used to estimate nonverbal intelligence.

The Number Recall subtest of the Kaufman Assessment Battery for Children (K–ABC; Kaufman & Kaufman, 1983) provided a measure of short-term verbal memory. This subtest requires participants to repeat increasingly longer sequences of digits presented at a rate of one digit per sec. The Spatial Memory subtest from the K–ABC was also included in the testing protocol but the comparison group performed at ceiling levels. Thus, it was excluded from further consideration.

Working memory was assessed with the Counting Span Test, an experimental measure adapted from Case, Kurland, and Goldberg (1982). Participants were shown an array of large blue and yellow dots arranged randomly on a page and asked to touch and count all of the blue dots on a page (e.g., 5). They were then shown another page of blue and yellow dots and again asked to count (beginning at 1) all of the blue dots on the page (e.g., 3). Finally, the participant was shown a page with a question mark and asked to recall the number of blue dots on each page in the order they were presented (e.g., 5, 3). Testing began with a block of five two-page trials. Additional pages were added for subsequent blocks until trials included a maximum of five pages. Testing was terminated when participants failed two or more trials within a block.

Procedure

Participants were tested at their convenience, either in the research laboratory of a children's hospital, at meetings of the Williams Syndrome Association, or at home. Testing took place in a quiet room that was free from distractions. Tasks were administered in a fixed order. Matrices and the RP task were administered first. Number Recall and Spatial Memory were tested during rest periods of the RP task. The final three tests were Counting Span, the AGL task, and PPVT–R. Testing took approximately 75 min to complete. For 1 participant with WS, results from the second half of the AGL task were unavailable because he became fatigued and refused to complete the second half of the task. For 1 participant in the comparison group, RP scores were excluded because of technical difficulties.

RESULTS

Preliminary Analyses

A set of preliminary analyses examined differences between the WS and comparison groups on the raw scores obtained on the supplementary measures.

Descriptive statistics are provided in Table 1. The comparison group performed better than the WS group on each measure, PPVT–R: $t(52) = 3.26, p = .002$; Matrices: $t(51) = 10.31, p < .001$; Number Recall: $t(52) = 5.41, p < .001$; Counting Span: $t(51) = 8.16, p < .001$. Whereas group membership accounted for only 17% of the variance (i.e., eta-squared) in PPVT–R scores, it explained at least 36% of the variance in each of the other three measures (Number Recall 36%; Counting Span 57%; Matrices 68%). This pattern is consistent with other results showing that the vocabulary knowledge of individuals with WS is relatively spared compared to their marked impairments in other domains. Indeed, the WS group had higher standard scores on our test of receptive vocabulary (PPVT–R) than on our test of nonverbal reasoning (Matrices), $t(22) = 2.10, p = .048$. By contrast, the comparison group performed better on Matrices than on PPVT–R, $t(26) = 2.19, p = .038$.

Implicit Learning: Artificial Grammar

Scores on the AGL task represent the total number of correct responses (maximum = 40). Descriptive statistics are provided in Table 2. One-sample *t* tests (one-tailed) were used to compare performance with chance levels (20 correct). The comparison group performed significantly better than chance, $t(26) = 8.39$, $p < .001$, with performance levels (66% correct) similar to that reported in other AGL studies with normal individuals (Knowlton et al., 1992; McAndrews & Moscovitch, 1985; A. S. Reber & Allen, 2000). The WS group was only marginally better than chance, $t(25) = 1.36, p = .093$. Whereas 56% of participants in the comparison group (15 of 27) performed significantly better than chance as individuals (binomial test), only 15% did so in the WS group (4 of 26). An independent-samples *t* test confirmed that the difference among groups was reliable,

TABLE 1
Descriptive Statistics for Scores on the Supplementary Measures

	Williams Syndrome Group		*Comparison Group*	
	M	*SD*	*M*	*SD*
PPVT–R: raw score	111.9	28.2	135.8	25.8*
PPVT–R: standard score	73.6	16.0	97.3	18.6*
Matrices: raw score	19.5	4.3	34.0	5.8*
Matrices: standard score	66.2	13.2	103.8	11.5*
Number Recall: raw score	9.3	2.5	13.3	2.9*
Counting Span: raw score	6.4	3.8	14.1	3.0*

Note. PPVT–R = Peabody Picture Vocabulary Test–Revised.
*Williams syndrome and comparison groups significantly different, *ps* < .005.

$t(51) = 4.46$, $p < .001$, accounting for 28% of the variance in the data. This between-group effect size is similar in magnitude to the effect size for PPVT–R and for Number Recall, but significantly smaller than the effect size for Matrices, $z = 3.28$, $p = .001$, and for Counting Span, $z = 2.36$, $p = .018$.

AGL performance in the WS group was investigated further by comparing the first block of 20 trials with the second block. During the first block, 26% of individuals in the WS group (7 of 27) performed significantly better than chance. As a group, performance was better than chance (10 correct) on the first block, $t(25) = 2.87$, $p = .004$, but not on the second block. The decrement in performance from the first to the second block was significant, $t(25) = 2.71$, $p = .012$. In other words, implicit learning was evident among the WS group only for the first half of the AGL procedure. The comparison group exceeded chance levels for the first and second blocks, $ts(26) = 8.28$ and 5.51, respectively, $ps < .001$, and outperformed the WS group in both cases, $t(52) = 3.80$ and $t(51) = 3.65$, respectively, $ps < .001$. The difference among groups accounted for 22% of the variance in the first-block data and for 21% in the second block. Nonetheless, the comparison group also exhibited a significant decrement in performance over time, $t(26) = 2.85$, $p = .008$. Moreover, a 2 × 2 mixed-design analysis of variance (ANOVA) with one within-subjects variable (first vs. second block) and one between-subjects variable (group) did not uncover a two-way interaction, $F < 1$. In short, the comparison group performed better than the WS group throughout the procedure, and the performance of the two groups deteriorated similarly from the first to the second half of the testing protocol.

The next set of analyses investigated the effects of age on AGL performance. Scatterplots are provided in Figure 2. A general linear model with one dichotomous variable (group), one continuous variable (age), and an interaction term (Group × Age) yielded no significant results (Figure 2, top panel); identical null findings were observed when the analysis was limited to the first block (Figure 2, bottom panel). Indeed, tests of simple associations between age and AGL performance revealed correlations that were unlikely to be significant even with much larger samples of participants (WS group: $r = -.091$; comparison group: $r = .118$; groups combined: $r = -.007$; $ps > .5$). Again, separate analysis of the first block yielded identical results. Because many of the participants in both groups were adults, associations between age and AGL performance could be curvilinear. A rigorous set of tests failed, however, to uncover any nonlinear associations.[1]

The next set of analyses tested whether the comparison group was more sensitive than the WS group to the presence of chunks (i.e., specific reoccurring

[1]Tests of nonlinearity were twofold: (a) We used nonparametric tests (Spearman correlations) to test for monotonic associations of any type and (b) we successively added more and more higher order nonlinear terms to regression equations that were used to analyze the implicit-learning measures (i.e., age, age + age^2, age + age^2 + age^3, and age + age^2 + age^3 + age^4).

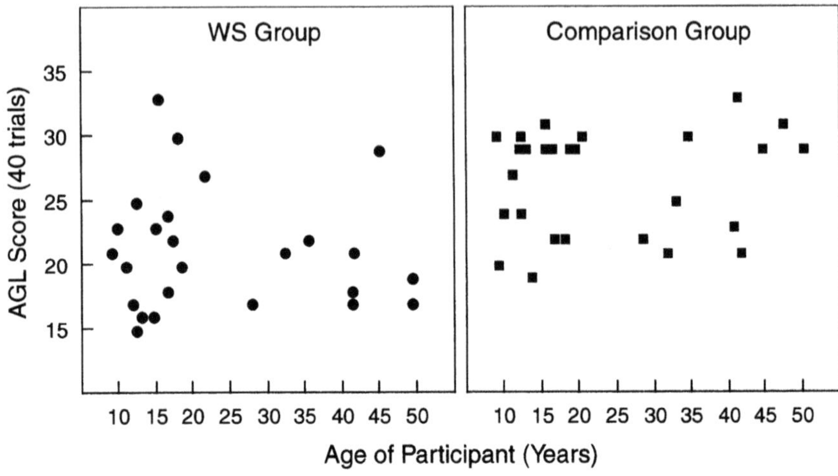

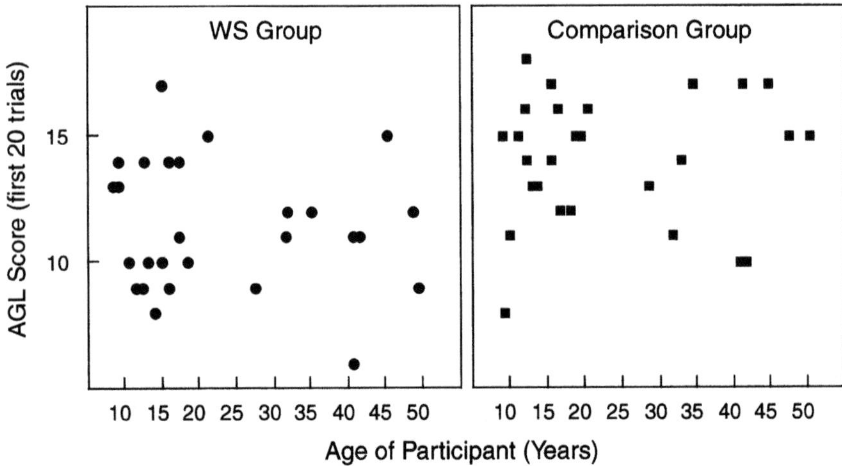

FIGURE 2 Scatterplots illustrating scores on the artificial grammar learning (AGL) task (number correct) as a function of age. The upper panel shows total scores derived from the first and second blocks of trials (maximum score = 40, chance = 20). The lower panel shows scores from the first block (maximum score = 20, chance = 10).

strings of letters) in the AGL targets and foils. A mixed-design 2 × 2 × 2 ANOVA had one between-subjects variable (group) and two within-subjects variables, which represented the chunk strength of the targets (high or low) and the chunk strength of the foils (high or low). In addition to the reported overall advantage for the comparison group, the analysis revealed a significant main effect of the chunk strength of the targets, $F(1, 52) = 10.97$, $p = .002$, with better performance for high-chunk-strength compared to low-chunk-strength targets. By contrast, the decrement in performance for high-chunk-strength compared to low-chunk-strength foils was only marginally significant, $F(1, 52) = 8.96$, $p = .096$. Our prediction of a larger effect of chunk strength for the comparison group over the WS group received partial support. Specifically, the two-way interaction between group and the chunk strength of the targets approached conventional levels of significance, $F(1, 52) = 3.16$, $p = .081$. Moreover, separate analysis of the comparison and WS groups revealed that performance was reliably better with high-chunk-strength compared to low-chunk-strength targets for the comparison group, $F(1, 26) = 15.58$, $p < .001$, but not for the WS group.

To confirm that overall responding on the AGL task did not rely on recognizing familiar strings of letters, we conducted additional analyses of the 20 trials in which the target and the foil items had equal chunk strength. The comparison group performed better than chance (10 correct) in these conditions ($M = 13.52$), $t(26) = 9.68$, $p < .001$ (one-tailed), but the WS group did not ($M = 10.33$). The difference among groups was significant, $t(52) = 4.64$, $p < .001$, and accounted for 29% of the variance in the data. When we examined the 10 equal-chunk trials that occurred during the first block of trials, however, we found that the WS group did indeed perform better than chance (5 correct; $M = 5.67$), $t(26) = 1.88$, $p = .035$.

Additional analyses explored in more detail the differences among groups that we observed on the AGL task. Specifically, a series of four analyses of covariance (ANCOVAs) was conducted, one for each of the supplementary measures. In each case, the independent variable was the group (WS or comparison), the dependent variable was the total number of correct responses, and the covariate was one of the supplementary measures. Because the main effect of group was tested multiple (four) times, we used the Bonferroni multistage procedure (Howell, 1997) to ensure that the alpha level for this family of tests did not rise above .05. Differences among groups on the AGL task remained significant when group differences in receptive vocabulary (as measured by the PPVT–R) were partialed out, $F(1, 50) = 12.80$, corrected $p = .003$, and when differences in Number Recall were held constant, $F(1, 50) = 7.64$, corrected $p = .024$. Between-group differences on the AGL task were no longer significant, however, when Counting Span or Matrices scores were included as covariates.

Implicit Learning: Rotor Pursuit

Scores on the RP task are illustrated in Figure 3 and summarized in Table 2. Initial analysis of our main outcome measure (duration of contact on the final block) uncovered a finding consistent with analyses of the AGL data: The WS group's

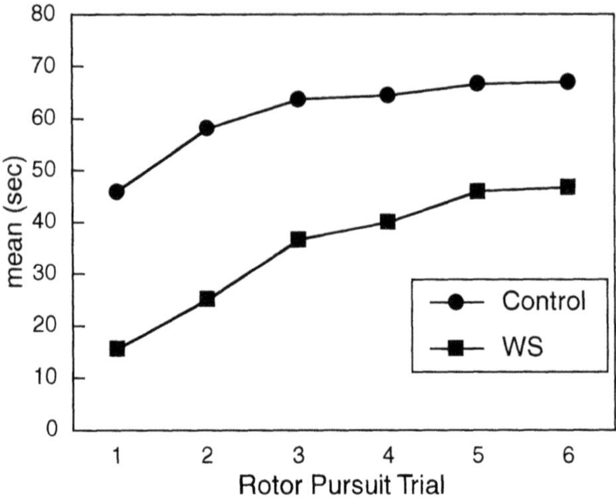

FIGURE 3 Scores (duration of contact) on the six trials of the rotor pursuit task.

TABLE 2
Descriptive Statistics for Scores on the Implicit-Learning Measures

	Williams Syndrome Group			*Comparison Group*		
	M	*SD*	*Range*	*M*	*SD*	*Range*
Artificial grammar learning						
All 40 trials	21.23	4.62	15–33	26.56	4.06	19–33
First block	11.41	2.55	6–17	14.04	2.53	8–18
Second block	9.96	2.72	6–16	12.52	2.38	6–16
Rotor pursuit						
Final (sixth) block (sec)	46.69	17.69	1.46–72.02	66.97	6.56	40.02–75.17
Change (block 6–block 1)	32.29	12.61	−1.69–48.33	21.28	7.52	11.65–38.27

performance was significantly below that of the comparison group, $t(51) = 5.49$, $p < .001$. Between-group differences accounted for 37% of the variance in the data. In contrast to our predictions, this effect size was similar in magnitude to the effect size observed on the AGL task. It was significantly smaller, however, than the between-group effect size reported for our measure of nonverbal intelligence (Matrices), $z = 2.27$, $p = .023$, but no different from the effect sizes reported for our three other supplementary measures.

Improvement in performance across the six RP blocks was examined with a multivariate repeated-measures ANOVA that included one within-subjects factor (blocks 1–6) and one between-subjects factor (group). As shown in the figure, the comparison group outperformed the WS group throughout the procedure, $F(1, 50) = 63.51$,

$p < .001$. Performance also improved across blocks, $F(5, 46) = 66.78, p < .001$, and a significant interaction indicated that the pattern of change differed across groups, $F(5, 46) = 7.58, p < .001$. To investigate the interaction in more detail, a rotor change score was calculated for each participant by subtracting their score on the first block from their score on the final (sixth) block. Whereas duration of contact for the WS group increased, on average, by 32.29 sec from the first to the sixth block ($SD = 12.61$ sec), the comparison group increased by 21.28 sec ($SD = 7.52$ sec). The between-group difference in rotor-change scores was statistically significant, $t(40.8) = 3.82, p < .001$ (separate variances test). As can be seen in the figure, however, the comparison group reached their plateau (near ceiling levels for the test) by the third block, whereas the WS group began their plateau on the fifth block. Moreover, the performance of the WS group plateaued at a level approximately equivalent to the initial level witnessed for the comparison group.

To investigate the association between age and implicit learning on the RP task, we calculated correlations between age and duration of contact on the final RP block (see Figure 4, upper panel). The correlation was not significant for the WS group, the comparison group, or for the groups combined, $rs = .122$, .165, and .095, respectively, $ps > .4$.

Analyses of rotor-change scores yielded a slightly different pattern (see Figure 4, lower panel). Whereas change scores of the groups combined and the WS group analyzed separately did not have a reliable association with age, $rs = -.177$ and .001, respectively, $ps > .2$, the comparison group exhibited a significant negative correlation, $r = -.586, p = .002$. In other words, younger participants in the comparison group tended to have larger improvements over the six RP blocks than did their older counterparts. Rotor-change scores for younger participants in the comparison group (median split) were still relatively low ($M = 26.60$), however, compared to those of the WS group (see Figure 4, lower panel). Indeed, Figure 4 makes it clear that individual differences in change scores for the comparison group—due to age as well as to other factors—were smaller than they were for the WS group, $F(25, 25) = 2.81, p = .012$ (test of equal variance). Moreover, a linear association between age and performance on the RP task was evident for the comparison group during the first RP block, $r = .487$, $p = .012$, but not for any subsequent blocks. Rigorous investigation of the possibility of nonlinear associations based on age yielded no additional findings (see footnote 1). In sum, the RP data provided partial support for A. S. Reber's (1992) hypothesis that implicit learning is independent of age. The only exception was that the comparison group showed a significant positive association with age on the first of six blocks, and, thus, relatively large improvement from the first to the final block for younger participants.

As with the AGL analyses, the next set of analyses explored further the between-group differences in performance evident on the RP task. Specifically, a series of four ANCOVAs was conducted (Bonferroni-corrected for four tests),

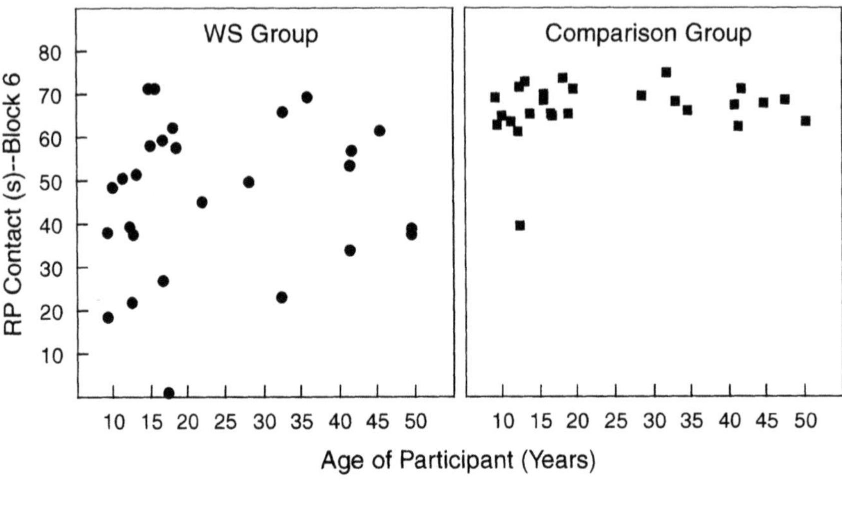

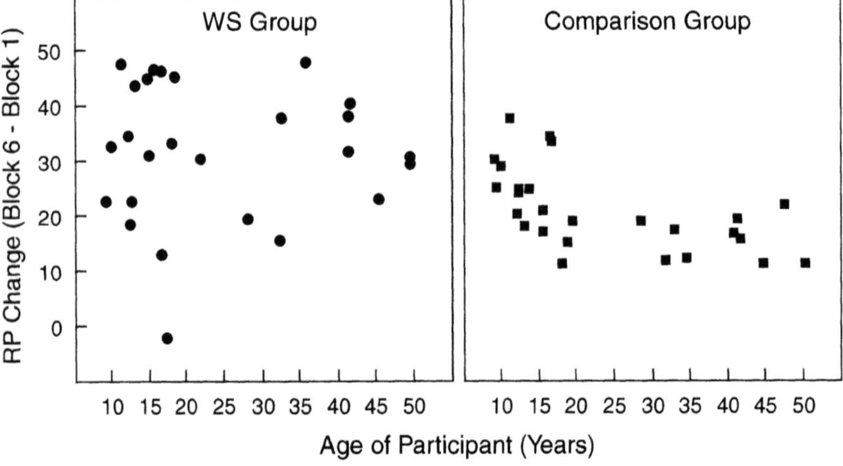

FIGURE 4 Scatterplots illustrating scores (duration of contact) on the rotor pursuit (RP) task as a function of age. The upper panel shows scores on the final (sixth) block. The lower panel shows RP-change scores, which represent improvement from the first to the final block.

with group (WS or comparison) as a between-subjects factor and one of the supplementary measures as a covariate. The outcome variable was the score on the final (sixth) block. In each analysis, our goal was to determine whether the advantage for the comparison group over the WS group would still be evident when group differences on the particular covariate were held constant. As with the AGL task, the advantage for the comparison group remained significant when differences in PPVT–R scores, $F(1, 50) = 20.74$, corrected $p < .001$, and Number Recall scores, $F(1, 50) = 7.58$, corrected $p = .025$, were held constant, but not when Counting Span or Matrices scores were partialled out.

Associations Between the Implicit-Learning Tasks and the Supplementary Measures

Partial correlations for all pairwise combinations of the two implicit-learning measures and the four supplementary measures are provided in Table 3. In each case, variance due to differences in age is held constant. Because negative correlations were unexpected and uninterpretable, tests of statistical significance were one-tailed. As shown in the table, the correlation between the two implicit-learning tasks was significant for the WS group but essentially zero for the comparison group. Correlations between implicit-learning measures in the comparison group may have been depressed, however, because performance on the RP task was near ceiling levels for this group.

In general, the 15 partial correlations were higher for the WS group than for the comparison group, $p = .007$ (sign test). Moreover, the eight correlations among the implicit-learning and supplementary measures were lower than the six correlations

TABLE 3
Partial Correlations Between Measures (Raw Scores) With Chronological Age Held Constant

	AGL	*RP*	*PPVT–R*	*Matrices*	*Number Recall*
Williams syndrome group (*ns* = 25–27)					
RP	.359**				
PPVT–R	.448**	.148			
Matrices	.085	.287***	.591*		
Number Recall	.288***	.576*	.538*	.350**	
Counting Span	.395**	.431**	.706*	.721*	.553*
Comparison group (*ns* = 26–27)					
RP	.012				
PPVT–R	.163	.055			
Matrices	.252	–.041	.683*		
Number Recall	.209	.432**	.380**	.265***	
Counting Span	.112	.250	.455*	.481*	.220

Note. AGL = Artificial grammar learning; RP = rotor pursuit; PPVT–R = Peabody Picture Vocabulary Test–Revised.

*$p < .01$. **$p < .05$. ***$p < .1$ (one-tailed).

among all possible pairwise combinations of supplementary measures, a pattern evident for both groups of participants (WS group: $p = .020$; comparison group: $p = .014$; Mann–Whitney tests). In other words, despite the weak (i.e., in the WS group) or null (i.e., in the comparison group) association between the implicit-learning measures, the two measures were somewhat dissociated from the four supplementary measures, which, by contrast, exhibited relatively strong and consistent pairwise associations.

DISCUSSION

We examined implicit learning in a group of individuals with WS and in a comparison group of normal individuals matched for chronological age. The results indicated that individuals with WS are capable of implicit learning in at least two contexts: (a) a categorization task in which stimulus grammaticality depends on a complex, probabilistic, and unstated set of rules (artificial grammar learning, AGL), and (b) a simple, repetitive motor-learning task (RP). On both tasks, however, performance of participants with WS was well below performance of the comparison group. The results speak not only to the issue of age and IQ independence of implicit learning, but more generally to the issue of cognitive dissociations and preservations in mental retardation. At the outset, however, it is important to acknowledge that our study did not include a comparison group matched for mental age (IQ) to the WS group. As such, it is impossible to determine whether the patterns we observed are specific to WS or more generally applicable to other populations with mental retardation.

Both groups of our participants spanned a wide range of age, which allowed for adequate tests of whether implicit learning varies as a function of age. In general, our results supported A. S. Reber's (1992) contention that implicit learning is relatively invariant across differences in age and maturity. Specifically, the age of the participants in the WS group did not affect their performance on either of our implicit-learning measures. Moreover, for the comparison group, there was no association between age and performance on the AGL task. On the RP task, however, younger participants in the comparison group tended to perform relatively poorly on the very first block of trials, but there were no age effects on subsequent blocks. Because age differences were noted for the initial block only, it is problematic to interpret our finding as evidence of a deficit in implicit learning in younger participants because learning may have not yet begun. Moreover, this initial decrement in performance may be attributable to age differences in attending, fine motor skills, or understanding the experimental instructions. Nonetheless, the decrement in performance on the first block of trials meant that younger participants tended to show greater improvement across the six blocks, which could be interpreted as an advantage in implicit learning.

More importantly, the relative lack of variability in implicit learning as a function of age appears to generalize across a broad range of intellectual abilities. Specifically, our WS group showed marked impairments on measures of vocabulary (PPVT–R) and nonverbal reasoning (K–BIT matrices), whereas our comparison group performed well within the normal range on both tasks. Our results also extend the age range for previously reported findings of age invariance on AGL tasks. Although the results for the RP are slightly less clear, it seems that for individuals 9 years of age and older, effects of age and maturity on implicit learning are very weak if they exist. Of course, our data do not address whether performance on other tests of implicit learning could vary reliably with age, or whether children younger than 9 years of age would show age-related differences in performance on the AGL and RP tasks.

By examining differences between the WS and comparison groups, we tested the hypothesis that implicit learning is independent of individual differences in intellectual functioning. Although previous studies yielded conflicting results, our findings revealed no ambiguity in this regard. Rather, the performance of the WS group was inferior to that of the comparison group on both implicit-learning measures. Moreover, because previous findings make it clear that individuals with WS have better grammar than individuals with Down syndrome (Bellugi, Lichtenberger, Jones, Lai, & St. George, 2000), we expect that deficits on the AGL task would be at least as great in the latter group as they are in the former.

The difference in performance between the WS and comparison groups on both implicit-learning measures was eliminated when the groups were equated by including either K–BIT Matrices (a measure of nonverbal intelligence) or Counting Span (a measure of working memory) as a covariate in the analyses. By contrast, partialing out group differences in vocabulary and short-term memory (as measured by PPVT–R and Number Recall, respectively) did not eliminate the effect. Preliminary analyses showed that our two groups of participants differed more in nonverbal intelligence and working memory than they did in receptive vocabulary and short-term verbal memory. In other words, statistically equating groups on the measures that best distinguish them eliminated the WS deficit in implicit learning.

Previous research makes it clear that cognitive deficits in WS are widespread, yet it is equally clear that the cognitive profile associated with WS is markedly uneven, with some abilities (e.g., language and music) better preserved than others (e.g., Don et al., 1999). Although deficits in implicit learning were apparent for the WS group, the effect size for between-group differences on our AGL task was similar in magnitude to those for vocabulary (PPVT–R) and short-term memory (Number Span) and much smaller than the effect size for nonverbal reasoning (Matrices) and working memory (Counting Span). Similar findings were obtained for effect sizes on the RP task, except that the difference in magnitude between the RP task and Counting Span was not significant. In other words, implicit learning may be an area of *relative* strength in WS, which is consistent with the spirit of A. S. Reber's (1992) proposals.

Interestingly, individual differences in nonverbal intelligence were not significantly correlated with performance on either implicit-learning measure for the comparison group (see Table 3; effects of age held constant). For the WS group, the partial association was not significant for the AGL task and very small and only marginally significant for the RP task. (The association of nonverbal intelligence with working memory was reliable for both groups.) In other words, our results suggest that large between-group differences in nonverbal intelligence are predictive of implicit-learning abilities, whereas relatively small individual differences within groups are not. This hypothesis is consistent with the results of Fletcher et al. (2000). On a contextual-learning task, these researchers (Maybery et al., 1995) found no evidence of an association between performance and IQ when their sample was restricted to children in the borderline to normal range (i.e., a narrow range of IQ). When they included participants with mental retardation (i.e., a large range of IQ), however, a reliable association with IQ was evident.

By contrast, our measure of working-memory capacity (Counting Span) was associated with individual differences in implicit learning among participants in the WS group as well as with differences among groups. For the comparison group, however, working memory was not associated with either of our measures of implicit learning. This result differs from that reported by P. J. Reber and Kotovsky (1997), who suggested that working memory serves as a necessary resource for implicit learning in the normal population. This discrepancy may be explained, however, by the different experimental design (dual task interference) and the different implicit-learning task used by those researchers. Our results suggest that large between-group differences in working-memory abilities are predictive of implicit learning, whereas individual differences within groups are predictive for some populations but not for others. Whether these findings extend to other groups with mental retardation could be addressed in future research.

Although the WS group showed deficits relative to the comparison group on the RP task, they also demonstrated greater improvement over the course of the six RP trials (Figure 3). The very poor performance of the WS participants on the initial trials is likely to be the primary reason for this finding; the WS group simply had more room to improve. Moreover, the comparison group improved rapidly to ceiling levels of task performance. Nonetheless, our findings make it clear that individuals with WS can implicitly acquire some motor skills over time. It seems unlikely, however, that their skills in this domain would ever catch up to those of normally developing individuals.

Our study is the first to use a two-alternative forced-choice response format for AGL tasks (i.e., which of two strings is grammatical?). Nonetheless, levels of performance for our comparison group (approximately 65% correct) were similar to those reported in studies that used a stimulus-categorization task (i.e., is a specific string grammatical or ungrammatical?). A higher proportion of correct responses might have been expected for our forced-choice method, but our task was unique in limiting our stimulus strings to five letters and presenting a smaller number of training stimuli. Both of these factors may have hindered performance (A. S. Reber, 1992, 1993) and offset potential gains from our choice of response format. Our comparison group also demonstrated expected effects of stimulus chunk strength, with superior performance for high-chunk-strength than for low-chunk-strength targets. As predicted, such effects, which rely on explicit memory, were nonexistent in the WS group. It is important to note, however, that the comparison group performed better than chance when targets and foils were matched for chunk strength, as did the WS group during the first block of trials. In short, patterns of responding on our forced-choice AGL task were very similar to patterns reported with other versions of the task (Knowlton & Squire, 1994).

Differences between the AGL and RP results raise the possibility that the various tests of implicit learning do not make up a homogeneous set. Indeed, our two measures showed no association in the comparison group, although they were correlated in the WS group. Different implicit-learning tasks may have distinct processing demands, or they may rely on distinct neurobiological substrates, which means that they could be differentially impaired in different disorders. For example, participants with WS showed a deterioration in performance over time on the AGL task but not on the RP task. In a previous study (Beatty et al., 1990), response patterns for adults with Parkinson's disease on an AGL task were similar to those observed for participants with WS in this study. Specifically, both groups performed at above-chance levels in the first half of AGL testing but deteriorated to chance levels as testing continued. Note, however, that our comparison group also deteriorated from the first to the second block of trials, and the WS and comparison groups did not differ in this regard. In short, chance levels of performance for the WS cohort in the second half of AGL testing may reflect a general deterioration of performance over time, starting from a level that was only slightly above chance. It may be premature, therefore, to relate the WS pattern of performance to the neuropathologic condition of the basal ganglia that is found in both WS and Parkinson's disease.

Indeed, decrements in performance for both of our participant groups on the AGL task may stem from proactive interference. Meulemans and Van der Linden (1998) speculated that the decrements in performance in their Parkinson patients were a consequence of attentional difficulties, yet deteriorations in performance were evident in both of our groups, and our comparison group appeared to be attentive throughout the task. Hence, a simpler explanation is that proactive interference caused the general decrement in performance that we observed. This hypothesis could be tested in the future by adding a third set of trials containing the foils and grammatical items of the original series as well as novel foils. If proactive interference plays a role in the performance decrement, foils from the prior set should be chosen more frequently than novel foils.

Despite the deterioration in performance over time, our data suggest that individuals with WS are capable of implicit learning on the AGL task. In the first half of testing, their performance was above chance levels even when targets and foils were matched for chunk strength. Obviously, this study is an initial and preliminary exploration of implicit learning in WS. Further investigation is required to determine whether other cognitive factors may contribute to the implicit-learning deficits in WS and whether such deficits are specific to WS or generalizable to other groups of individuals with mental retardation. Additional investigation could confirm whether implicit learning in WS is sufficient to be useful in other developmental tasks and whether other implicit-learning skills are better preserved or more severely impaired in WS.

Initial accounts of WS made claims of "islands of preservation" for specific cognitive skills (Bellugi et al., 1994). By contrast, recent reports tend to emphasize (a) the need for closer scrutiny of cognitive processes to avoid overinterpreting performance on specific tasks (Karmiloff-Smith, 1997) and (b) the need to study developmental changes in the deficits and relative assets associated with WS (Paterson, Brown, Gsödl, Johnson, & Karmiloff-Smith, 1999). It is now generally accepted that many of the apparently preserved skills of individuals with WS are accomplished by nonstandard processing mechanisms. Nevertheless, our findings provide additional evidence that individuals with WS have a very "unusual neuropsychological profile" (Bellugi et al., 1994). On the one hand, cognitive deficits in WS are widespread, and individuals who do relatively well (or particularly poorly) on one task tend to perform similarly on other tasks. Indeed, correlations among the measures we administered were higher in the WS group than they were in the comparison group. Other investigators have reported similarly high intertask correlations in WS (Mervis et al., 1999), and Detterman and Daniel (1989) suggested that low-IQ groups will typically show higher intertask correlations than their high-IQ counterparts. On the other hand, group deficits for individuals with WS are much smaller on some tasks (language, music, short-term memory, implicit learning) than they are on others (nonverbal reasoning, spatial abilities). In other words, our results provide support for islands of relative preservation. Moreover, our finding that implicit learning is relatively dissociated from other abilities implies that the various islands are not necessarily subserved by a common mechanism. More detailed examination of the relative strengths and weaknesses associated with WS could improve our understanding of WS in particular and of cognitive functioning in general.

ACKNOWLEDGMENTS

This study was supported by a grant from the National Institutes of Health (K08 HD01174) and by a Basil O'Connor Award from the March of Dimes Foundation (funding awarded to P.P.W.). The authors thank the study participants and their families. William C. Heindel, provided the initial suggestion to study rotor-pursuit learning in Williams syndrome.

REFERENCES

Abrams, M., & Reber, A. S. (1988). Implicit learning: Robustness in the face of psychiatric disorders. *Journal of Psycholinguistic Research, 17,* 425–439.

Altmann, G. T. M., Diennes, Z., & Goode, A. (1995). On the modality independence of implicitly acquired grammatical knowledge. *Journal of Experimental Psychology: Learning, Memory, and Cognition, 21,* 899–912.

Beatty, W. W., Goodkin, D. E., Monson, N., & Beatty, P. A. (1990). Implicit learning in patients with chronic progressive multiple sclerosis. *International Journal of Clinical Neuropsychology, 12,* 166–172.

Bellugi, U., Lichtenberger, L., Jones, W., Lai, Z., & St. George, J. (2000). The neurocognitive profile of Williams syndrome: A complex pattern of strengths and weaknesses. *Journal of Cognitive Neuroscience, 12*(Suppl.), 7–29.

Bellugi, U., Wang, P. P., & Jernigan, T. (1994). Williams syndrome: An unusual neuropsychological profile. In F. Broman & J. Grafman (Eds.), *Atypical cognitive deficits in developmental disorders: Implications for brain function* (pp. 23–56). Hillsdale, NJ: Lawrence Erlbaum Associates, Inc.

Brooks, D. N., & Baddeley, A. D. (1976). What can amnesic patients learn? *Neuropsychologia, 14,* 111–122.

Case, R., Kurland, D. M., & Goldberg, J. (1982). Operational efficiency and the growth of short-term memory span. *Journal of Experimental Child Psychology, 33,* 386–404.

Charness, N., Milberg, W., & Alexander, M. P. (1988). Teaching an amnesic a complex skill. *Brain and Cognition, 8,* 253–272.

Corkin, S. (1968). Acquisition of motor skill after bilateral medial temporal-lobe excisions and bilateral hippocampal lesions. *Neuropsychologia, 3,* 255–265.

Curran, T. (1997). Effects of aging on implicit sequence learning: Accounting for sequence structure and explicit knowledge. *Psychological Research, 60,* 24–41.

Detterman, D. K., & Daniel, M. H. (1989). Correlations of mental tests with each other and with cognitive variables are highest for low IQ groups. *Intelligence, 13,* 349–359.

Dilts, C. V., Morris, C. A., & Leonard, C. O. (1990). Hypothesis for development of a behavioral phenotype in Williams syndrome. *American Journal of Medical Genetics* Supplement, *6,* 126–131.

Don, A. J., Schellenberg, E. G., & Rourke, B. P. (1999). Music and language skills of children with Williams syndrome. *Child Neuropsychology, 5,* 154–170.

Dunn, E. S., & Dunn, L. M. (1981). *Manual: Peabody Picture Vocabulary Test–Revised.* Circle Pines, MN: American Guidance Service.

Ewart, A. K., Morris, C. A., Atkinson, D., Jin, W., Sternes, K., Spallone, P., et al. (1993). Hemizygosity at the elastin locus in a developmental disorder, Williams syndrome. *Nature Genetics, 5,* 11–16.

Fischer, J. P. (1997). L'Apprentissage d'une grammaire artificielle par des enfants de 9 a 11 ans [English abstract]. *L'Annee psychologique, 97,* 207–236.

Fletcher, J., Mayberry, M. T., & Bennett, S. (2000). Implicit learning differences: A question of developmental level? *Journal of Experimental Psychology: Learning, Memory, and Cognition, 26,* 246–252.

Gomez, R. L., & Gerkin, L. A. (1999). Artificial grammar learning by 1-year-olds leads to specific and abstract knowledge. *Cognition, 70,* 109–135.

Grafton, S. T., Mazziotta, J. C., Presty, S., Friston, K. J., Frackowiak, R. S., & Phelps M. E. (1992). Functional anatomy of human procedural learning determined with regional cerebral blood flow and PET. *Journal of Neuroscience, 12,* 2542–2548.

Harrington, D. L., Haaland, K. Y., Yeo, R. A., & Marder, E. (1990). Procedural memory in Parkinson's disease: Impaired motor but not visuoperceptual learning. *Journal of Clinical and Experimental Neuropsychology, 12,* 323–339.

Heindel, W. C., Butters, N., & Salmon, D. P. (1988). Impaired learning of a motor skill in patients with Huntington's disease. *Behavioral Neuroscience, 102,* 141–147.

Howard, J. H., & Howard, D. V. (1997). Age differences in implicit learning of higher order dependencies in serial patterns. *Psychology and Aging, 12,* 634–656.

Howell, D. C. (1997). *Statistical methods for psychology* (4th ed.). Belmont, CA: Duxbury.

Jernigan, T. L., Bellugi, U., Sowell, E., Doherty, S., & Hesselink, J. R. (1993). Cerebral morphological distinctions between WS and DS. *Archives of Neurology, 50,* 186–191.

Karmiloff-Smith, A. (1997). Crucial differences between developmental cognitive neuroscience and adult neuropsychology. *Developmental Neuropsychology, 13,* 513–524.

Kaufman, A. S., & Kaufman, N. L. (1983). *Kaufman Assessment Battery for Children: Administration and scoring manual.* Circle Pines, MN: American Guidance Service.

Kaufman, A. S., & Kaufman, N. L. (1990). *Kaufman Brief Intelligence Test: Manual.* Circle Pines, MN: American Guidance Service.

Knowlton, B. J., & Squire, L. R. (1994). The information acquired during artificial grammar learning. *Journal of Experimental Psychology: Learning, Memory, and Cognition, 20,* 79–91.

Knowlton, B. J., & Squire, L. R. (1996). Artificial grammar learning depends on implicit acquisition of both abstract and exemplar-specific information. *Journal of Experimental Psychology: Learning, Memory, and Cognition, 22,* 169–181.

Knowlton, B. J., Ramus, S. J., & Squire, L. R. (1992). Intact artificial grammar learning in amnesia: Dissociation of classification learning and explicit memory for specific instances. *Psychological Science, 3,* 172–179.

Kosslyn, S. M., & Koenig, O. (1992). *Wet mind.* New York: Free Press.

Manza, L., & Reber, A. S. (1997). Representing artificial grammars: Transfer across stimulus forms and modalities. In D. Berry (Ed.), *How implicit is implicit learning? Debates in psychology* (pp. 73–106). New York: Oxford University Press.

Marcus, G. F., Vijayan, S., Rao, S. B., & Vishton, P. M. (1999). Rule learning by seven-month-old infants. *Science, 283,* 77–80.

Matthews, R. C., Buss, R. R., Stanley, W. B., Blanchard-Fields, F., Cho, J. R., & Druhan, B. (1989). Role of implicit and explicit processes in learning from examples: A synergistic effect. *Journal of Experimental Psychology: Learning, Memory, and Cognition, 15,* 1083–1100.

Mattson, S. N., & Riley, E. P. (1999). Implicit and explicit memory functioning in children with heavy prenatal alcohol exposure. *Journal of the International Neuropsychological Society, 5,* 462–471.

Maybery, M., Taylor, M., & O'Brien-Malone, A. (1995). Implicit learning: Sensitive to age but not IQ. *Australian Journal of Psychology, 47,* 8–17.

McAndrews, M. P., & Moscovitch, M. (1985). Rule-based and exemplar-based classification in artificial grammar learning. *Memory & Cognition, 13,* 469–475.

Mecklenbraeuker, S., Wippich, W., & Schulz, I. (1998). Implicit memory in children: No age differences when solving picture puzzles [in German with English abstract]. Zeitschrift für *Entwicklungspsychologie und Paedagogische Psychologie, 30,* 13–19.

Mervis, C. G., Morris, C. A., Bertrand, J., & Robinson, B. F. (1999). Williams syndrome: Findings from an integrated program of research. In H. Tager-Flusberg (Ed.), *Neurodevelopmental disorders: Contributions to a new framework from the cognitive neurosciences* (pp. 65–110). Cambridge, MA: MIT Press.

Meulemans, T., & Van der Linden, M. (1998). Implicit sequence learning in children. *Journal of Experimental Child Psychology, 69,* 199–221.

Milner, B., Corkin, S., & Teuber, H. L. (1968). Further analysis of the hippocampal amnesic syndrome: Fourteen year follow-up study of H.M. *Neuropsychologia, 6,* 215–234.

Nissen, M. J., Willingham, D., & Hartman, M. (1989). Explicit and implicit remembering: When is learning preserved in amnesia? *Neuropsychologia, 27,* 341–352.

Paterson, S. J., Brown, J. H., Gsödl, M. K., Johnson, M. H., & Karmiloff-Smith (1999). Cognitive modularity and genetic disorders. *Science, 286,* 2355–2357.

Perruchet, P., & Pacteau, C. (1990). Synthetic grammar learning: Implicit rule abstraction or explicit fragmentary knowledge? *Journal of Experimental Psychology: General, 119,* 264–275.

Reber, A. S. (1992). The cognitive unconscious: An evolutionary perspective. *Consciousness and Cognition, 1,* 93–113.

Reber, A. S. (1993). *Implicit learning and tacit knowledge: An essay on the cognitive unconscious.* London: Oxford University Press.

Reber, A. S., & Allen, R. (2000). Individual differences in implicit learning: Implications for the evolution of consciousness. In R. G. Kunzendork & B. Wallace (Eds.), *Individual differences in conscious experiences* (pp. 228–247). Philadelphia: John Benjamin.

Reber, A. S., Walkenfeld, F. F., & Hernstadt, R. (1991). Implicit and explicit learning: Individual differences and IQ. *Journal of Experimental Psychology: Learning, Memory and Cognition, 17,* 888–896.

Reber, P. J., & Kotovsky, K. (1997). Implicit learning in problem solving: The role of working memory capacity. *Journal of Experimental Psychology: General, 126,* 178–203.

Reber, P. J., & Squire, L. R. (1994). Parallel brain systems for learning with and without awareness. *Learning and Memory, 2,* 217–229.

Reber, P. J., & Squire, L. R. (1997). Intact learning of artificial grammars and intact category learning by patients with Parkinson's disease. *Behavioral Neuroscience, 113,* 235–242.

Saffran, J. R., Aslin, R. N., & Newport, E. L. (1996). Statistical learning by 8-month-old infants. *Science, 274,* 1926–1928.

Sagar, H. J., Gabrielli, J. D. E., Sullivan, E. V., & Corkin, S. (1990). Recency and frequency discrimination in the amnesic patient H.M. *Brain, 113,* 581–602.

Seger, C. A. (1994). Implicit learning. *Psychological Bulletin, 115,* 163–196.

Servan-Schreiber, E., & Anderson, J. R. (1990). Learning artificial grammars with competitive chunking. *Journal of Experimental Psychology: Learning, Memory, and Cognition, 16,* 592–608.

Squire, L. R., Knowlton, B., & Musen, G. (1993). The structure and organization of memory. *Annual Review of Psychology, 44,* 453–495.

Udwin, O., & Yule, W. (1990). Expressive language of children with Williams syndrome. *American Journal of Medical Genetics Supplement, 6,* 108–114.

Udwin, O., & Yule, W. (1991). A cognitive and behavioral phenotype in Williams syndrome. *Journal of Clinical and Experimental Neuropsychology, 13,* 232–244.

Vicari, S., Bellucci, S., & Carlesimo, G. A. (2000). Implicit and explicit memory: A functional dissociation in persons with Down syndrome. *Neuropsychologia, 38,* 240–251.

Vokey, J. R., & Brooks, L. R. (1992). Salience of item knowledge in learning artificial grammars. *Journal of Experimental Psychology: Learning, Memory, and Cognition, 18,* 328–344.

Wyatt, B. S., & Connors, F. A. (1998). Implicit and explicit memory in individuals with mental retardation. *American Journal on Mental Retardation, 102,* 511–526.

Dethroning the Myth: Cognitive Dissociations and Innate Modularity in Williams Syndrome

Annette Karmiloff-Smith, Janice H. Brown, Sarah Grice, and Sarah Paterson

ICH Neurocognitive Development Unit
London, England

Despite increasing empirical data to the contrary, it continues to be claimed that morphosyntax and face processing skills of people with Williams syndrome are intact. This purported intactness, which coexists with mental retardation, is used to bolster claims about innately specified, independently functioning modules, as if the atypically developing brain were simply a normal brain with parts intact and parts impaired. Yet this is highly unlikely, given the dynamics of brain development and the fact that in a genetic microdeletion syndrome the brain is developing differently from the moment of conception, throughout embryogenesis, and during postnatal brain growth. In this article, we challenge the intactness assumptions, using evidence from a wide variety of studies of toddlers, children, and adults with Williams syndrome.

Neurocognitive studies of developmental disorders never turn out to be as straightforward as they first promise. Studies of Williams syndrome (WS) are no exception. The pioneering work of Bellugi, Lichtenberger, Jones, Lai, and St. George (2000) seemed to point to some clear-cut dissociations in the cognitive architecture of WS. Language and face processing appeared to be preserved in the face of both general retardation and particularly serious problems with visuospatial cognition, number skills, planning, and problem solving (Bellugi, Wang, & Jernigan, 1994). Researchers in the field of WS have been cautious about these claims, couching them in terms of relative strengths and weaknesses rather than absolute ones (Bellugi et al., 2000; Karmiloff-Smith, 1998; Karmiloff-Smith

Requests for reprints should be sent to Annette Karmiloff-Smith, Neurocognitive Development Unit, Institute of Child Health, 30 Guilford Street, London WC 1N 1EH, United Kingdom. E-mail: annette@cdu.ucl.ac.uk

et al., 1997; Klein & Mervis, 1999; Mervis, 1999; Vicari, Carlesimo, Brizzolara, & Pezzini, 1996; Volterra, Capirci, Pezzini, Sabbadini, & Vicari, 1996). By contrast, secondary sources regarding WS data, cited in writings by linguists, psychologists, and philosophers, have often used WS to bolster claims about innate and independently functioning modules, some of which are intact and others impaired (e.g., Bickerton, 1997; Pinker, 1994, 1999). This emanates from a view, held explicitly or implicitly, that behavioral deficits found in the phenotypic outcome of individuals with genetic disorders are direct windows on the initial state, that is, the innate modular structure of the cognitive system (Baron-Cohen, 1998; Leslie, 1992; Temple, 1997; see Karmiloff-Smith, 1998, for critical discussion). As Baron-Cohen (1998) put it,

> I suggest that the study of mental retardation would profit from the application of the framework of cognitive neuropsychology. In cognitive neuropsychology, one key question running through the investigator's mind is 'is this process or mechanism intact or impaired in this person'?

The notion that an ability is necessarily intact in a genetic disorder when behavior falls within the normal range fails to consider the psychological processes underlying overt behavior. This kind of reasoning negates the role of development in producing phenotypic outcomes and treats the end-state cognitive system as if it were a normal system with some components missing and others intact. In other words, it is based on the neuropsychology model of brain damage to previously normal adults and can, in our view, be very misleading when applied to developmental disorders. Further, as far as WS is concerned, the nativist literature frequently misrepresents the empirical findings, treating relative strengths as absolute strengths. In the first part of this article, data relating to the phenotypic outcome of two areas hailed as intact in WS—language and face processing—are examined. In the second part, we look at the early cognitive state in toddlers with WS and consider its relationship to the adult end state.

LANGUAGE AND WILLIAMS SYNDROME

In our view, it remains questionable as to whether any aspect of language—syntax, semantics, phonology, or pragmatics—is intact in WS. Yet a number of researchers have tried to demonstrate that language, in particular morphosyntax, is preserved in WS and functions independently of other cognitive systems. Rossen, Jones, Wang, and Klima (1995), for example, claimed that "Williams syndrome presents a remarkable juxtaposition of impaired and intact mental capacities: linguistic functioning is preserved in WS while problem solving ability and visuospatial cognition are impaired." Likewise, Pinker (1991) claimed that:

> Although IQ is measured at around 50, older children and adolescents with WS are described as hyperlinguistic with selective sparing of syntax, and grammatical abilities are close to normal in controlled testing. This is one of several kinds of dissociation in which language is preserved despite severe cognitive impairments.

Not all researchers make such sweeping claims, but many linguists of a Chomskyan persuasion nonetheless try to find an aspect of WS language that is spared and, by extension, innately specified. For example, Clahsen and Almazan (1998) argued for a double dissociation of innate mechanisms, on the basis of their claim that in WS lexical memory is impaired and syntax is intact, whereas in specific language impairment (SLI) the opposite obtains. These authors used evidence from a number of syntactic elicitation and comprehension tasks. These included tests of past tense formation, expressive language, and the interpretation of passive sentences and of anaphoric and reflexive pronouns. Performance of the individuals with WS on the latter two tasks was at ceiling. However, ceiling effects are notoriously difficult to interpret because they can simply suggest that a task is not sensitive enough. Furthermore, Clahsen and Almazan's arguments were based on a very small sample of children with WS ($n = 2$ for mental age [MA] 5 years and $n = 2$ for MA = 7 years), together with considerable interindividual variation among the few participants. Strong claims about the cognitive architecture of a syndrome cannot be made on the basis of such sparse data.

The main claim of the Clahsen and Almazan (1998) study was that individuals with WS have a specific deficit in forming irregular past tenses (e.g., creep–crept) but intact performance in forming the regular past tense (e.g., walk–walked). Because this important claim was based on such a small sample with individual variation, we carried out a much broader, in-depth study of past tense formation (Thomas et al., 2001), comparing the performance of 21 participants with WS on two past tense elicitation tasks with that of four typically developing control groups at ages 6 years, 8 years, 10 years, and adult. Given that WS language is seriously delayed initially, Thomas et al. (2001) argued that it is not sufficient to show that irregular past tense formation is poorer than regular past tense formation, because this is also true of some stages of typical development. Rather it is necessary to demonstrate that the level of past tense formation is poorer than would be expected in individuals with WS for their actual level of language development. The study showed that when performance was related to chronological age (CA) using regression analyses, individuals with WS showed a somewhat greater disparity between irregular and regular verbs compared to the controls. However, when verbal MA was controlled for, the WS group displayed no selective deficit in irregular past tense formation. Moreover, we could not replicate the Clahsen and Almazan (1998) control data. At no age did our controls show high levels of irregularization of novel verbs that rhyme with irregular verbs (see also van der Lely & Ullman [2001] for similar control data results to ours). Furthermore, our results also highlighted how potentially misleading small samples such as in the Clahsen and Almazan (1998) study can be. As individuals, a few of our participants with WS performed very poorly on both regular and irregular verbs, whereas a few others displayed very high performance on both. If these high performers had by chance constituted the very small *N* of the Clahsen and Almazan study, then the authors would have had to draw totally different conclusions from the ones drawn. Our findings on a much larger population of 21 individuals with WS are inconsistent with the view that people with WS are selectively impaired on irregular past tense forms. Indeed, as a group, there was no selective deficit for irregulars and the WS results could be placed on the typical developmental pathway found in younger individuals. The results were in fact consistent with the hypothesis that the WS language system is delayed because it has developed under different constraints. Mervis and her collaborators (e.g., Klein & Mervis, 1999) have also concluded that the best way to characterize WS language is that it is delayed, revealing patterns typical of younger children.

A number of findings now suggest, however, that the WS language system is not only delayed but also develops along a different trajectory compared to controls, with individuals with WS placing relatively more weight on phonological information and relatively less weight on semantic information. For example, during the early acquisition of language, the naming spurt in WS precedes fast-mapping ability, whereas in typical development these two are closely associated (Mervis & Bertrand, 1997). These same authors also showed that the naming spurt in WS does not coincide with exhaustive category sorting, an index of children's maturing semantic representations, which suggests that vocabulary growth relies less on semantics than in the typically developing case (Mervis & Bertrand, 1997). Further, although local semantic organization looks normal in WS in terms of priming effects (Tyler et al., 1997) and in terms of category fluency (Scott et al., 1995), global semantic organization remains at the level of young children and never reaches the mature state even in relatively high functioning adults with WS (Johnson & Carey, 1998).

A number of other studies of oral and written language also point to a reduced contribution of semantics in language development in WS. For example, Karmiloff-Smith et al. (1997) found that when participants with WS were monitoring sentences for a target word, they did not show sensitivity to subcategory violations, suggesting that in WS semantic information may become available too slowly to be integrated with the online processing of syntax. A recent study of reading in WS came to similar conclusions about the role of phonology over semantics. The group with WS displayed equal levels of reading for both concrete and abstract words (Laing, Hulme, Grant, & Karmiloff-Smith, 2001). By contrast, the controls found concrete, imageable words much easier to read. In addition, the study showed that imageability effects are weaker in people with WS. Finally, Grant et al. (1997) used the Children's Nonword Repetition task (Gathercole,

Willis, Baddeley, & Emslie, 1994) with participants with WS. They showed that, despite a vocabulary test age of 8 years, when learning new words people with WS behaved like 4- to 5-year-olds and did not show the pattern seen from 6 years onward in the typically developing population. Like very young children, the participants with WS were less influenced by the semantics of the words that the nonce terms resembled and relied more on phonology. Taken together, these different studies suggest that, unlike typical development, semantics seems to place somewhat less of a constraint compared to phonology in the way in which WS language develops over time.

We have so far suggested that semantics may play a somewhat less important role in WS lexical development than in typical controls and that this aspect of WS language develops atypically. However, it remains possible that WS syntax is intact, as many have claimed (e.g., Bickerton, 1997; Clahsen & Almazan, 1998; Pinker, 1999). There are, however, a number of lines of evidence that cast doubt on this. First, vocabulary levels are usually better than syntactic levels in WS on various standardized tasks, and both are significantly below CA (Karmiloff-Smith et al., 1997). Second, even in very simple imitation tasks, participants with WS show impairment with complex syntactic structures like embedded relative clauses. A recent study by Grant, Valian, and Karmiloff-Smith (2002) showed that despite having a mean vocabulary test age of 9 years, the participants with WS performed significantly worse on relative clauses than the 6- and 7-year-old controls and worse than even the 5-year-olds on three of the four sentence types. Length of sentence did not explain the results because the shortest of the sentence types was the most difficult for the WS group who performed at ceiling on non-embedded filler sentences of varying length. These findings are inconsistent with the view that WS syntax is intact. Even in an area of relatively simple syntax–grammatical concord over sentence elements—which normal French-speaking children acquire easily and early—people with WS show impairment. Karmiloff-Smith et al. (1997) studied the ability of a group of French-speaking participants with WS to use grammatical gender agreement. The results showed that although the children with WS learned the local gender marker (correct article) for a nonce term easily (in fact, more easily than control children), their capacity for gender agreement across sentence elements such as agreement on adjectives or pronouns was seriously impaired. Even for known words, the WS group made double the number of errors of the young controls. This suggests that memory for local verbal material (article + noun) is good, but processing of sentential syntax (gender agreement across sentence elements) is not. Studies of Italian-speaking children have also revealed that grammatical gender is a particular problem, with children with WS displaying errors never encountered in typical development (Volterra et al., 1996). Several studies (e.g., Klein & Mervis, 1999) now suggest that the problems that people with WS have with semantics and syntax can often be camouflaged by their good verbal memory.

Despite these and numerous other linguistic data from studies of WS, the myth that WS morphosyntax is intact continues to thrive. This is clear from the following quotation from Pinker's (1999) recent book, where he contrasts individuals with SLI and WS, respectively: "The genes of one group of children impair their grammar while sparing their intelligence; the genes of another group of children impair their intelligence while sparing their grammar" (p. 262).

It is in our view theoretically misleading and empirically inaccurate to claim that grammar is spared in this clinical population. WS grammar is relatively good compared to some other clinical groups and relatively good compared to WS spatial deficits, but no better than their MA would predict. These are relative descriptions, not absolute ones. One of the crucial features of WS language is that in infancy and toddlerhood it is initially seriously delayed (Mervis, Morris, Bertrand, & Robinson, 1999; Mervis, Robinson, & Pani, 1999; Singer Harris, Bellugi, Bates, Jones, & Rossen, 1997). Now, if the WS infant brain presented with an intact morphosyntactic module, as many such quotations suggest, then this severe delay would surely be surprising. But given the empirical facts, it is not. The myth of intact WS language needs to be dethroned and buried once and for all. This does not mean that the WS cognitive architecture is uninteresting. On the contrary, we need to understand why the language of people with WS language is initially so delayed (Laing et al., 2002; Nazzi, Paterson, & Karmiloff-Smith, in press) and why it develops atypically. We will look at the issue of early development, with respect to language, number, and spatial cognition, in the third part of this article. Prior to doing so, we consider another aspect of the WS cognitive architecture—face processing—that is also claimed to be intact.

FACE PROCESSING SKILLS IN WILLIAMS SYNDROME

As with language, initial claims about face processing in WS suggested an innately specified face processing module that is intact. Indeed, Bellugi, Birhle, Jernigan, Trauner, and Doherty (1990) asserted, "we find in the WS population *normal* face processing capacities with at floor performance on spatial tasks," and Rossen et al. (1995) claimed to have found "*selective preservation* [italics added] of face recognition in Williams syndrome." There is no doubt that people with WS are very proficient at face processing. One might ask if face processing in adults with WS is modular, and the reply could be affirmative, that is, it has become modularized with development. One might also ask: Is it an intact module? But this is the wrong question because it negates development and the possibility that the cognitive processes underlying proficient WS face processing are different from those of typically developing controls. Indeed, several studies (Deruelle, Mancini, Livet, Cassé-Perrot, & de Schonen, 1999; Karmiloff-Smith, 1998; Udwin & Yule, 1991) have replicated Bellugi's earlier work and revealed normal or near-normal behavioral scores on standardized tasks like the Benton Facial Recognition Test (Benton, Hamsher, Varney, & Spreen, 1983) and the Rivermead Behavioural Memory Test (Wilson, Cockburn, & Baddeley, 1985). But these same studies have seriously challenged the notion that the behavioral success displayed in WS face processing capacities is normal. It has been shown that whereas typically developing controls use predominantly configural processes to recognize faces, people with WS tend to use predominantly componential or featural processes and do less well when a task forces configural processing (Wang, Doherty, Rourke, & Bellugi, 1995). Under certain circumstances, they are capable of using global or configural processing, particularly in low-level perceptual tasks (Birhle, Bellugi, Delis, & Marks, 1989; Mervis et al., 1999; Pani, Mervis, & Robinson, 1999), but they show a stronger tendency toward featural processing in many low-level and higher level visuospatial tasks, including face processing.

In an elegant set of studies using faces, buildings, and geometric shapes, Deruelle et al. (1999) showed that when faces and buildings are inverted, typically developing controls display a significant inversion effect for faces (they are faster and more accurate for upright faces) but not for buildings. By contrast, although the performance of the group with WS decreased slightly with inverted faces, this decrease was not significantly greater than that observed for buildings. The lack of the face inversion effect is not attributable to a floor effect because the WS accuracy scores were similar to those of their MA matches who did exhibit an inversion effect with faces. Furthermore, although the WS group ranged from 7 to 23 years, there was no trend with age toward the typical pattern. This finding was also supported using another set of geometric stimuli. Deruelle et al. gave participants the choice between similarity on the basis of configuration or similarity on the basis of features. For example, a square composed of four tiny circles might be placed with a square composed of four tiny squares (same configuration, different features) or a rectangle composed of four tiny circles (same features, different configuration). Control participants of either the same CA or the same MA tended to choose patterns of the same configuration, whereas the WS group showed no such preference. With a match-to-sample design using a set of schematic faces in which either configuration or features were changed, the WS group did not differ in the number of errors made on local features, but showed severe deficits compared to the controls in the configural trials. The authors conclude that individuals with WS display a selective configural processing deficit compared to both CA and MA matches. Their face processing proficiency stems from a deviant developmental pathway and does not reveal the functioning of a so-called normal, intact module. So, it is not the case that people with WS have an intact face processing module and an impaired space processing module. Both follow atypical developmental trajectories.

Imaging studies focusing on the electrophysiology of face processing in WS also support the notion of a differently developing expertise rather than an intact module. In a face recognition (match/mismatch) event-related potentials (ERP) study of 18 adults with WS, Mills et al. (2000) found abnormalities in the early waveform (100 and 200 msec post stimulus onset) of each of the participants with WS. This was not found in any of the controls. The authors suggest that these differences index abnormalities in face perception that may be specific to WS. Another study also points to abnormalities in face processing in WS. Using high-density ERP and a simplified task of face perception, Grice et al. (2001) tested 18 individuals with WS (*M* CA = 21.4 years) and also found waveform differences compared to CA-matched controls that indicated both deviance and delay. The N170 face-sensitive component was abnormal in the WS group and, unlike controls, was not increased in amplitude to inverted faces. There was also less right lateralization than for controls. In addition, unlike the control group, there was no difference in the N170-equivalent component to human faces or monkey faces. This finding suggests that the individuals in the WS group are not specialized for human faces in the same way as are controls. These data again refute the idea of an 'intact' module. Rather, they suggest that people with WS have either an incomplete or a different form of modularization for face processing.

EARLY DEVELOPMENT IN WILLIAMS SYNDROME

We now turn to early development with respect to these two areas of relative proficiency in WS language and face processing. Our aim (Paterson, 2000; Paterson, Brown, Gsödl, Johnson, & Karmiloff-Smith, 1999) is to challenge some of the deeply engrained assumptions in cognitive neuropsychology and developmental cognitive neuroscience about the use of developmental disorders for bolstering nativist claims. The assumption—which we will call the Modular Continuity Hypothesis—often remains implicit in writings, but is in fact part and parcel of the logic of the argument and stems, as we suggested in the Introduction, from adult neuropsychology models. It holds that the brain is organized into innate (genetically determined) mental/neural modules that have the same potential for dissociation across the human lifespan. In other words, it is assumed that there is a transparent relationship between phenotypic outcomes and genes, with the expectation that the same dissociations observed in the adult steady state hold during the period in which these abilities emerge.

Is the inference that the WS phenotypic end state supports the case for innate modularity justified? In other words, can one assume the state of early development simply from the pattern of proficiencies and impairments in the phenotypic outcome in the adult, without studying their developmental trajectories? It is known that WS and Down syndrome (DS) display different cognitive profiles in the end state (Jernigan, Bellugi, Sowell, Doherty, & Hesselink, 1993; Klein & Mervis, 1999; Wang, Doherty, Hesselink, & Bellugi, 1992), although, using more subtle measures, Klein and Mervis (1999) discovered a number of hitherto neglected similarities between WS and DS at 9 to 10 years of age. In adulthood, however, it remains clear that vocabulary levels of people with WS are better than those with DS and that both syndromes show serious impairment in the domain of number (Bellugi et al., 1994; Paterson, 2000).

Paterson (2000; Paterson et al., 1999) purposely chose two tasks—one language-related, one number-related—which could be designed to be as similar as possible for both very young children and adults. For number, numerosity judgments were required; for language, receptive vocabulary measures were taken. The domains of vocabulary and number were purposely chosen because in the phenotypic end state it had been claimed that individuals with WS show greater proficiency in vocabulary than individuals with DS, and that both syndromes are seriously impaired in number. If the phenotypic end state can be directly used to assume the pattern obtaining in infancy, then the infant profiles should resemble the adult profiles across these two syndromes. Paterson (2000) first examined adult abilities. She tested participants with WS and DS who were matched on CA and on MA from the British Ability Scales, $t(13) = 2.05, p > .06$. She showed that these adults had significantly different scores on a vocabulary test, the British Picture Vocabulary Scales (BPVS), with a smaller discrepancy between CA and test age on the BPVS for adults with WS than for those with DS, $t(6) = 2.55$, $p < .05$, as had been demonstrated in previous work. Numerosity judgment tasks had not been hitherto used with adults with either WS or DS. Participants were required to judge which of two numbers (either Arabic numerals 1–10 or dots displays) displayed on a computer screen is the larger. Reaction times and accuracy were measured. In the normal case, a distance effect is always apparent: Numbers very close (like 7 and 8) take longer for a decision as to which is the larger than numbers that are far apart (like 7 and 2). Paterson demonstrated that adults with WS and DS performed differently on the numerosity judgment tasks. The adults with DS, although slower overall, showed a clear-cut effect as evidenced by typically developing controls. By contrast, the adults with WS performed significantly worse than the matched adults with DS on several number tasks and, although there was a trend in the right direction, this WS group did not show the distance effect. There was a significant difference between the WS and DS groups for the discrepancy between reaction times to close and far pairs (Mann–Whitney $U = -11, p < .05$). So the phenotype in the adult end state was DS significantly worse than WS on vocabulary, WS significantly worse than DS on numerosity judgments.

An attempt was made to devise similar number tasks with adults and toddlers. In both cases, the tasks involved making a comparison between two numerosities. In the toddler case, an implicit same/different judgment was required, whereas the adults had to decide which of the numerosities was the larger. Likewise, vocabulary comprehension was measured in both adults and toddlers.

Paterson et al. (1999) used a preferential looking paradigm to examine numerosity and vocabulary in 65 toddlers between 13 and 36 months, divided into groups of toddlers with WS, atypical controls with DS matched for CA and MA on the Bayley Infant Scales II (Bayley, 1993), typically developing MA controls (also matched on the Bayley), and typically developing CA controls. If the use of the so-called Modularity Continuity Hypothesis were justified, then these young children should show a similar profile of cognitive abilities and impairments to adults in each of the syndromes. However, this was not the case. The toddlers with WS and DS were equally impaired and performed significantly worse than CA controls on the language task, despite the fact that adults with WS were significantly better than the adults with DS. For vocabulary, then, both atypical groups of toddlers performed like the MA controls, that is, at approximately half their CA. By contrast, although the adults with WS were more impaired than the adults with DS with numerosity judgments, the toddlers with WS showed unimpaired performance on the numerosity judgment task. They performed like the CA controls, whereas the toddlers with DS were seriously impaired and did not even reach the level of the MA controls. Again, the pattern in early development differed considerably from that observed in adulthood. Caution must therefore be exercised when making claims about innate modules based on phenotypic outcomes. These data suggest either that the learning trajectories of the two syndromes are different in development or, in the language example, that children with DS are subject to increasing deficit in linguistic skills compared to their counterparts with WS, who retain a relatively stable pattern of delay throughout development. Whichever turns out to be the case, it is only via developmental studies following infants and toddlers from the initial state through childhood and adulthood that this question can be properly addressed. Alas, in WS, a syndrome characterized by initial feeding problems and failure to thrive, it is very hard to test infants in the very early phases of postnatal life. Even as late as 20 months, however, the toddler profile is different from the resulting adult profile. This again stresses the need to focus on the process of development itself when studying developmental disorders (Karmiloff-Smith, 1998) and that claims regarding starting states cannot necessarily be based on patterns found in phenotypic outcomes. In other words, although it is always possible that in some cases early developmental patterns turn out to show the same profile of abilities and impairments as the adult end state, this cannot be taken for granted without empirical verification. Furthermore, although the adult profile concerns higher level cognitive domains, it is probable that impairments in infancy are related to much lower level processing mechanisms.

With respect to language, we are left with an intriguing question as to why onset in WS is so delayed, given the relative proficiency in later life. We have argued that this may in part be due to an imbalance between semantics and phonology leading to weak semantic representations. It may also in part be due to abnormality of nonlinguistic precursors to language. For instance, Mervis and Bertrand (1997) showed that, unlike typical development, in WS naming precedes pointing. Thus, early naming in WS may be more like sound production and less like language production. Results from recent work in our lab also suggest that pointing and joint attention, which underpin certain aspects of normal language acquisition, are significantly reduced and atypical in toddlers with WS compared to MA and CA controls (Laing et al., in press). We are also examining early speech perception and have shown that infants with WS have deficits in early speech segmentation abilities (Nazzi et al., in press). It is in our view crucial to examine the array of prelinguistic abilities that the typically developing child brings to the language-learning task. It is clear that throughout development, however, from the early stages through to the adult end state, WS language is not intact at any level that researchers have hitherto seriously examined. Let us reiterate, the myth of intact language should be buried and the search for intact modules ceased, so that more subtle research can be pursued to discover the developmental language trajectories followed by individuals with WS. The lack of intactness is unsurprising if we recall that the WS brain is qualitatively different from the normal brain in terms of brain anatomy (Bellugi, Lichtenberger, Mills, Galaburda, & Korenberg, 1999), brain chemistry (Rae et al., 1998), and computational processing (Grice et al., 2001; Mills et al., 2000). Nor is it therefore surprising that seemingly normal behavioral outcomes even in adults turn out to be underpinned by different linguistic processes from the normal case (Karmiloff-Smith, 1998).

What about face processing in early development? Can that provide clues to the atypical processing style used by adults with WS? First, it is known that normally developing infants already show a right hemisphere superiority for configural face processing from 4 to 5 months of age onward (Deruelle & de Schonen, 1998; de Schonen & Mathivet, 1990). So the right hemisphere bias in normal adults is already present early in infancy. Second, by 1 month of age, typically developing infants show a novelty preference for new faces over old faces in a preferential looking task. By 3 months of age, not only do they display a novelty preference, but they also show a prototype effect (de Haan, Johnson, Maurer, & Perrett, 2001). Take the following experimental situation. Four faces are displayed one after another and then the infant is given a choice between a fifth face (not previously seen by the infant, but a prototype morphed from the previous four faces) and one of the already-seen faces. In this situation, 3-month-olds (but not yet 1-month-olds) treat the morphed face as more familiar than the already seen face. This means that by 3 months, infants do not simply learn the details of exemplars, but build up a prototypical representation of the configuration of previously processed faces. In a pilot study, Brown (2000) found that infants with WS did not show the prototypical effect. This suggests that infants and toddlers with WS tend to learn exemplars and may lack the generalization processes necessary to form prototypes. If this preliminary finding holds, the WS lack of prototype extraction could well be due to a tendency early in development toward featural rather than configural processing. Because it has been shown that toddlers with WS spend more time than typically developing or DS controls fixated on faces (Mervis et al., 2003), the early infant processing style may explain the phenotypical outcome in WS adult face processing. It may also be a clue as to why infants with WS succeed in discriminating small numerosities compared to infants with DS: The former group's seemingly normal performance may actually rely on a focus on qualitative detail rather than quantity.

Yet again we need to bury the myth of what at first blush seemed like an intact face processing module in adults with WS. Face processing follows a different developmental trajectory in this clinical population.

It has always been recognized that children and adults with WS show clear behavioral deficits in visuospatial tasks outside face processing. Our lab has also pursued spatial cognition in infancy (see also Atkinson et al., 1997). In a study of saccade planning, Brown and colleagues (Brown, 2000; Brown et al., in press) showed that toddlers with WS (with a mean CA of 29 months, range 23–37 months) have atypical spatial representations for planning visually guided actions. Saccades in healthy controls and in CA/MA-matched toddlers with DS (with a mean CA of 29 months, range 24–37 months) are executed within body-centered spatial coordinates. By contrast, toddlers with WS displayed evidence of deficits in saccade planning, suggesting in their case a greater reliance on subcortical processing mechanisms than the other groups. So once again, be it face processing or visuospatial processing, the WS brain proceeds along an atypical developmental pathway. Moreover, in both the prototype face processing and saccade planning studies, toddlers with WS displayed sticky fixation, that is, they looked longer at all the displays than participants with DS and the CA- and MA-matched typically developing controls. It is therefore possible that subsequent focus on features is the result of an early inability to disengage. To reiterate, it is not that one module—face processing—is spared and the other module—visuospatial processing—is impaired. Both domains develop atypically in WS.

CONCLUDING COMMENT

In our view, the notion of direct impairment to higher level cognitive modules is unlikely to explain the phenotypic outcome in WS or other genetic disorders. We anticipate that impairments will be in the form of lower level mechanisms traceable back to early infancy. There may be cases where infant and adult impairments turn out to be similar, but our new work stresses the importance of not taking for granted the idea that the infant start state will display the same profile as the adult end state. As we stated in the Introduction, neurocognitive studies of developmental disorders never turn out to be as straightforward as they first promise. We have shown that studies of WS are no exception, and that it is time that the myths of static, intact modules be dethroned in favor of studying the complex dynamics of developmental trajectories.

ACKNOWLEDGMENTS

The studies reported in this article were funded by Programme Grant No. G9715642 and Project Grant No. 9809880 to A. K.-S. by the U.K. Medical Research Council, by a joint grant from the European Science Foundation, and by PhD studentships from the Medical Research Council and the Down's Syndrome Association.

REFERENCES

Atkinson, J. A., King, J., Braddick, O. J., Nokes, L., Anker, S., & Braddick, F. (1997). A specific deficit of dorsal stream function in Williams syndrome. *NeuroReport, 8,* 1919–1922.

Baron-Cohen, S. (1998). Modularity in developmental cognitive neuropsychology: Evidence from autism and Gilles de la Tourette syndrome. In J. A. Burack, R. M. Hodapp, & E. Zigler (Eds.), *Handbook of mental retardation and development* (pp. 335). Cambridge, England: Cambridge University Press.

Bayley, N. (1993). *Bayley Scales of Infant Development* (2nd ed.). San Antonio, TX: Psychological Corporation.

Bellugi, U., Birhle, A., Jernigan, T., Trauner, D., & Doherty, S. (1990). Neuropsychological, neurological, and neuroanatomical profile of Williams syndrome. *American Journal of Medical Genetics, 6,* 115–125.

Bellugi, U., Lichtenberger, L., Jones, W., Lai, Z., & St. George, M. (2000). The neurocognitive profile of Williams syndrome: A complex pattern of strengths and weaknesses. *Journal of Cognitive Neuroscience, 12*(1), 7–29.

Bellugi, U., Lichtenberger, L., Mills, D., Galaburda, A., & Korenberg, J. R. (1999). Bridging cognition, the brain and molecular genetics: Evidence from Williams syndrome. *Trends in Neurosciences, 22*(5), 197–207.

Bellugi, U., Wang, P. P., & Jernigan, T. (1994). Williams syndrome: An unusual neuropsychological profile. In S. H. Broman & J. Grafman (Eds.), *Atypical cognitive deficit in developmental disorders: Implications for brain function* (pp. 23–56). Hillsdale, NJ: Lawrence Erlbaum Associates, Inc.

Benton, A. L., Hamsher, K. de S., Varney, N. R., & Spreen, O. (1983). *Contributions to neuropsychological assessment.* New York: Oxford University Press.

Bickerton, D. (1997). Constructivism, nativism, and exploratory adequacy. *Behavioral and Brain Sciences, 20,* 557–558.

Birhle, J. M., Bellugi, U., Delis, D., & Marks, S. (1989). Seeing either the forest or the trees: Dissociation in visuospatial processing. *Brain and Cognition, 11,* 37–49.

Brown, J. (2000). *The development of visual cognition in infants with Williams and Down syndromes.* Unpublished doctoral thesis, University College London.

Brown, J., Johnson, M. H., Paterson, S., Gilmore, R., Gsödl, M., Longhi, E., et al. (in press). Spatial representation and attention in toddlers with Williams syndrome and Down syndrome. *Neuropsychologia.*

Clahsen, H., & Almazan, M. (1998). Syntax and morphology in Williams syndrome. *Cognition, 68,* 167–198.

de Haan, M., Johnson, M. H., Maurer, D., & Perrett, D. I. (2001). Recognition of individual faces and average face prototypes by 1- and 3-month-old infants. *Cognitive Development, 16,* 659–678.

Deruelle, C., & de Schonen, S. (1998). Do the right and the left hemispheres attend to the same visual information within a face in infancy? *Developmental Neuropsychology, 14,* 535–554.

Deruelle, C., Mancini, J., Livet, M. O., Casse-Perrot, C., & de Schonen, S. (1999). Configural and local processing of faces in children with Williams syndrome. *Brain and Cognition, 41,* 276–298.

de Schonen, S., & Mathivet, E. (1990). Hemispheric asymmetry in a face discrimination task in infants. *Child Development, 61,* 1992–1205.

Gathercole, S. E., Willis, C. S., Baddeley, A. D., & Emslie, H. (1994). The children's test of nonword repetition: A test of phonological working memory. *Memory, 2,* 103–127.

Grant, J., Karmiloff-Smith, A., Gathercole, S. E., Paterson, S., Howlin, P., Davies, M., et al. (1997). Phonological short-term memory and its relationship to language in Williams syndrome. *Journal of Cognitive Neuropsychiatry, 2*(2), 81–99.

Grant, J., Valian, V., & Karmiloff-Smith, A. (2002). A study of relative clauses in Williams syndrome. *Journal of Child Language, 29,* 403–416.

Grice, S., Spratling, M. W., Karmiloff-Smith, A., Halit, H., Csibra, G., de Haan, M., et al. (2001). Disordered visual processing and oscillatory brain activity in autism and Williams syndrome. *NeuroReport, 12,* 2697–2700.

Jernigan, T. L., Bellugi, U., Sowell, E., Doherty, S., & Hesselink, J. R. (1993). Cerebral morphologic distinctions between Williams and Down syndromes. *Archives of Neurology, 50,* 186–191.

Johnson, S., & Carey, S. (1998). Knowledge enrichment and conceptual change in folk biology: Evidence from Williams syndrome. *Cognitive Psychology, 37,* 156–184.

Karmiloff-Smith, A. (1998). Development itself is the key to understanding developmental disorders. *Trends in Cognitive Sciences, 2,* 389–398.

Karmiloff-Smith, A., Grant, J., Berthoud, I., Davies, M., Howlin, P., & Udwin, O. (1997). Language and Williams syndrome: How intact is "intact"? *Child Development, 68,* 246–262.

Klein, B. P., & Mervis, C. B. (1999). Contrasting patterns of cognitive abilities of 9- and 10-year-olds with Williams syndrome or Down syndrome. *Developmental Neuropsychology, 16,* 177–196.

Laing, E., Butterworth, G., Gsödl, M., Panagiota, G., Paterson, S., Longhi, E., et al. (2002). Preverbal communication in infants with Williams Syndrome. *Developmental Science, 5*(2), 233–246.

Laing, E., Hulme, C., Grant, J., & Karmiloff-Smith, A. (2001). Learning to read in Williams syndrome: Looking beneath the surface of atypical reading development. *Journal of Child Psychology and Psychiatry, 42,* 729–739.

Leslie, A. M. (1992). Pretence, autism, and the theory-of-mind-module. *Current Directions in Psychological Science, 1,* 18–21.

Mervis, C. B. (1999). The Williams syndrome cognitive profile: Strengths, weakness, and interrelations among auditory short-term memory, language, and visuospatial constructive cognition. In E. Winograd, R. Fivush, & W. Hirst (Eds.), *Ecological approaches to cognition: Essays inhonor of Ulric Neisser* (pp. 193–227). Mahwah, NJ: Lawrence Erlbaum Associates, Inc.

Mervis, C. B., & Bertrand, J. (1997). Developmental relations between cognition and language: Evidence from Williams syndrome. In L. B. Adamson & M. A. Romski (Eds.), *Research on communication and language disorders: Contributions to theories of language development* (pp. 75–106). New York: Brookes.

Mervis, C. B., Morris, C. A., Bertrand, J., & Robinson, B. F. (1999). Williams syndrome: Findings from an integrated program of research. In H. Tager-Flusberg (Ed.), *Neurodevelopmental disorders* (pp. 65–110). Cambridge, MA: MIT Press.

Mervis, C. B., Morris, C. A., Klein-Tasman, B. P., Bertrand, J., Kwitny, S., Appelbaum, L. G., et al. (2003). Additional characteristics of infants and toddlers with Williams syndrome during triadic interactions. *Developmental Neuropsychology, 23,* 243–268.

Mervis, C. B., Robinson, B. F., & Pani, J. R. (1999). Cognitive and behavioral genetics '99: Visuospatial construction. *American Journal Human Genetics, 65,* 1222–1229.

Mills, D. L., Alvarez, T. D., St. George, M., Appelbaum, L. G., Bellugi, U., & Neville, H. (2000). Electrophysiological studies of face processing in Williams syndrome. *Journal of Cognitive Neuroscience, 12*(Suppl.), 47–64.

Nazzi, T., Paterson, S., & Karmiloff-Smith, A. (in press). Early word segmentation by infants and toddlers with Williams syndrome. *Infancy.*

Pani, J. R., Mervis, C. B., & Robinson, B. F. (1999). Global spatial organization by individuals with Williams syndrome. *Psychological Science, 10,* 453–458.

Paterson, S. (2000). *The development of language and number understanding in Williams syndrome and Down syndrome: Evidence from the infant and mature phenotypes.* Unpublished doctoral thesis, University College London.

Paterson, S. J., Brown, J. H., Gsödl, M. K., Johnson, M. H., & Karmiloff-Smith, A. (1999). Cognitive modularity and genetic disorders. *Science, 286,* 2355–2358.

Pinker, S. (1991). Rules of language. *Science, 253,* 530–535.

Pinker, S. (1994). *The language instinct.* London: Penguin.

Pinker, S. (1999). *Words and rules.* London: Weidenfeld & Nicolson.

Rae, C., Karmiloff-Smith, A., Lee, M. A., Dixon, R. M., Blamire, Thompson, et al. (1998). Brain biochemistry in Williams syndrome: Evidence for a role of the cerebellum in cognition? *Neurology, 51,* 33–40.

Rossen, M., Jones, W., Wang, P. P., & Klima, E. S. (1995). Face processing: Remarkable sparing in Williams syndrome. *Genetic Counseling, 6,* 138–140.

Scott, P., Mervis, C. B., Bertrand, J., Klein, B. P., Armstrong, S. C., & Ford, A. L. (1995). *Semantic organization and word fluency in 9- and 10-year-old children with Williams syndrome.* Paper presented at the meeting of the Society for Research in Child Development, Indianapolis, IN.

Singer Harris, N. G., Bellugi, U., Bates, E., Jones, W., & Rossen, M. (1997). Contrasting profiles of language development in children with Williams and Down syndromes. *Developmental Neuropsychology, 13,* 345–370.

Temple, C. M. (1997). Cognitive neuropsychology and its applications to children. *Journal of Child Psychology and Psychiatry, 38,* 27–52.

Thomas, M. S. C., Grant, J., Barham, Z., Gsödl, M., Laing, E., Lakusta, L., et al. (2001). Past tense formation in Williams syndrome. *Language and Cognitive Processes, 2*(16), 143–176.

Tyler, L., Karmiloff-Smith, A., Voice, J. K., Stevens, T., Grant, J., Udwin, O., et al. (1997). Do individuals with Williams syndrome have bizarre semantics? Evidence for lexical organization using an on-line task. *Cortex, 33,* 515–527.

Udwin, O., & Yule, W. (1991). A cognitive and behavioural phenotype in Williams syndrome. *Journal of Clinical and Experimental Neuropsychology, 13,* 232–244.

van der Lely, H. K. J., & Ullman, M. T. (2001). Past tense morphology in specifically language-impaired and normally-developing children. *Language and Cognitive Processes, 16*(2), 177–217.

Vicari, S., Carlesimo, G., Brizzolara, D., & Pezzini, G. (1996). Short-term memory in children with Williams syndrome: A reduced contribution of lexical-semantic knowledge to word span. *Neuropsychologia, 34,* 919–925.

Volterra, V., Capirci, O., Pezzini, G, Sabbadini, L., & Vicari, S. (1996). Linguistic abilities in Italian children with Williams syndrome. *Cortex, 32,* 663–677.

Wang, P. P., Doherty, S., Hesselink, J. R., & Bellugi, U. (1992). Callosal morphology concurs with neurobehavioral and neuropathological findings in two neurodevelopmental disorders. *Archives of Neurology, 49,* 407–411.

Wang, P. P., Doherty, S., Rourke, S. B., & Bellugi, U. (1995). Unique profile of visuo-perceptual skills in a genetic syndrome. *Brain and Cognition, 29,* 54–65.

Wilson, B., Cockburn, J., & Baddeley, A. (1985). *Rivermead Behavioural Memory Test.* Reading, England: Thames Valley Test Co.

Attentional Characteristics of Infants and Toddlers With Williams Syndrome During Triadic Interactions

Carolyn B. Mervis
University of Louisville

Colleen A. Morris
University of Nevada School of Medicine

Bonita P. Klein-Tasman
Emory University

Jacquelyn Bertrand
Centers for Disease Control

Susanna Kwitny, Lawrence G. Appelbaum, and Catherine E. Rice
Emory University

Two studies were conducted to consider the looking behavior of infants and toddlers with Williams syndrome (WS). In Study 1, the looking behavior of a 10-month-old girl with WS during play sessions with her mother and with a stranger was compared to that of 2 groups of infants who were developing normally (ND), 1 matched for chronological age and the other for developmental age. The infant with WS spent more than twice as much time looking at her mother as the infants in either contrast group did. She also spent twice as much time looking at the stranger. In addition, during 78% of this time, her gaze at the stranger was coded as extremely intense. Looks of this intensity were virtually never made by the ND infants. In Study 2, the looking behavior of 31 individuals with WS ages 8 to

Requests for reprints should be sent to Carolyn B. Mervis, Department of Psychological and Brain Sciences, University of Louisville, Louisville, KY 40292. E-mail: cbmervis@louisville.edu

43 months during a genetics evaluation was compared to that of 319 control children in the same age range (242 with developmental delay due to causes other than WS). Twenty-three of the 25 participants with WS aged 33 months or younger demonstrated extended and intense looking at the geneticist. In contrast, none of the control participants looked extensively or intently at the geneticist. Findings are discussed in the context of previous research on arousal and focused attention during normal development and on temperament and personality of older children and adults with WS. It is argued that the unusual looking patterns evidenced by infants and toddlers with WS presage the unusual temperament and personality of older individuals with WS, and the possibility of a genetic basis for these behaviors is addressed.

Imagine the following scenario: Your colleague, Fred, who had never met a person with Williams syndrome (WS) before, has just been to a party attended by Julie, a 12-year-old who has WS. Fred knows that you are interested in WS, so he comes by your office the next day to describe his experience to you. His dominant impression was how very sociable Julie was. She had simply walked up to him and started a conversation, as though the two were already well acquainted. Fred had never met a person who was that friendly—Julie seemed almost too friendly. She showed no reticence at all, asked a number of personal questions, and continued to try to prolong the conversation even after he had given her repeated hints that he wanted to end it. Then, when Fred had finally succeeded in extracting himself, he walked partway across the room, only to stub his toe on a table leg. He responded with a quiet expression of pain. Julie noticed his distress immediately and reappeared to inquire, with a great deal of concern, about his pain and to reassure him that his toe would stop hurting soon.

Although this pattern of behavior by children and adults with WS has been noted repeatedly, there has been no research on early manifestations of this overly sociable behavior during the infant and toddler years. The absence of research on very young individuals is understandable, given how rare WS is (1/20,000 live births) and the fact that at least until recently, it typically was not diagnosed until after infancy. In this article we present two studies that begin to fill this gap. These studies focus on the quantity and quality of infants' and toddlers' attention to strangers. The first involves a case study of the attention behavior of a single infant with WS when playing with a stranger, relative to that of control participants who are developing normally. In the second study, we take a very different approach, reporting on the looking behavior of a large sample of 8- to 43-month-olds with WS during a genetics evaluation, relative to that of more than 300 controls, the majority of whom had developmental delay. In the remainder of the introduction, we briefly review the literature on personality and social behavior of individuals with WS and then turn to a very different topic, the early development of attention by normally developing (ND) infants. Finally, we describe the single previous case study of looking behavior of a toddler with WS when playing with her mother and with a stranger.

PERSONALITY AND SOCIAL BEHAVIOR OF INDIVIDUALS WITH WILLIAMS SYNDROME

We began this article by describing a hypothetical initial interaction between a person with WS and a stranger. Implied in this description are personality characteristics such as highly approaching, extremely or overly friendly, and empathic. These characteristics have been reported repeatedly in behavioral descriptions of individuals with WS. Psychologists who have studied individuals with WS have described them as highly sociable (e.g., Dilts, Morris, & Leonard, 1990), never going unnoticed in a group (e.g., Dykens & Rosner, 1999), highly approaching (e.g., Tomc, Williamson, & Pauli, 1990), overly friendly (e.g., Gosch & Pankau, 1997), and highly empathic (e.g., Gosch & Pankau, 1994; Tager-Flusberg & Sullivan, 1999). This combination of characteristics has not been ascribed to any other syndrome or to ND individuals and is often summed up by the word "delightful" (Morris & Mervis, 2000).

Several studies have been conducted comparing individuals with WS to chronological age (CA)- and IQ-matched individuals with other syndromes or mental retardation of unknown etiology with regard to these characteristics. The results have consistently indicated that individuals with WS manifest these attributes to a significantly greater extent than any of the comparison groups. Dykens and Rosner (1999) found that parents rated adolescents and adults with WS as much more likely than matched individuals with Prader–Willi syndrome or mental retardation of unknown etiology to "never go unnoticed in groups," "often initiate interactions," and "feel terrible when others are hurt." Gosch and Pankau (1997), in another rating study, found that children with WS were significantly less reserved toward strangers than were matched children with Down syndrome or Brachmann–de Lange syndrome. In the only experimental study addressing personality characteristics of WS, Tager-Flusberg and Sullivan (1999) found that children with WS showed much more concern than matched children with Prader–Willi syndrome when an experimenter appeared to have hurt her knee. The children with WS were also significantly more likely to offer comfort or validation.

In summary, WS is associated with an unusual personality profile, involving high sociability and overfriendliness, high approach to other people, and high empathy. Evidence regarding this profile has been obtained primarily from older children, adolescents, and adults. The question of the early antecedents of these characteristics in WS has not yet been addressed.

NORMAL PATTERN OF DEVELOPMENT OF ATTENTION DURING ADULT–INFANT INTERACTION: DEVELOPMENT OF ATTENTION IN COMMUNICATIVE INTERACTIONS

Adamson (1995) divided the development of attention during communicative interactions into three periods: shared attentiveness, interpersonal engagement, and joint object involvement (see also Bruner, 1975; Schaeffer, 1984). During the first period (typically ages birth–2 months) the infant and his or her parents gradually adjust their patterns of behavior to increase the amount of time when they are attentive simultaneously. In the second period, (typically ages 2–5 months), the infant and his or her parents share both attention and affect. During periods of interpersonal engagement, the undivided attention of both the infant and the parent is directed to the partner.

At the end of the interpersonal engagement period, episodes of face-to-face interaction have become familiar to the infant, and he or she suddenly becomes fascinated by objects. The infant, now almost 6 months old, has entered the third period, joint object involvement. The amount of time infants spend looking at objects increases steadily from ages 6 to 18 months (Bakeman & Adamson, 1984; Ruff & Saltarelli, 1993). At the start of this period, infants are able to attend to either objects or their partner, but not to both simultaneously. Beginning at about 12 months, infants are able to coordinate their attention to both object and partner, leading to episodes of joint attention (e.g., Bruner, 1975). These episodes increase from 4% of the time during mother–infant play sessions at age 12 months to 27% at 18 months (Bakeman & Adamson, 1984).

ATTENTION PATTERNS OF A TODDLER WITH WILLIAMS SYNDROME

The development of attention in communicative interactions has been addressed in only one study involving an individual with WS: a longitudinal case study of a toddler ("Peggy," a pseudonym) between the ages of 20 and 29 months, conducted as an honors thesis in the first author's laboratory (Rice, 1992). This study focused on Peggy's development of joint attention. Developmental changes in this pattern of distribution of attention were similar to those of the ND infants studied by Bakeman and Adamson (1984), but much delayed. Bakeman and Adamson found that 12-month-olds spent a mean of 3.6% of the time during mother–infant play sessions engaged in joint attention; this figure increased to 11.2% at age 15 months and 26.6% at age 18 months. In contrast, at age 20 months, Peggy was engaged in episodes of joint attention for just 4.7% of the play session with her mother. This percentage remained relatively steady until age 27 to 29 months, when it increased suddenly to 19.41%. Thus, like ND children, Peggy showed a sudden increase in percentage of time spent in joint attention with objects and her mother. However, this burst occurred at a much later age.

During our first visits with Peggy, we noted that she was extremely interested in our faces, spending most of her time staring at us. Peggy was the first child under age 2 years that most of us had seen with WS. In contrast, we had seen a large number of toddlers with Down syndrome, and although they had been interested in us, they had not stared at us in the same manner, nor had they looked at us for extremely long periods of time. Because we felt Peggy's behavior with strangers was unusual, we decided to conduct a case study of her play behavior with an older child she had not seen previously, in comparison to her play behavior with her mother. This study took place when Peggy was 22 months old. She played first with her mother for about 30 min and then played with Ari, an 8-year-old boy who enjoyed interacting with younger children. Peggy's mother remained in the room for a few minutes (to make sure Ari was comfortable; Peggy had paid no attention to her once Ari had entered the room), then left without Peggy noticing. Despite Ari's multiple creative attempts to engage her with the toys, Peggy continued to simply stare at him with such intensity that viewers of the videotape described her gaze as "It looks as though her eyes are boring into him." Peggy spent 70.83% of her time looking at Ari's face and only 6.50% looking at toys. In contrast, in the play session with her mother, Peggy spent 9.83% of the time looking at her mother's face and 67.74% looking at toys. The percentage of time Peggy spent looking at Ari was much greater than the percentage reported in any previous study for toddlers, even with disabilities, when toys were available. Note that even the percentage of time Peggy spent looking at her mother's face was substantially higher than would be expected for an ND 12-month-old and more than double that for a 15-month-old.

Peggy's play sessions were coded using Bakeman and Adamson's (1984) coding system. This system does not include codes for intensity of gaze; none of the children (ages 6–18 months) in the study for which the coding system was developed had produced gazes of unusual intensity (L. B. Adamson, personal communication, June 1991). Thus, although the results provide clear evidence that Peggy spent considerably more time looking at her partner's face than would be expected for a toddler her age (or her developmental age, which was estimated as 14 months based on the Bayley Scales of Infant Development [Bayley, 1969]), the most unusual aspect of her interactive behavior with strangers was not addressed: the extreme intensity with which she looked at their faces. Furthermore, because the stranger was a child and the play session with him was not the primary focus of the thesis, no control participants were tested.

These limitations are addressed by the two studies reported in this article. Study 1 is a case study of an older infant with WS. This time the stranger was an adult. Both CA-matched and developmental age (DA)-matched ND infants were included as controls. A new coding system was developed, which took into account intensity of gaze. In Study 2, we address remaining limitations of Study 1: the inclusion of only a single participant with WS and the lack of control participants with developmental delay. In that study, we consider the behavior of a large group of very young children with WS in comparison to control children during a genetics evaluation.

STUDY 1

Study 1 is a case study of the looking behavior of a 10-month-old infant with WS relative to that of ND infants matched for either CA or DA. Infants played first with their mother and then with an adult female whom they had not seen previously. The videotapes from the play sessions were coded using a new coding system, which took into account intensity of gaze. This study provides an opportunity to replicate and extend the findings from the Rice (1992) study.

Method

Participants

Participants included one infant girl with WS (hereafter referred to as "Jenny," a pseudonym), 10 infant girls of the same CA, 10 infant girls of the same DA,[1] and the infants' mothers. Jenny was diagnosed with supravalvar aortic stenosis (SVAS) at age 1 month. At that time, the cardiologist referred her to a geneticist because of the possibility of WS. At the genetics evaluation, which took place when Jenny was 3.5 months old, the geneticist told her parents that because Jenny had only a few of the facial features characteristic of WS, he was not sure if she had WS or instead had only SVAS. (Although most individuals with SVAS have WS, about 10% do not; the latter individuals often have a few of the WS facial features as infants [Frangiskakis et al., 1996].) Jenny entered our longitudinal study at age 5 months. At that time, the fluorescence *in situ* hybridization (FISH) test for WS was not available commercially. We offered Jenny's parents the opportunity to have the test performed as part of a research protocol, and several months later, they chose to have Jenny tested. The results from the FISH test indicating that

---

[1]Jenny's DA as determined based on performance on the Bayley Scales of Infant Development–II (Bayley, 1993) was 6 months. We are well aware of the problems involved in using DA (Mental age) as a control variable (see Mervis & Robinson, 1999). However, both Jenny's physical abilities and her vocal abilities were consistent with the DA obtained from the Bayley–II. For example, she was able to sit unsupported but had not yet begun to crawl, she reached for and manipulated objects she found interesting but was not yet proficient at manipulation, and she produced canonical babble but not variegated babble. Thus, we decided that Jenny's DA was the best measure available for determining an appropriate CA for a younger comparison group.

Jenny has WS were obtained about 1 month after her participation in this cross-sectional study. Jenny was 10 months, 11 days old at the time of this study. She was able to sit without support, but had not begun to crawl. She produced canonical babbles and looked at you if you called her name, but did not understand other words and had not begun to talk. She did not comprehend or produce pointing gestures. Her DA was estimated by interpolating between her raw scores on the Bayley Scales of Infant Development–II (Bayley, 1993) at CAs of 6 and 12 months. The resulting raw score corresponded to a DA of 6 months.

Each of the infants in the CA-matched group was within 10 days of Jenny's CA. Mean CA for this group was 10 months, 15 days (*SD* = 5.90 days). The CA of each infant in the DA-matched group was within 7 days of Jenny's DA (6 months). These infants had a mean CA of 6 months, 1 day (*SD* = 5.29 days).

Setting and Materials

The study was conducted in a comfortable laboratory playroom equipped with two remote-control cameras mounted in diagonally opposed corners of the room. Cameras were operated from an adjoining control room. The person operating the cameras was able to monitor both camera views and recorded the view that provided the most information about where the infant was looking. Split-screen capability was also available and was used as appropriate.

A standard set of age-appropriate toys was used during the play sessions. The toys included two stuffed animals (kitty, dog); a large baby doll; a spider pull toy; a toy bus with removable people; a wooden rattle; a cloth hammer that rattled when shaken; a string of large wooden beads made into a necklace; a slinky; a toy mirror; a clear plastic ball containing a butterfly that rotated on a rod; a weighted plastic ball with a clear top half containing a rocking horse and other small rocking figures, which rattled when shaken; and a set of very large Lego-type blocks in a plastic crate. A long, sausage-shaped pillow was available to provide support for the few infants in the DA group who needed assistance in maintaining a sitting position (e.g., when reaching for toys).

Procedure

Play sessions. The procedure was first explained to the mother during the phone call in which she was invited to participate in the study. When the mother and the infant arrived at the laboratory, the procedure was again explained to the mother while she and the infant were in the waiting room and any questions she had were answered. Once the mother indicated that she understood the procedure and was comfortable participating in the study, she was invited to sign the informed consent form. A researcher then reminded the mother that she should play with her infant as she did at home, and mother and infant went into the playroom and played together for 20 min. After 20 min, a female researcher (henceforth referred to as "stranger") whom the infant had never seen before entered the room, and the mother tried to leave the room unobtrusively. The mothers of 8 of the 10 infants in the DA group and 2 of the 10 infants in the CA group were able to leave without upsetting their infants. If an infant was upset, her mother was asked to remain in the playroom, but to sit in a corner and interact with her infant as little as possible other than to offer reassurance if needed. The same female researcher served as the stranger for all the infants.

Coding. Videotapes were coded for the focus and intensity of the infant's gaze on a second-by-second basis. Both coders were blind as to which infant had WS.

The following codes were used for focus of attention:

1. Partner: Infant is looking at the face of her primary adult partner (mother in the mother–infant play session; stranger in the stranger–infant play session).
2. Toy: Infant is looking at one of the toys or at another object that she is treating as a toy (e.g., fabric of the stranger's skirt, which the infant is fingering; mother's hand during a clapping game).
3. Other Object: Infant is looking at an object that is not a toy and that the infant is not using as a toy (e.g., the floor).
4. Nothing: Infant is not looking at anything in particular or is looking off into space.
5. Adult Other Than Primary Partner: Infant is looking at her mother's face during the stranger–infant play session.
6. Undetermined: Focus of the infant's gaze cannot be determined (e.g., the infant is off camera or is blocked by the adult partner).
7. Crying: Infant is not looking at anything because she is crying.

For analysis purposes, the toy and other object codes were combined into a single object code.

The following codes were used for intensity of gaze:

1. Weak: Infant is looking toward a person or object, but is not attending to it (i.e., infant appears to be looking through the person or object).
2. Typical: Infant is looking at a person or object in a typical manner (i.e., normal range of intensity).
3. Intense: Infant is focused extremely intently on a person or object (i.e., infant's eyes seem to be boring through the person or object).

The primary coder coded all of the videotapes. To assess reliability, the tapes of Jenny's play sessions and those of two randomly chosen infants from each of the control groups were coded independently by a second person. Both coders were blind as to which infant had WS. The focus codes that are important for the statistical analyses to be reported in the Results section are partner, object, and nothing (unengaged). For the eight play sessions involving the ND infants, the percentage of time assigned to these codes by the two coders was quite similar: Mean difference between the two coders for percentage of time assigned was 0.65 for partner, 1.28 for object, and 2.70 for unengaged. For Jenny, the two coders agreed almost perfectly: Differences in percentage of time assigned to each code ranged from 0.16 to 0.35. (Close agreement on Jenny's play sessions is critical because her percentage of time for each code was used as the test value for the statistical analyses, as described in the Results section.) For intensity, agreement was 100% for the infants in the control groups. For Jenny, agreement was 100% for the Level 1 code. The second coder assigned the Level 2 code 3% less often than the original coder and the Level 3 code 5% more often. The analyses reported here are based on the primary (more conservative) coder.

Results

To provide a basis for comparing how infants distributed their gaze during the play sessions, we began by adjusting the total amount of time of the play session to include only the time that the coder was able to determine the focus of the infant's attention and that the infant was in a state conducive to play. Thus, we subtracted the amount of time coded as undetermined, crying, and adult other than primary partner from the total time of the play session. This adjusted length of time for the play session was used as the denominator for converting the partner, object, and nothing looking times to percentages. For each of these percentages, we also determined the proportion of time assigned to each of the three intensities of looking behavior. Mean percentages of codable time assigned to the partner, object, and nothing codes are presented in Table 1, along with standard deviations and ranges. To compare the percentage of time that Jenny spent looking at her partner, at objects, or either (henceforth, "engaged") to that spent by the infants in each of the control groups, we began by conducting one-sample t tests using Jenny's percentage as the test value. All reported p values are two-tailed.

Focus of Attention

Adjusted percentage of time spent looking at partner. Mean adjusted percentages of time spent looking at the partner are presented in Figure 1 separately for each group and each partner. In the mother play session, Jenny spent a significantly larger percentage of time looking at her mother than did either the DA matches,

TABLE 1
Means, Standard Deviations, and Ranges for Percentage of Adjusted Total Time Spent Looking at Partner, Looking at an Object, or Looking at Nothing, as a Function of Group and Play Partner

	Looking at Partner			*Looking at Object*			*Looking at Nothing*		
Group	*M*	*SD*	*Range*	*M*	*SD*	*Range*	*M*	*SD*	*Range*
Jenny									
Mother	21.39			68.84			9.77		
Stranger	27.17			72.32			0.50		
DA control									
Mother	9.86	7.74	2.03–23.83	71.19	11.32	54.66–84.38	18.95	7.95	9.58–30.74
Stranger	14.11	13.48	1.87–48.07	76.65	13.43	49.19–89.83	9.23	5.18	2.74–20.63
CA control									
Mother	5.27	2.93	1.22–9.62	82.90	8.55	61.89–91.68	11.83	7.00	3.73–28.48
Stranger	14.37	4.50	8.60–20.67	73.93	6.46	65.98–82.65	11.69	4.42	5.73–20.53

Note. DA = developmental age; CA = chronological age.

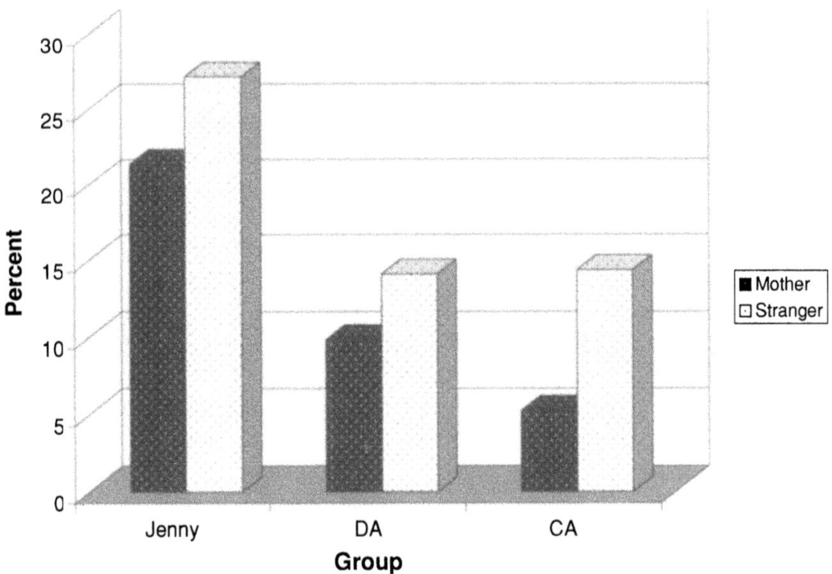

FIGURE 1 Mean adjusted percentage of time spent looking at partner as a function of group and partner.

$t(9) = 4.71$, $p = .001$, or the CA matches, $t(9) = 17.41$, $p < .001$. Jenny's percentage was more that twice as large as the mean of the DA group and four times as large as the mean for the CA group. The partner percentages of only 2 of the infants in the DA group and none in the CA group were as large as Jenny's. In the stranger play session, Jenny spent a significantly larger percentage of time looking at the stranger than did the infants in the CA group, $t(9) = 4.78$, $p = .001$. Although the difference between Jenny's percentage of looking and the DA group's percentage of looking was not significant ($p = .13$), the DA group included a clear outlier whose percentage of looking time at the stranger was more than twice that of any of the other ND infants in the study and more than 2.5 *SD* greater than the mean for the DA group. When this infant was excluded from the analysis, Jenny's percentage of looking time at the stranger was significantly larger than that of the DA group, $t(8) = 7.51$, $p < .001$. The mean percentages (including the outlier) for both of the control groups were only half that of Jenny's. None of the infants in the CA group and only one infant in the DA group (the outlier) evidenced Partner percentages as large as Jenny's.

Adjusted percentage of time spent looking at objects. In Figure 2, the mean adjusted percentages of time spent looking at objects are presented as a function of group and partner. During the mother play session, Jenny and the DA

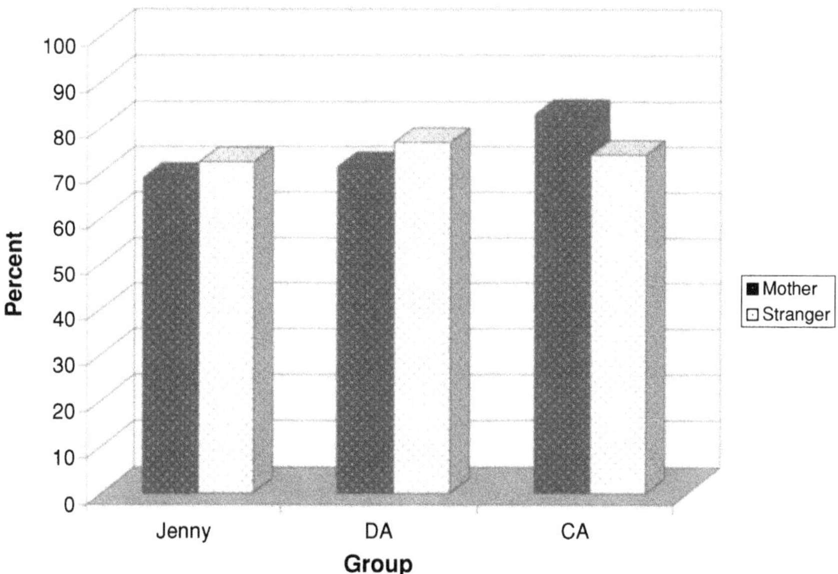

FIGURE 2 Mean adjusted percentage of time spent looking at objects as a function of group and partner.

group spent equivalent percentages of time looking at objects ($p = .53$). However, the CA group spent a significantly larger percentage of time looking at objects than Jenny did, $t(9) = -5.20$, $p = .001$. During the stranger play session, Jenny's percentage of time spent looking at objects was equivalent to the percentages for both the DA group ($p = .33$) and the CA group ($p = .45$).

Adjusted percentage of time engaged. To determine what percentage of the play sessions the infants were engaged, we summed the percentages of time coded as partner and as object. (This is equivalent to subtracting the percentage of time coded as nothing from 100.) In Figure 3, we present the adjusted percentage of time spent engaged as a function of group and partner. During the mother play session, Jenny's percentage engaged was significantly higher than the DA group's, $t(9) = 3.65$, $p = .005$, and equivalent to the CA group's, $p = .38$. Only 2 of the infants in the DA group had equivalent percentages of time engaged as Jenny, whereas 5 of the infants in the CA group had higher percentages of time engaged than Jenny did. Jenny was engaged during virtually the entire stranger play session (99.50%), a significantly larger percentage of time than either the DA group, $t(9) = 5.32$, $p < .001$, or the CA group, $t(9) = 8.01$, $p < .001$. Jenny was engaged a larger percentage of time than any of the control infants.

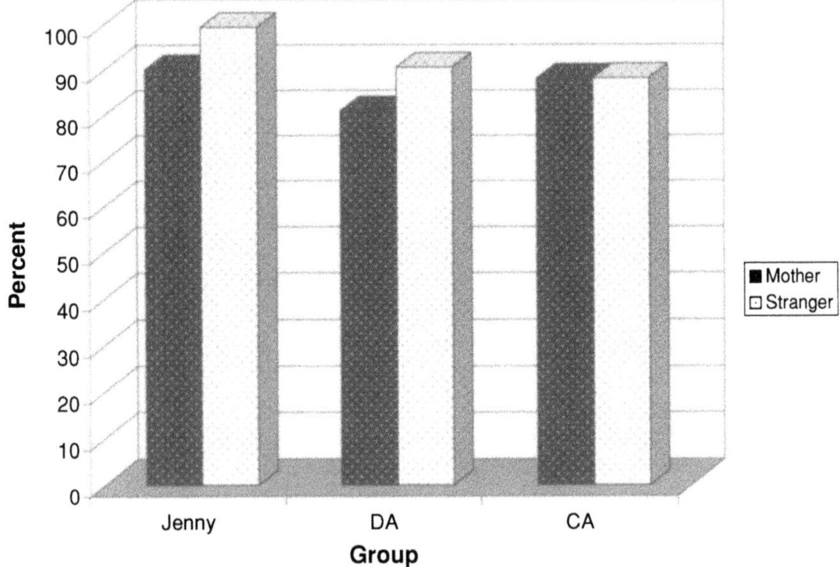

FIGURE 3 Mean adjusted percentage of time spent engaged as a function of group and partner.

Intensity of Looking

Across the 42 play sessions, the weak intensity code (seems to be looking through the partner or object) was used only once. This was for a short look at an object by 1 of the infants in the DA group during the play session with her mother. In the remainder of this section, we consider looks at the typical and intense levels.

Mother play session. For all of the infants in the study, all looks (whether at the partner or an object) during the mother play session were coded as typical (i.e., within the normally expected range of intensity).

Stranger play session. The proportions of looking time coded as intense during the stranger play session are shown in Figure 4 for looking time at partner and Figure 5 for looking time at objects, as a function of group. It is immediately clear from these figures that Jenny's behavior was radically different from that of the infants in either control group. Statistics confirmed the obvious: Jenny spent a significantly larger portion of her partner looking time gazing intensely than either the DA group, $t(9) = 507.95$, $p < .001$, or the CA group, $t(9) = 64.60$, $p < .001$. Nine of the 10 infants in each control group never produced an intense

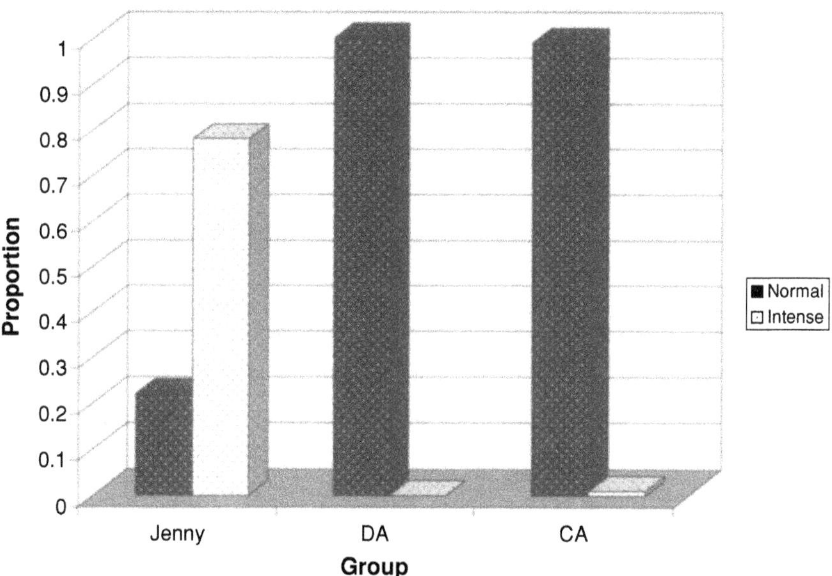

FIGURE 4 Mean proportion of partner looking time coded as normal or intense during play session with stranger.

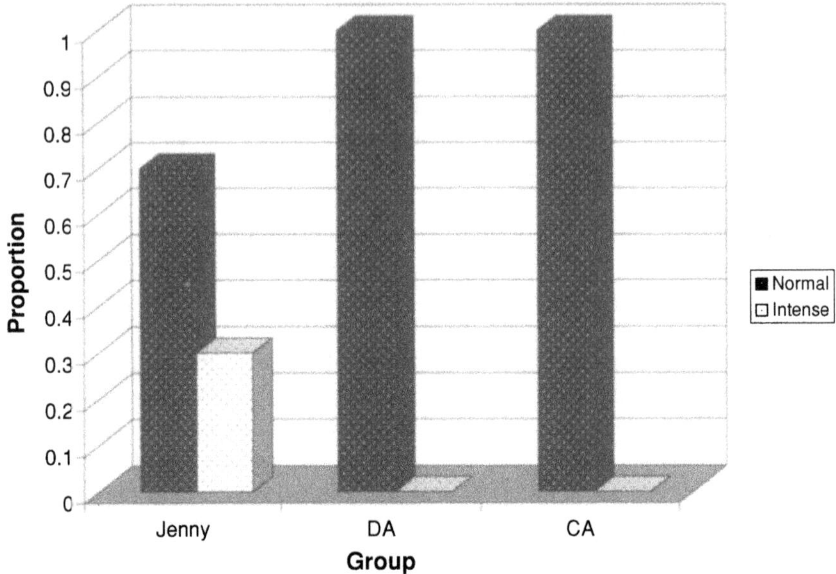

FIGURE 5 Mean proportion of object looking time coded as normal or intense during play session with stranger.

look at her partner. The proportion of partner looking time spent looking intensely was .02 for the remaining infant in the DA group and .12 for the remaining infant in the CA group. In dramatic contrast, the proportion for Jenny was .78.

Although Jenny's proportion of object looking time spent gazing intensely was much lower than her proportion of partner looking time spent gazing intensely, her proportion for objects was still very different from either control group. Jenny's proportion of object looking time spent gazing intensely was significantly greater than that of the DA group, $t(9) = 930.30$, $p < .001$. One infant in the DA group produced one brief intense look at an object, yielding an intense proportion of .0003. None of the other children in the DA group and none of the children in the CA group produced any intense looks at objects.

Brief Discussion

From a quantitative perspective, Jenny's looking behavior differed in two important ways from that of the infants in the control groups. First, Jenny spent far more time looking at her partner, regardless of whether the partner was her mother or the stranger, than the infants in either control group. Second, when the stranger was the partner, Jenny was engaged throughout virtually the whole (99.50%) play session, a higher percentage than any other infant in the study. During the mother session, Jenny's rate of engagement was similar to that of the CA group and significantly greater than that of the MA group.

However, the most dramatic difference between Jenny and the control groups was the qualitative difference in intensity of looking behavior during the stranger session. During the mother play session, none of the infants, including Jenny, ever looked Intensely at either the mother or an object. Thus, although Jenny spent more of the play session looking at her partner than did either of the control groups, and was more engaged overall, there was no qualitative difference in looking behavior. The infants in the control groups maintained their level of looking behavior at the typical level throughout the stranger play session as well. In stark contrast, 78% of the time that Jenny spent looking at the stranger and 30% of the time that Jenny spent looking at objects during the stranger play session were coded as intense. This intense looking behavior was never shown toward objects by any infant in the control group, and was only shown toward the stranger—and only very briefly—by two control infants (one in each group). On several occasions when Jenny was looking intensely at her, the stranger tried to get Jenny to break her gaze by waving a stuffed kitty in front of her face. Although she would occasionally glance briefly at the kitty, Jenny returned almost immediately to looking intently at the stranger's face. Jenny showed this behavior regardless of whether the stranger was talking or not. This behavior was also typical of her interaction with strangers outside of the laboratory, regardless of whether they were talking to her. When Jenny was 9 months old, her mother wrote in a journal she kept regarding Jenny's development that whenever Jenny saw a stranger, "She can just stare you [the stranger] down!!"

These differences between Jenny and the infants in the control groups likely are early signs of the extreme interest individuals with WS show, across the lifespan, in other people. As mentioned in the Introduction, individuals with WS have been described as extremely social in virtually every article reporting behavioral data on the syndrome. Possible reasons for these differences between Jenny and the ND infants, especially those involving Intensity of looking behavior, are addressed in the General Discussion.

These results replicate those of Rice (1992) but with better control. Like Peggy, Jenny spent a much greater proportion of her mother play session looking at her mother than did ND infants matched for either CA or DA. For both Peggy and Jenny, looks at the mother were of normal intensity. Jenny looked much longer at the stranger than the control groups did. Although no control data were available for Peggy, the percentage of time she spent looking at Ari was so high that we can be virtually certain that no control group would have matched it. Most of the looks that Jenny made to the stranger were extremely intense. Although Peggy's looks at Ari were not coded for intensity, everyone who has viewed the videotape has commented spontaneously on the unusual quality of her gaze when it was directed at him.

In summary, we have provided evidence of intense looking behavior by both of the participants we have studied who have WS. In contrast, ND participants did not demonstrate this type of looking behavior. To determine if this type of looking behavior is characteristic of, and largely restricted to, older infants and toddlers with WS, we need to examine both its occurrence in a larger sample of children with WS and in a more varied sample of control participants. Therefore, in Study 2 we take a very different approach to amassing a large sample of infants and toddlers with WS and of similarly aged, and more varied, controls.

STUDY 2

Study 1 took place in a laboratory setting with good experimental control, but suffers from the obvious weakness of small sample size plus the lack of a developmentally delayed control group. In Study 2, we take the opposite approach. This study includes a very large sample of young patients evaluated by a clinical geneticist (Colleen A. Mervis; hereafter, "CAM"). The trade-off is that some experimental control had to be sacrificed. It was not possible to videotape the examinations or to measure looking time precisely. Nevertheless, the extremely large sample size should permit us to determine better how common intense looking behavior is among infants and very young children with a variety of disabilities, many involving developmental delay.

Method

Participants

Participants included 31 children with WS between the ages of 8 and 43 months who were evaluated by CAM. All had genetic deletions of the classic length. Also included were 319 children in this age range who did not have WS who were evaluated by CAM from 1996 through 1999. Thus, there was a total of 350 participants, of whom 273 had developmental delay (31 due to WS and 242 due to other causes). The remaining 87 participants did not have developmental delay. Five of these individuals had familial SVAS caused by mutations of the elastin gene, 4 had small deletions in the WS region but did not have WS, and 78 had been referred for genetic evaluation for a reason not related to developmental delay. The distribution of participants by diagnosis, CA, and sex is shown in Table 2.

TABLE 2
Distribution of Participants by Diagnosis, Chronological Age, and Sex

	Number of Participants							
	8–11 Months		*12–23 Months*		*24–35 Months*		*36–43 Months*	
Diagnosis	*Girls*	*Boys*	*Girls*	*Boys*	*Girls*	*Boys*	*Girls*	*Boys*
Developmental delay								
Williams syndrome	2	1	6	9	4	4	3	2
Other	19	24	55	58	24	30	11	21
No delay								
Familial supravalvar aortic stenosis	0	1	1	2	0	0	0	1
Small deletion	1	1	1	1	0	0	0	0
Other	10	10	18	21	1	7	5	6

Setting

For participants who were seen in Nevada, testing occurred in a typical doctor's examining room, which included chairs for parents and children and an examining table as well as several toys. Participants who were assessed elsewhere were seen in as comparable a setting as possible.

Procedure

Parent(s) and child were taken to the examining room by a staff member or a researcher. The geneticist entered the room, greeted the family, and then began to interview the parents regarding the child's and family's medical history. When the family history was completed, the geneticist asked the mother to seat the child on her lap (if the child was not already sitting there). The geneticist then began the physical exam, which included examining and measuring the child's hands and feet. During this part of the exam, the geneticist noted whether the child consistently looked at her face or instead looked briefly (if at all) at her and then looked at something else, for example, the part of the body the geneticist was examining, the stethoscope that was hanging around her neck, or the child's parents. The geneticist also noted whether the child looked at her intensely or normally.

For 9 participants with WS, 3 with familial SVAS, and 3 with small deletions in the WS region, an additional researcher was present during the physical exam to record the measurements as the geneticist dictated them. This researcher also observed the participant's looking behavior during the hand and foot exam. In most of these cases, the second researcher was not aware of the participant's deletion status. Agreement regarding intensity of looking at the geneticist was 100%. During most of the exams for the remaining participants, a second person (who was not a researcher and generally was not aware of the child's diagnosis) was also present to record measurements. No assistant ever mentioned that any of the participants who did not have WS showed unusual looking behavior. However, it is important to note that these assistants were not explicitly asked to observe looking behavior. One of these assistants also had observed several of the toddler-aged participants with WS while they were in the waiting room and commented spontaneously that these individuals spent a great deal of time looking intensely at her, whereas none of the participants with other diagnoses did so.

Results and Discussion

The proportion of children who looked intensely at the geneticist is indicated in Figure 6, as a function of diagnosis and CA. All of the children who looked intensely at the geneticist also looked primarily at her throughout the examination of their hands and feet. As is clear from the figure, all of the participants who looked intensely had WS; none of the other participants ever looked intensely at the geneticist.[2] Further, these participants looked only briefly (or not at all) at the geneticist while she was measuring their hands and feet. In contrast, a large proportion of the older infant and toddler participants with WS evidenced intense looking behavior. Thus, these findings replicate those of Study 1 for a much larger sample but in a less controlled format.

Intense looking behavior was shown by 23 of the 25 infants and toddlers with WS in the 8- to 11; 12- to 23-, and 24- to 35-month age groups. The most extreme form of intense looking behavior was shown by a 30-month-old, who looked intensely at CAM throughout the genetics exam, including during venipuncture. The finding that almost all of the individuals with WS in this age range showed intense looking behavior to a stranger provides a strong replication of the results of Study 1 in a very different type of situation. Similarly, the finding that none of the control children in Study 2 showed intense looking behavior replicates and extends to children of a wider age range and children with diverse forms of developmental delay the finding from Study 1 that ND infants do not demonstrate unusual intensities of looking.

---

[2]Prior to the interval covered by this study (1996–1999), CAM had evaluated a 14-month-old boy with Kabuki syndrome who evidenced looking behavior that was similar in length to that shown by infants of this age who have WS but was not as intense. He also showed this type of looking behavior at a follow-up visit at age 23 months. Two participants with Kabuki syndrome were included in Study 2; neither showed either extensive or intense looking at CAM.

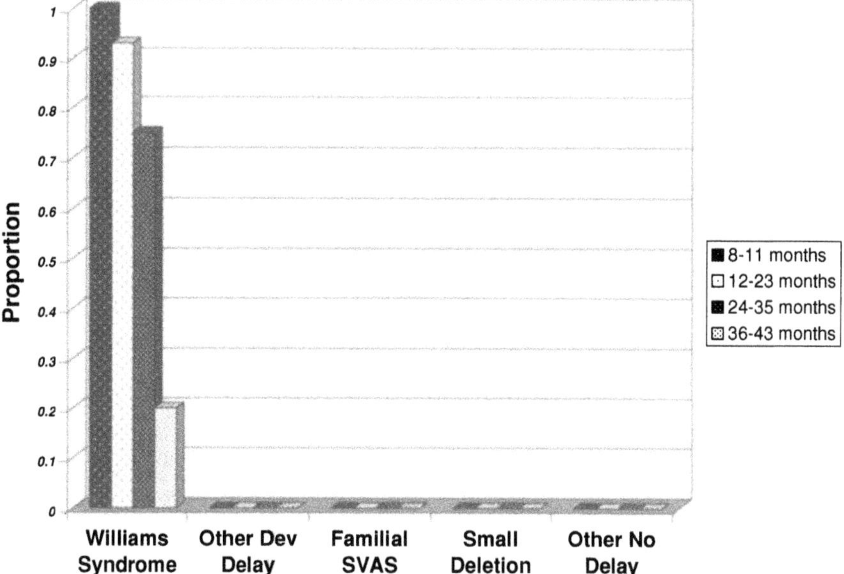

FIGURE 6 Proportion of children who looked intensely at the geneticist as a function of diagnosis and chronological age.

In the 24- to 35-month WS group, the 2 oldest children who showed intense looking behavior were 32 and 33 months old. The group also included a 34-month-old, who did not look intensely at CAM. The 36- to 43-month group included three 36-month-olds; none of them looked intensely at CAM. This pattern of findings suggests the possibility that the end of the period of intense looking at strangers may be relatively sudden. The only child in the 36- to 43-month group who looked intensely at CAM was much more delayed than any of the other 24- to 43-month-olds with WS. Even though they no longer produce intense looks at strangers, however, most individuals with WS continue to spend a great deal of time looking at people.

GENERAL DISCUSSION

The results of the two studies presented in this article clearly show that the looking behavior of infants and young children with WS differs both from ND individuals of the same CA or DA and also from same-CA individuals with developmental delay due to other causes. First, individuals with WS spend considerably more time looking at both their mother (Study 1) and at strangers (Studies 1 and 2) than do individuals who do not have WS. Second, and more dramatically, older infants and toddlers with WS look at strangers with an intensity that is almost never shown by anyone else. We first consider these findings within the framework of previous research on arousal and focused attention by ND infants and young children. We then consider our findings within the context of what is known about temperament and personality of individuals with WS. Finally, we consider the possibility of a genetic basis for the extremely intense looking behavior of infants and toddlers with WS in the presence of strangers.

Arousal and Focused Attention

Attention is controlled by two systems: a lower level orienting/investigative system and a higher level control system. The lower level system is partially functional at birth. At age 1 month, ND infants typically evidence "obligatory attention" (Stechler & Latz, 1996) leading to great difficulty in disengaging from even an unengaging stimulus; often crying is the only way that the infant is able to disengage (Johnson, 1997). However, by age 3 months, ND infants easily disengage from one stimulus (even if it is facelike) to look at another stimulus (Atkinson, 2000). The orienting system is fully functional by age 6 months.

The control system begins to be available between ages 9 and 12 months, but this system is very weak at least until age 18 to 24 months (Ruff & Rothbart, 1996). Thus, all of the participants in Study 1 and most of the participants in Study 2 should have been relying primarily on the orienting/investigative system. This system draws attention to the most salient entity in the environment and maintains attention there until something else becomes more salient. Attention to an entity is a function of arousal. This arousal serves to sustain engagement and to make a person more active and alert toward the target of attention. Jenny and Peggy both demonstrated very high levels of engagement throughout the play sessions with their unfamiliar partner; these levels were significantly higher than those of the MA- and CA-matched groups. Highly increased arousal also is likely responsible for the intense manner in which Jenny and Peggy looked at their unfamiliar play partners.

When arousal during social interaction becomes too high, people typically will look away (Ruff & Rothbart, 1996). This looking-away behavior was shown by all of the ND infants in Study 1 and all of the non-WS participants in Study 2. It also was shown by the stranger in Study 1 and by Ari in our previous study of the looking behavior of a toddler with WS (Rice, 1992). However, it was not shown by either Jenny or Peggy or by most of the younger participants with WS in Study 2, suggesting that they did not find this level of arousal overwhelming.

The behavior of Jenny and Peggy and most of the 8- to 33-month-old participants with WS in Study 2 demonstrates an extreme form of focused attention.

Between ages 5 and 12 months, ND infants show focused attention primarily when an object is new, and for a maximum of 2 to 3 min (Ruff, 1986). In contrast, infants and toddlers with WS maintain focused attention for much longer. Highly focused attention requires blocking of attention to other possible foci. When attention is maintained to the same target for an extended period of time, the intensity of attention increases, leading to attentional inertia (Anderson, Choi, & Lorch, 1987), which in turn makes it likely that attention will continue to be maintained to the same target, even if there is a potentially salient change in the environment (Ruff & Rothbart, 1996). Three examples of highly focused attention leading to high-intensity looking and attentional inertia stand out from these studies. In Study 2, 1 toddler kept her eyes locked on the geneticist's face throughout the genetics evaluation, not even breaking gaze when her blood was being drawn. In Study 1, Jenny locked her eyes onto the stranger's from the time the stranger entered the room. After the stranger was repeatedly unable to entice Jenny to attend to something else, she tried to force Jenny to direct her attention elsewhere by waving a stuffed kitty in front of her face. Jenny glanced briefly at the kitty but then immediately looked around the kitty to resume staring at the stranger. When the stranger moved to a different location, Jenny disengaged attention briefly but then began searching for the stranger; upon finding her, Jenny immediately resumed looking at her intensely. In the pilot study (Rice, 1992), Peggy looked so intensely at Ari that he lay down on the floor and hid his face. Peggy became extremely upset, walked over to him, and crouched down next to his face. When he picked up his head, she cheered up and immediately resumed gazing at him intensely. This cycle was repeated several times. It is possible that these episodes of intense looking are due to obligatory attention leading to difficulty disengaging attention ("sticky fixation"). However, the strategies that older infants and toddlers with WS use to maintain intense attention to people's faces suggest that much of this behavior is voluntary and deliberate. Further, if another novel person enters the child's visual field, the child will disengage attention from the first person and focus intently on the second person. People's faces, especially those of strangers, are considerably more motivating to young children with WS than are toys that ND children find extremely attractive.

Unfortunately, the cost of such highly focused attention, whether deliberate or due to difficulty disengaging attention, is great: This type of attentional behavior leads to a substantial reduction in the individual's ability to monitor the rest of his or her environment. Accordingly, highly focused attention is adaptive only in situations that require attention to detail and to highly organized but nonroutine action (Ruff & Rothbart, 1996). Highly focused attention is detrimental in situations that depend on broad perception of the environment or on flexible responding. By devoting so much of their attention to people's faces rather than to what the person is doing or to other objects in the environment, individuals with WS significantly reduce their opportunities to learn about their world. For example, the insistence of very young children with WS on focusing on their communicative partner's face rather than the object or action to which the partner is pointing (Mervis & Bertrand, 1997) reduces their opportunities to pair labels with their referents, likely leading to a slower rate of vocabulary acquisition.

Temperament and Personality

Motivation, which is tightly tied to emotional reactions, plays a critical role in deploying and maintaining focused attention (Ruff & Rothbart, 1996). This finding, coupled with the attention patterns shown by the participants in this study, indicates that even in infancy, individuals with WS find other people more motivating than do matched ND individuals or individuals who have developmental disability that is not due to WS. In Study 1, Jenny spent twice as much time looking at the stranger as either the group of ND 6-month-olds (DA match) or the group of ND 10-month-olds (CA match) did. Furthermore, most of the time that Jenny spent looking at the stranger was coded as intense, rather than typical. In Study 2, the infants and toddlers with WS spent a large portion of a genetics examination looking at the geneticist, typically very intensely. In contrast, of the more than 300 infants and toddlers who did not have WS, none looked more than briefly at the geneticist, and none looked at her intensely. This very large contrast group included both individuals with developmental delay of other origins and individuals whose intellectual development was normal.

The motivating role of people for infants and toddlers with WS is not limited to people they have not seen before. When playing with her mother, Jenny spent about twice as much time looking at her as infants in the DA group spent looking at their mothers, and more than four times as much as the infants in the CA group did. Similarly, Peggy spent far more time looking at her mother than the older toddlers (who were 4 months younger than her) in Bakeman and Adamson's (1984) study had spent looking at theirs. The percentage of time that Peggy spent looking at her mother was greater even than that spent by considerably younger participants in the Bakeman and Adamson study.

The attention patterns of infants and toddlers with WS presage the patterns of temperament and personality shown by somewhat older children with WS and that continue into adulthood. A result that consistently emerges from studies of temperament and personality is that children and adults with WS are extremely people-oriented. Adjectives that have been used to describe this orientation for children with WS include high in approach (Tomc et al., 1990), overly friendly (Gosch & Pankau, 1996, cited in Gosch & Pankau, 1997), and not reserved toward strangers (Gosch & Pankau, 1997). For adolescents and adults, Dykens and Rosner (1999) described a combination of "often initiates interactions," "never goes unnoticed in groups," and "feels terrible when others are hurt." In all of these studies, the researchers showed that the listed adjectives were significantly more characteristic of people with WS than of people in the comparison groups. These findings provide strong evidence that children and adults with WS are highly motivated to pay attention to other people.

Klein-Tasman and Mervis (this issue) addressed the question of the sensitivity and specificity of the temperamental and personality patterns of 8-, 9-, and 10-year-olds with WS. Their results provide clear evidence that the differences among individuals with WS and individuals with other developmental disabilities continue into middle childhood with regard to pattern of attention to other people. In this study, parental ratings of child temperament on the Children's Behavior Questionnaire (CBQ; Rothbart, Ahadi, & Hershey, 1994) were used to define a temperament profile for children with WS. The resulting profile had a sensitivity of .96 and a specificity of .85. Thus, 96% of the participants with WS, but only 15% of CA- and IQ-matched individuals with other forms of developmental disability fit this profile. The profile is based on ratings from two of the CBQ scales: Sociability (Shyness, reverse-coded) and Empathy. The Sociability factor is transparently related to the attention behavior shown by older infants and toddlers in the research reported here. Empathy has not been directly considered in studies of toddlers with WS. However, their consistent focus on other people would be expected to yield frequent opportunities to notice another person's distress. Parents have reported numerous anecdotes suggesting that toddlers with WS already are often aware of other people's distress and offer comfort when they realize someone is upset.

Genetic Basis for the Attention Patterns of Infants and Toddlers with Williams Syndrome

WS is caused by a microdeletion of about 1.5 megabases of the long arm of chromosome 7 (7q11.23). So far, 17 genes have been assigned to the deleted region (Osborne et al., 2001). More than 98% of individuals with WS have the same deletion breakpoints; the resulting deletion is referred to as the "classic" or "common" WS deletion (Morris & Mervis, 2000). Deletion breakpoints have been determined for both Peggy and Jenny and for the participants in Study 2; in all cases, deletions have been found to be classic. Virtually all of the participants with WS between the ages of 8 and 33 months evidenced an unusual attention pattern, characterized by extreme interest in other people as measured by both amount of time spent looking at a partner and intensity of gaze at strangers. In contrast, this pattern was not shown by any of the ND participants. Further, the pattern was not shown by any of the infants or toddlers with other developmental disabilities, including those who had been clinically diagnosed with WS but did not have a deletion. This set of findings strongly suggests that there is a genetic substrate to the attention patterns shown by infants and toddlers with WS, involving one or more of the deleted genes (in interaction with multiple genes from outside the deleted region and with environmental factors).

All of the participants with WS had the same deletion and thus were missing copies of the same genes, and almost all of the 8- to 33-month-old participants with WS evidenced unusual looking behavior. Thus, we know that when all of these genes are missing, the phenotype includes unusual interest in people and intense looking during infancy and toddlerhood. To determine if this phenotype would also result from smaller deletions in the region, it is necessary to examine the looking behavior of individuals with such deletions. Thus, consideration of these individuals should be helpful in determining which genes in the classic deletion region might be involved in biasing the development of infants and toddlers with WS such that they show these unique attention patterns. Nine relevant infants or toddlers were included in Study 2; none of these participants showed unusual looking behavior. Five of these participants had SVAS caused by subtle mutations of the *elastin* gene (*ELN*). Two participants had deletions of part of *ELN* and all of the *LIM-kinase1* (*LIMK1*) gene; one had deletion of *ELN, LIMK1*, and the *replication factor C subunit 2* (*RFC2*) gene. (These deletions are described in Frangiskakis et al., 1996.) Although characterization of the remaining participant's deletion is not yet complete, it has been determined that his deletion includes *ELN, LIMK1*, and *RFC2*, plus additional genes. The penetrance of the unusual-looking-behavior phenotype is close to 100% for children with WS in the age range of the participants with small deletions. Thus, given that none of the participants with small deletions has shown unusual looking behavior, it is likely that hemizygosity of only the genes included in their deletions does not bias development in the direction of unusual looking behavior. As individuals with different small deletions are identified, it may be possible to determine which genes are involved in biasing development in the direction of extreme interest in looking at people, accompanied by unusually intense looking behavior. We have argued that this looking behavior is an early manifestation of the WS personality phenotype. Thus, hemizygosity of the same genes is likely involved in biasing development toward these personality characteristics.

We are not suggesting that there is a gene or genes for intense looking or for the WS personality phenotype. These behavioral characteristics are manifestations of a developmental process involving cascades of genes and transactions with the environment at all levels (e.g., cellular, whole organism, external). We believe that the typical cascades and transactions involved in shaping the organism such that the development of normal looking patterns ensues are altered by the hemizygous deletion of one or more of the genes deleted in WS, yielding the unusual looking patterns and extreme interest in other people associated with WS.

In conclusion, our findings indicate that infants and toddlers who have WS manifest an extreme interest in looking at other people (whether novel or familiar).

Further, looks directed at strangers are characteristically very intense. This pattern was not shown by either same-CA individuals who had developmental delays of other etiologies or same-MA or same-CA ND individuals, suggesting that these looking patterns may be unique to WS. Further, these looking behaviors are likely an early manifestation of the WS personality phenotype, which is shaped by the effects of hemizygosity for one or more genes in the deleted region on the genetic and environmental cascades that affect the structure and functioning of the developing brain.

ACKNOWLEDGMENTS

This research was supported by Grant No. HD29957 from the National Institute of Child Health and Human Development and by Grant No. NS35102 from the National Institute of Neurological Disorders and Stroke. We thank all of the participants and their families. Some of the research presented in this article was included in Cathy Rice's and Susanna Kwitny's honors theses submitted to Emory University. Portions of the research were presented at the 11th Biennial International Conference on Infancy Studies, Atlanta, Georgia, in April 1998 and at the David W. Smith Workshop on Malformations and Morphogenesis, Whistler, British Columbia, in August 1998.

REFERENCES

Adamson, L. B. (1995). *Communication development during infancy*. Madison, WI: WCB Brown & Benchmark.

Anderson, D. R., Choi, H. P., & Lorch, E. P. (1987). Attentional inertia reduces distractibility during young children's TV viewing. *Child Development, 58,* 798–806.

Atkinson, J. (2000). *The developing visual brain*. Oxford, England: Oxford University Press.

Bakeman, R., & Adamson, L. B. (1984). Coordinating attention to people and objects in mother–infant and peer–infant interaction. *Child Development, 55,* 1278–1289.

Bayley, N. (1969). *Bayley Scales of Infant Development*. New York: Psychological Corporation.

Bayley, N. (1993). *Bayley Scales of Infant Development* (2nd ed.). San Antonio, TX: Psychological Corporation.

Bruner, J. (1975). From communication to language: A psychological perspective. *Cognition, 3,* 255–287.

Dilts, C., Morris, C. A., & Leonard, C. O. (1990). Hypothesis for development of a behavioral phenotype in WS. *American Journal of Medical Genetics Supplement, 6,* 126–131.

Dykens, E. M., & Rosner, B. A. (1999). Refining behavioral phenotypes: Personality-motivation in Williams and Prader–Willi syndromes. *American Journal on Mental Retardation, 104,* 158–169.

Frangiskakis, J. M., Ewart, A. K., Morris, C. A., Mervis, C. B., Bertrand, J., Robinson, B. F., et al. (1996). LIM-kinase1 hemizygosity implicated in impaired visuospatial constructive cognition. *Cell, 86,* 59–69.

Gosch, A., & Pankau, R. (1994). Social–emotional and behavioral adjustment in children with Williams–Beuren syndrome. *American Journal of Medical Genetics, 53,* 335–339.

Gosch, A., & Pankau, R. (1997). Personality characteristics and behaviour problems in individuals of different ages with WS. *Developmental Medicine and Child Neurology, 39,* 327–533.

Johnson, M. H. (1997). *Developmental cognitive neuroscience.* Cambridge, MA: Blackwell.

Klein-Tasman, B. P., & Mervis, C. B. (2003/this issue). Distinctive personality characteristics of 8- 9-, and 10-year-olds with Williams syndrome. *Developmental Neuropsychology, 23,* 271–292.

Mervis, C. B., & Bertrand, J. (1997). Developmental relations between cognition and language: Evidence from Williams syndrome. In L. B. Adamson & M. A. Romski (Eds.), *Communication and language acquisition: Discoveries from a typical development* (pp. 75–106). New York: Brookes.

Mervis, C. B., & Robinson, B. F. (1999). Methodological issues in cross-syndrome comparisons: Matching procedures, sensitivity (*Se*), and specificity (*Sp*). *Monographs of the Society for Research in Child Development, 64* (Serial no. 256), pp. 115–130.

Morris, C. A., & Mervis, C. B. (2000). WS and related disorders. *Annual Review of Genomics and Human Genetics, 1,* 461–464.

Osborne, L. R., Li, M., Pober, B., Chitayat, D., Bodurtha, J., Mandel, A., et al. (2001). A 1.5 million-base pair inversion polymorphism in families with Williams–Beuren syndrome. *Nature Genetics, 29,* 321–325.

Rice, C. E. (1992). *The development of joint attention by a young child with WS.* Unpublished honors thesis, Emory University, Atlanta, GA.

Rothbart, M. K., Ahadi, S. A., & Hershey, K. L. (1994). Temperament and social behavior in childhood. *Merrill-Palmer Quarterly, 40,* 21–39.

Ruff, H. A. (1986). Components of attention during infants' manipulative exploration. *Child Development, 57,* 105–114.

Ruff, H. A., & Rothbart, M. K. (1996). *Attention in early development: Themes and variations.* New York: Oxford University Press.

Ruff, H. A., & Saltarelli, L. M. (1993). Exploratory play with objects: Basic cognitive processes and individual differences. In M. H. Bornstein & A. W. O. Reilly (Eds.), *New directions for child development: Vol. 59. The role of play in the development of thought* (pp. 5–15). San Francisco: Jossey-Bass.

Schaffer, H. R. (1984). *The child's entry into a social world.* London: Academic.

Stechler, G., & Latz, E. (1966). Some observations on attention and arousal in the human infant. *American Academy of Child Psychiatry, 5,* 517–525.

Tager-Flusberg, H., & Sullivan, K. (1999, April). *Are children with WS spared in theory of mind?* Paper presented at the biennial meeting of the Society for Research in Child Development, Albuquerque, NM.

Tomc, S. A., Williamson, N. K., & Pauli, R. M. (1990). Temperament in WS. *American Journal of Medical Genetics, 36,* 345–352.

Distinctive Personality Characteristics of 8-, 9-, and 10-Year-Olds With Williams Syndrome

Bonita P. Klein-Tasman
University of Wisconsin-Milwaukee

Carolyn B. Mervis
University of Louisville

Although previous research and clinical observation have indicated that individuals with Williams syndrome have a distinctive personality, an empirically derived personality profile has not been developed. The objective of the current investigation was to develop a personality profile that is descriptive of and distinctive to children with Williams syndrome. Participants were 23 8- to 10-year-old children with Williams syndrome and 20 8- to 10-year-old children with developmental disabilities of other etiologies. Participant groups had equivalent intellectual abilities. Parents completed measures of childhood temperament (Children's Behavior Questionnaire [CBQ]) and personality (parent report, short form of Multidimensional Personality Questionnaire [MPQ]). Using group comparisons and signal detection theory, we contrasted the personality characteristics of children with Williams syndrome and children with developmental disabilities of other etiologies. On the CBQ, high mean ratings on shyness (reverse-coded) and empathy together characterized 96% of the children in the Williams syndrome group, but only 15% of the mixed etiology group. On the MPQ, high ratings on items measuring certain characteristics combined (gregarious, people-oriented, tense, sensitive, and visible) were characteristic of 96% of the Williams syndrome group but only 15% of the mixed etiology group. The personality profiles emerging from the CBQ and MPQ provide a crucial step toward investigations of genotype/phenotype relations.

"They show outstanding loquacity and a great ability to establish interpersonal contacts. This stands against a background of insecurity and anxiety" (von Arnim

Requests for reprints should be sent to Bonita P. Klein-Tasman, Department of Psychology, University of Wisconsin-Milwaukee, P.O. Box 413, Milwaukee, WI 53201. E-mail: bklein@uwm.edu

& Engel, 1964, p. 376). This early description of the personality of individuals with Williams syndrome effectively captures the current conceptualization that the distinctive personality of individuals with Williams syndrome is characterized by a strong interest in social interaction with others with an undercurrent of anxiety. Now that the genetic basis of Williams syndrome is known, the search for an empirically validated method by which to measure the Williams syndrome personality is more critical. Such a method would facilitate genotype–phenotype investigations of the Williams syndrome personality. In this investigation, we asked parents of 8-, 9-, and 10-year-old children with Williams syndrome (Williams syndrome group) or other developmental disabilities (mixed etiology group) to complete the Children's Behavior Questionnaire (CBQ; Rothbart & Ahadi, 1994) and a modified parent-report version of the Multidimensional Personality Questionnaire (MPQ; Tellegen, 1985), measures of temperament and personality. These questionnaires were chosen because they reflect biologically minded theories of personality and together cover the lifespan. We examined parent responses for evidence of unique personality characteristics typical of children with Williams syndrome within this age range.

MODELS OF TEMPERAMENT AND PERSONALITY

Most contemporary approaches to the study of personality converge on three to five main dimensions for the description of personality (often referred to as the Big Three or Big Five), seen as applicable across the lifespan (Digman, 1990; Goldberg, 1993). In the following subsections we briefly outline two of the three-factor theories that provide a framework for the measures included in this investigation. Both approaches are emotion-based conceptualizations of personality and are consistent with Gray's (1987) neuropsychological approach to personality. Together, these approaches have the potential to assess temperament and personality across the lifespan.

Tellegen's Three-Factor Model

Tellegen's (1985) interest lies in the relation between mood and personality. His model has traditionally been used with adult populations. The factors included in Tellegen's model are Positive Emotionality, Negative Emotionality, and Constraint. Tellegen discussed the correspondence between his model of personality and Gray's (1987) neuropsychological personality theory. In particular, Tellegen (1985) posits that his Positive Emotionality construct reflects reward-signal sensitivity (Gray's Behavioral Activation System) and his Negative Emotionality construct reflects punishment-signal sensitivity (Gray's Behavioral Inhibition

System). Sociability is seen as a reflection of high Positive Emotionality, whereas impulsivity is seen as a reflection of low Constraint. Tellegen et al. (1988) found that the Positive Emotionality construct appears to be made up of two somewhat separable constructs: Agentic Positive Emotionality and Communal Positive Emotionality. Communal Positive Emotionality reflects interpersonal aspects of personality and affect. Agentic Positive Emotionality is more strongly a measure of desire for achievement.

Rothbart's Psychobiological Approach

At the core of Rothbart's (1986) approach is a commitment to developmental theory. Rothbart defines temperament as "constitutionally based individual differences in reactivity and self-regulation with 'constitutional' referring to the relatively enduring biological makeup of the individual, influenced over time by heredity, maturation, and experience" (p. 356). Similarly to Tellegen (1985) behaviors are seen as reflective of the child's biological system (individual differences in susceptibility of primary emotions), shaped by maturation and experience. Rothbart's (1994) childhood model of personality (Rothbart & Ahadi, 1994) grew out of the study of infant temperament and an interest in developmental continuity of temperament. Rothbart and colleagues (Rothbart, 1981; Rothbart & Derryberry, 1981) focused on variables likely to have an inherited basis and to show consistency over time, and showed convergence between parent questionnaire and observational findings. In later research, Rothbart and colleagues (Rothbart, 1994; Rothbart & Ahadi, 1994; Rothbart, Ahadi, & Hershey, 1994) expanded and extended the infancy research to assess personality in childhood. Analysis of parental ratings of their children's behavior using the CBQ yielded a three-factor model of personality, which is shown in Table 1. Surgency refers to expressions of positive emotion such as smiling and laughter, approach behavior, and activity level. Negative Affectivity refers to expressions of negative emotions such as discomfort, fear, and anger. Effortful Control refers to regulatory mechanisms of attention and inhibitory control.

PERSONALITY CHARACTERISTICS OF CHILDREN WITH WILLIAMS SYNDROME

Tomc, Williamson, and Pauli (1990) examined the temperament of 204 children who had been diagnosed with Williams syndrome (aged 1–12 years) by comparing parents' ratings to norms for children developing normally. Parents completed one of three temperament questionnaires, depending on the child's age. Each of the questionnaires yielded scores for nine temperamental characteristics, based on

TABLE 1
Children's Behavior Questionnaire Scales and Factor Structure

Higher Order Factor	*Scale*
Surgency	Approach
	High-Intensity Pleasure
	Smiling and Laughter
	Activity
	Impulsivity
	Shyness (reverse-coded)
Negative Affectivity	Discomfort
	Fear
	Anger/Frustration
	Sadness
	Falling Reactivity and Soothability (reverse-coded)
Effortful Control	Inhibitory Control
	Attentional Focusing
	Low-Intensity Pleasure
	Perceptual Sensitivity (reverse-coded)
Scales not included in the factor scores	Aggression
	Empathy
	Guilt and Shame
	Help-Seeking
	Negativism
	Motor Activation
	Waking
	Drowsy

Thomas and Chess's (1977) approach to temperament. Relative to chronological age (CA) norms, the children with Williams syndrome were rated as significantly more approaching, significantly higher in intensity, distractibility, negative mood, and significantly lower in persistence and threshold of excitability. The researchers also estimated the mental age of the children with Williams syndrome and compared the children to the norms for those ages. The same pattern of findings held. Given that no contrast group of individuals with other etiologies of mental retardation was included, it is difficult to determine whether these findings are characteristic of individuals with mental retardation in general or particularly of individuals with Williams syndrome.

Studies in which ratings of individuals with Williams syndrome are compared to those of CA-matched individuals with other developmental disabilities are especially critical in delineating the characteristics that are specific to a particular syndrome, rather than more generally related to the developmental disability (see Dykens & Rosner [1999] for a more comprehensive discussion.) Children with Williams syndrome have been shown to be more anxious, more fearful, more curious, and less reserved toward strangers in comparison to children with Down syndrome or Brachman–de Lange syndrome (Gosch & Pankau, 1996, cited in Gosch & Pankau, 1997). Van Lieshout, De Meyer, Curfs, and Fryns (1998) administered a Dutch translation of the California Q-set (Block & Block, 1980) to parents of children with Prader–Willi syndrome, fragile-X syndrome, Williams syndrome, or CA-matched children developing normally. The Williams syndrome group, composed of individuals aged 2.5- to 19-years-old, was rated higher on measures of Agreeableness than the Prader–Willi syndrome group, but similarly to normally developing controls. The Williams syndrome group evidenced less Conscientiousness than either the normal or the fragile-X groups. There were no differences among the four groups on Extraversion. All three syndrome groups showed less Emotional Stability, less Openness, and more Irritability than normal controls.

Dykens and Rosner (1999) compared the personality and motivational profiles of adolescents and adults with Williams syndrome, Prader–Willi syndrome, or developmental disability of mixed etiology, using the Reiss Profiles of Fundamental Goals and Motivation Sensitivities for Persons with Mental Retardation (Reiss & Havercamp, 1998). Although there were significant differences across groups on 11 of 15 motivational domains, domain scores did not yield characteristics that were specific to individuals with Williams syndrome. Based on group comparisons, the Williams syndrome group was rated higher on the items "often initiates interactions with others," "never goes unnoticed when in a group," and "has many fears." In addition, the Williams syndrome group was rated significantly higher than the other groups on the item "feels terrible when others are hurt," which Dykens and Rosner (1999) discussed as reflecting particularly high empathy. Both the Williams syndrome and the Prader–Willi syndrome groups showed "strong desires to help others" and were "very happy when others do well." Discriminant analysis of ratings at the item level indicated that the groups could be distinguished based on a set of nine items together. These items correctly classified 89% of the individuals with Williams syndrome.

Tager-Flusberg and colleagues have conducted experimental research related to the social relatedness of individuals with Williams syndrome. Tager-Flusberg, Boshart, and Baron-Cohen (1998) found that adults with Williams syndrome are able to infer emotion from the eye region of a person's face as well as could adults developing normally and better than a matched group of adults with Prader–Willi syndrome. In an investigation of the capacity of children with Williams syndrome to read others' negative emotions and show empathy, Tager-Flusberg and Sullivan (1999) found that children with Williams syndrome showed much more concern than IQ-matched children with Prader–Willi syndrome when an experimenter appeared to have hurt her knee. The children with Williams syndrome were also significantly more likely to offer comfort or validation.

Studies examining the problem behaviors of children with developmental disabilities have also provided insight into the personality characteristics of individuals with Williams syndrome. Generally, children with Williams syndrome are seen as having attention problems compared with norms for children developing normally (Dilts, Morris, & Leonard, 1990; Greer, Brown, Pai, Choudry, & Klein, 1997; Pagon, Bennett, LaVeck, Steward, & Johnson, 1987). However, comparisons of children with Williams syndrome to children with other developmental disabilities indicate that these attention problems are likely not specific to Williams syndrome (e.g., Sarimski, 1997). Some findings that appear to be specific to Williams syndrome, relevant to the current investigation, are that children with Williams syndrome are more likely to be rated as worrying, talking too much, and being overfriendly to strangers (Sarimski, 1997). They are less likely than children with other developmental disabilities to be rated as self-conscious (Sarimski, 1997). Udwin and Yule (1991) also found that teachers reported that significantly more children with Williams syndrome than children with other developmental disabilities were fearful and fussy.

In sum, previous research is suggestive that there are personality characteristics that are more likely to be seen in children with Williams syndrome than in either children developing normally or children with other developmental disabilities. In particular, children with Williams syndrome are consistently rated as more approaching of others, more empathic, and less shy, and there is evidence for more worry and anxiety in children with Williams syndrome than in children with other developmental disabilities. With the exception of Dykens and Rosner (1999), studies have focused on evidence of broad group differences, rather than examining closely the effectiveness of personality characteristics at discriminating between individuals with different etiologies of developmental disability.

RATIONALE AND HYPOTHESES

The primary objective of the current investigation was to identify personality characteristics that together are both descriptive of and specific to individuals with Williams syndrome, as a necessary step toward investigations of genotype–phenotype relations. The CBQ, a measure of childhood temperament, and a short parent-report form of the MPQ, a measure of personality, were used to assess personality. On both measures, group differences at the broad, higher order factor level were not expected to provide the best basis on which to distinguish between the groups. By definition, the broad factors include many discrete personality characteristics; only some of these were expected to show group differences.

Given previous research, the following findings were expected for the measures used in this study. At the scale level on the CBQ, previous research suggests that children with Williams syndrome should be distinguishable from children with other developmental disabilities based on their lack of shyness (i.e., high sociability), high approach behavior, and high empathy. There is no direct measure of worry or anxiety on the CBQ; however, it is possible that children with Williams syndrome would differ from children in the contrast group in ratings of fear. Differences at the lower order factor level of the MPQ could be expected on Social Closeness and on Stress Reaction because the children with Williams syndrome would be expected to be rated higher on the majority of items on each of these scales. However, examination of ratings at the item level was expected to be more promising for the accurate description of the distinctive personality of children with Williams syndrome, given that such consideration enables exclusion of items not expected to be characteristic of children with Williams syndrome. At the item level of the MPQ, children with Williams syndrome were expected to differ from children with other developmental disabilities on the following items: Gregarious, Tense, People-Oriented, Sensitive, and Visible.

METHOD

Participants

Participants were twenty-three 8-, 9-, and 10-year-old children with Williams syndrome (11 girls, 12 boys) and twenty 8-, 9-, and 10-year-old children with developmental disabilities of other etiologies (8 girls, 12 boys). Parents of all of the children with Williams syndrome reported positive genetic testing results for Williams syndrome. Three additional children had been clinically diagnosed with Williams syndrome, but were included in the mixed etiology group because of negative genetic test results. The composition of the mixed etiology group is delineated in Table 2.

Parents of 1 child with Williams syndrome did not complete the CBQ, and parents of a different child with Williams syndrome did not complete the MPQ. Hence, there are 22 participants with Williams syndrome and 20 children with other etiologies of developmental disabilities in the analyses of the CBQ and MPQ. Mean chronological age for the Williams syndrome group was 9 years, 2 months (range = 8 years, 1 months–10 years, 11 months). For the mixed etiology group, mean chronological age was 9 years, 6 months (range = 8 years, 3 months–10 years, 10 months).

Participant recruitment was on a volunteer basis as follows. Participants for both groups were recruited at the 1998 National Williams Syndrome Association convention and at the 1998 Southeastern Williams Syndrome Association regional convention. (Individuals who have received a clinical diagnosis of Williams syndrome, but are later found not to meet genetic criteria for Williams syndrome, often attend these conventions.) The Williams syndrome group also

TABLE 2
Etiology of Developmental Disability for the Mixed Etiology Group

Number	*Etiology*
1	Down syndrome
1	Fetal alcohol syndrome
2	Fragile X syndrome
1	Sotos syndrome
1	4p-
1	9p-
1	Lactic acidosis
1	Neurofibromatosis
1	Autism
2	Pervasive Developmental Disorder–Not Otherwise Specified
8	Unknown etiology[a]

[a]Three of these children had previously been clinically diagnosed with Williams syndrome, but were later found not to have deletions of 7q11.23.

included all 8-, 9-, and 10-year-olds we were able to locate in Kentucky, Indiana, and Nevada and in the Chicago, Cleveland, and Atlanta areas. Children were identified based on Williams Syndrome Association, geneticist, and parent referrals. Participants in the mixed etiology group were also identified based on referrals from a collaborating clinical geneticist in Nevada, referrals from the Developmental Disorders Clinic at University of Chicago Hospitals, and recruitment from a school for English-speaking children with developmental disabilities in Montreal, Canada. Children who were referred for evaluation due to suspected Williams syndrome, but who were later found not to meet the genetic criterion, were also included in the mixed etiology group. These children came from midwestern or southeastern states. The native language of all participants in both groups was English.

Materials

Materials included a measure of intellectual abilities and two parent-report measures of temperament or personality.

Kaufman Brief Intelligence Test. The Kaufman Brief Intelligence Test (K–BIT; Kaufman & Kaufman, 1990) is a brief, individually administered measure of verbal and nonverbal intelligence. It consists of two subtests: Vocabulary, which assesses word knowledge and verbal concept formation, and Matrices, which measures ability to perceive relationships and complete analogies. The measure yields three standard scores: one for each subtest and an overall composite score (IQ). Normative data collected on a representative national sample are available for individuals aged 4 to 90 years.

Children's Behavior Questionnaire. The Long Form of the CBQ (Rothbart & Ahadi, 1994) contains 327 statements about child behaviors in typical situations. The CBQ was constructed to bridge the gap between typical infant/toddler measures of temperament and adult personality measures. The parent is asked to indicate how typical a given behavior is of their child, using a 7-point scale (1–7). Items omitted or marked "not applicable" by parents were not included in scale scores. Examples include, "My child laughs a lot at jokes and silly happenings" and "My child will move from one task to another without completing any of them." Factor structure and scale names are presented in Table 1. This measure has been developed for use with children developing normally aged 3 to 8 years.

Multidimensional Personality Questionnaire–Parent Version. The MPQ (Tellegen, 1985) was originally constructed as a self-report measure for adults. It was later shortened and modified for children, in order to be used as a parent-report measure in the Minnesota longitudinal twin project (S. O. Lilienfeld, personal communication, February 1996). Parents are presented with a series of adjectives and accompanying descriptions of individuals high and low on each adjective and are asked to rate their own child on a 4-point scale. Factor structure and item names are indicated in Table 3.

Procedure

Participants and their parents were first informed of the general purpose of the study and consent for participation was obtained. The parents of all participants were asked to complete several questionnaires including the CBQ and the parent-report short form of the MPQ. Children completed a battery of cognitive and language measures including an assessment of intellectual abilities (K–BIT). Data collection took place either at the home of the participant, in a quiet space at a conference hotel or school, or at university facilities.

RESULTS

In the following sections, we describe the results from analyses of the CBQ and the MPQ separately. Group comparison methods were used to examine differences between the Williams syndrome group and the mixed etiology group in personality characteristics that we expected would differ for the two groups. Informed by the group difference findings, signal detection theory was then used to develop a Williams Syndrome Personality Profile. More specifically, the factors

TABLE 3
MPQ Factor Structure and Scales (Four-Factor Model)

Higher Order Factor	*Lower Order Factor*
Communal Positive Emotionality	Well-Being
	Social Potency
	Social Closeness (doubled)
Agentic Positive Emotionality	Well-Being
	Social Potency
	Achievement (doubled)
Negative Emotionality	Stress Reaction
	Aggression
	Alienation
Constraint	Harm-Avoidance
	Control versus Impulsiveness
	Traditionalism
Not loading primarily on any factor	Absorption

or items that showed the strongest evidence of group difference were examined individually and in combination for sensitivity (i.e., probability of hits) and specificity (i.e., probability of correct rejections) for identifying children with Williams syndrome. Receiver operating characteristic (ROC) curves or "isosensitivity" curves (Levine & Parkinson, 1994) were examined to aid in the determination of the most effective cut points on a given dimension to maximize sensitivity and specificity. This method of analysis has been advocated for the development of diagnostic systems (Swets, 1988). In this study, we used the cut point that maximized sensitivity and specificity. A critical value of $p < .01$ was used.

Kaufman Brief Intelligence Test

Mean IQ for the mixed etiology group was 74.20 ($SD = 14.26$, range = 47–96) for all analyses. For the CBQ analyses, mean IQ in the Williams syndrome group was 70.59 ($SD = 13.79$, range = 49–98). The two groups did not differ in intellectual abilities, $t\,(40) = .83, p = .41$. For the MPQ analyses, mean IQ in the Williams syndrome group was 71.23 ($SD = 13.31$, range = 49–98). Once again, the groups had equivalent IQs, $t\,(40) = .70, p = .49$.

Children's Behavior Questionnaire

As discussed, higher order factors were not expected to distinguish best between the groups. Although differences were not hypothesized, independent-sample *t* tests were conducted to explore the possibility of meaningful group differences in CBQ higher order factor scores. Descriptive statistics, *t* values, and significance levels are indicated in Table 4. No significant group differences were found, but there was a trend toward higher Negative Affectivity for the Williams syndrome group.

Independent-sample *t* tests were conducted to explore group differences in CBQ scale scores. Descriptive statistics, *t* values, and *p* values are presented in Table 5. As predicted, the Williams syndrome group was rated significantly higher than the mixed etiology group on Empathy and Approach. Also as predicted, the Williams Syndrome group was rated significantly lower than the Mixed Etiology group on Shyness. A significant difference between groups was also found for Sadness.

The scales that distinguished well between the groups were then examined for evidence of sensitivity and specificity. As indicated in Table 6, the Empathy scale was most effective at identifying the Williams syndrome and the mixed etiology groups (sensitivity [*Se*] = .82, specificity [*Sp*] = .80), followed by the Shyness (*Se* = .82, *Sp* = .75) and then the Approach (*Se* = .73, *Sp* = .70) and the Sadness scales (*Se* = .73, *Sp* = .70).

To improve the potential for even better discrimination between the groups, composite scores composed of the mean of ratings on more than one scale were examined. The Shyness scale was transformed so that higher values were more characteristic of Williams syndrome and was renamed Sociability. We began first with the scales showing the strongest ability to distinguish between the groups, adding, one at a time based on the strength of *D* values, items showing weaker ability to distinguish between the groups. As indicated in Table 6, the combination of scales most effective at distinguishing between the groups was Empathy and Sociability together, which resulted, with a cut point of 5.1, in a specificity of .96 and a sensitivity of .85. Hence, the mean scale score of the Empathy and Sociability scale scores (CBQ Williams Syndrome Personality Profile) correctly identified 21 of 22 participants with Williams syndrome and 17 of 20 of the participants with other

TABLE 4
Mean Rating and Standard Deviations on CBQ Higher Order Factors[a]

	Williams Syndrome Group		*Mixed Etiology Group*			
Factor	*M*	*SD*	*M*	*SD*	*t value*	*p*
Surgency	5.06	0.37	4.84	0.54	1.62	.12
Negative Affectivity	4.55	0.44	4.19	0.51	2.46	.02
Effortful Control	4.28	0.58	4.25	0.53	0.21	.84

Note. CBQ = Children's Behavior Questionnaire.
[a]Ratings range from 1 to 7, with higher ratings reflecting stronger presence of characteristic.

TABLE 5
Mean Rating and Standard Deviations on CBQ Subscales[a]

	Williams Syndrome Group		*Mixed Etiology Group*			
Subscale	*M*	*SD*	*M*	*SD*	*t value*	*p*
Activity	4.52	1.00	4.89	0.68	−1.34	.19
Approach	5.88	0.62	5.35	0.62	2.81	.009
High-Intensity Pleasure	4.04	0.83	4.49	0.86	−1.72	.10
Impulsivity	4.51	0.47	4.65	0.53	−0.90	.31
Shyness	2.20	0.59	3.80	1.40	−4.92	<.001
Smiling and Laughter	5.62	0.44	5.44	0.73	0.96	.76
Anger/Frustration	4.90	0.63	4.68	0.73	1.05	.30
Discomfort	4.54	0.53	4.20	0.70	1.79	.08
Fear	4.50	0.75	4.25	1.08	0.84	.40
Sadness	4.77	0.69	4.16	0.72	2.82	.007
Attentional Focusing	3.12	0.98	3.50	0.77	−1.40	.17
Inhibitory Control	3.39	0.80	3.71	0.82	−0.88	.37
Low-Intensity Pleasure	5.34	0.52	4.90	0.83	2.09	.05
Perceptual Sensitivity	5.28	0.90	4.98	0.70	1.22	.23
Falling Reactivity and Soothability	3.96	0.78	4.36	0.76	−1.69	.10
Aggression	4.09	1.08	4.14	1.06	−0.14	.89
Empathy	5.79	0.62	4.58	0.76	5.64	<.001
Guilt/Shame	4.92	0.74	4.25	0.93	2.59	.01
Help-Seeking	5.26	0.61	4.86	0.49	2.28	.03
Negativism	4.47	0.81	4.41	0.78	0.02	.98
Motor Activation	3.90	1.00	3.88	0.98	0.08	.93
Waking	3.77	1.97	3.00	1.72	1.34	.18
Drowsy	4.32	1.82	4.60	1.99	−0.48	.63

Note. CBQ = Chidren's Behavior Questionnaire.
[a]Ratings range from 1 to 7, with higher ratings reflecting stronger presence of characteristic.

developmental disabilities. The participants in the mixed etiology group who were misclassified are one child with neurofibromatosis, one child with lactic acidosis, and one child with developmental disability of unknown etiology.

Multidimensional Personality Questionnaire

The MPQ comprises 34 items loading on 11 factors, which themselves load on three primary higher order factors: Positive Emotionality, Negative Emotionality, and Constraint. Tellegen et al. (1988) advocated a four-factor solution (see Table 3), with Positive Emotionality subdivided into Communal Positive Emotionality and Agentic Positive Emotionality. Factor scores were scored as the mean of the item ratings loading on the factor. Krueger et al. (1996) described Tellegen's (1985) instructions for composing the higher order factors. Specifically, Constraint was scored as Control + Harm Avoidance + Traditionalism, Negative Emotionality was scored as Stress Reaction + Alienation + Aggression, Agentic Positive Emotionality was scored as Well-Being + Social Potency + 2 × (Achievement), and Communal Positive Emotionality was scored as Well-Being + Social Potency + 2 × (Social Closeness). The mean higher order factor ratings for each group are indicated in Table 7. At the broad, higher order factor level, the Williams syndrome group was rated significantly higher in Communal Positive Emotionality than was the mixed etiology group. ROC analysis indicated that Communal Positive Emotionality was moderately successful at

TABLE 6
Results of ROC Analysis of CBQ Scales and Composite Scales

Scale	*D*[a]	*p*	*Cut Point*[b]	*Se*	*Sp*
Empathy	.90	<.001	5.3	.82	.80
Shyness[c]	.83	<.001	2.57	.82	.75
Approach	.75	.005	5.65	.73	.70
Sadness	.72	.016	4.4	.73	.70
Empathy, Sociability[d]	.96	<.001	5.1	.96	.85
Empathy, Sociability, Approach	.95	<.001	5.25	.91	.85
Empathy, Sociability, Sadness	.93	<.001	4.83	.91	.85
Empathy, Sociability, Approach, Sadness	.93	<.001	5.00	.91	.85

Note. ROC = receiver operating characteristic; CBQ = Children's Behavior Questionnaire; *Se* = sensitivity; *Sp* = specificity.
[a]*D* refers to the area under the ROC curve. [b]Ratings range from 1 to 7, with higher ratings reflecting stronger presence of characteristic. [c]On this scale, a low score is more indicative of Williams syndrome. [d]Sociability is Shyness reverse-coded.

TABLE 7
Mean Rating and Standard Deviations on MPQ Higher Order Factors[a]

	Williams Syndrome Group		*Mixed Etiology Group*			
Higher Order Factor	*M*	*SD*	*M*	*SD*	*t value*	*p*
Agentic Positive Emotionality	8.85	1.51	9.22	1.85	−0.71	.48
Communal Positive Emotionality	13.00	1.21	11.48	1.97	3.04	.004
Negative Emotionality	6.35	1.17	5.90	1.63	1.03	.31
Constraint	6.95	1.29	7.53	0.75	−1.75	.09

Note. MPQ = Multidimensional Personality Questionnaire.
[a]Possible range of scores for Agentic Positive Emotionality is 4 to 16, for Communal Positive Emotionality is 4 to 16, for Negative Emotionality is 3 to 12, and for Constraint is 3 to 12.

classifying the participants ($D = .75, p = .006$), but with inadequate sensitivity ($Se = .68$) and specificity ($Sp = .60$).

Next, the three lower order factors that included the items predicted to show group differences were examined: Social Closeness, Social Potency, and Stress Reaction. Independent-sample *t* tests were conducted to explore the possibility of meaningful group differences on these factors. Descriptive statistics, *t* values, and significance levels for all lower order factors are indicated in Table 8. Children with Williams syndrome were rated significantly higher than the children in the mixed etiology group on Social Closeness and Stress Reaction. The groups were not significantly different in Social Potency or on any other lower order factor. The sensitivity and specificity of each scale for which significant group differences were found were examined and then combinations of factors were examined. As indicated in Table 9, the Composite score composed of the mean of the Social Closeness and Stress Reaction factors was most effective at discriminating between the Williams syndrome and the mixed etiology groups ($D = .90$, $p < .001$, $Se = .86$, $Sp = .75$).

The distinctive characteristics of children with Williams syndrome were expected to be best captured by individual items on the MPQ rather than the factors; the latter include some items for which group differences would not be expected. Hence, group differences at the item level were examined. Descriptive statistics are presented in Table 10. Children with Williams syndrome were rated significantly higher on all five of the items expected to best distinguish between the groups: Gregarious, People-Oriented, Tense, Sensitive, and Visible.

TABLE 8
Mean Rating and Standard Deviations on MPQ Lower Order Factors[a]

	Williams Syndrome		*Mixed Etiology*			
Lower Order Factor	*M*	*SD*	*M*	*SD*	*t value*	*p*
Well-Being	3.17	.42	3.11	.62	0.310	.773
Social Closeness	3.68	.43	3.01	.56	4.36	<.001
Social Potency	2.47	.49	2.33	.70	0.74	.493
Achievement	1.61	.60	1.88	.56	−1.54	.123
Stress Reaction	3.14	.57	2.35	.68	4.08	<.001
Aggression	1.59	.49	1.87	.70	−1.49	.156
Alienation	1.62	.61	1.68	.70	−0.31	.806
Harm Avoidance	2.50	.57	2.70	.43)	−1.27	.211
Control vs. Impulsivity	1.82	.58	2.07	.44	−1.55	.126
Traditionalism	2.64	.70	2.77	.39	−0.73	.448
Absorption	2.85	.66	2.70	.71	0.70	.472

Note. MPQ = Multidimensional Personality Questionnaire.
[a]Ratings range from 1 to 4, with higher ratings reflecting stronger presence of characteristic.

TABLE 9
Results of ROC Analysis of MPQ Scales

Scale	*D*[a]	*p*	*Cut Point*[b]	*Se*	*Sp*
Social Closeness	.84	<.001	3.1	.91	.65
Stress Reaction	.81	.001	2.5	.86	.60
Social Closeness, Stress Reaction	.90	<.001	2.9	.86	.75

Note. ROC = receiver operating characteristic; MPQ = Multidimensional Personality Questionnaire; *Se* = sensitivity; *Sp* = specificity.
[a]*D* refers to the area under the ROC curve. [b]Ratings range from 1 to 4, with higher ratings reflecting stronger presence of characteristic.

Composite ratings were then computed by calculating the mean of two or more item scores. First, the items showing the strongest ability to distinguish between the groups were examined, adding, one at a time based on strength of *D* values, items showing weaker ability to distinguish between the groups. As illustrated in Table 11, the combination of items most effective at discriminating between the groups was Gregarious, People-Oriented, Tense, Sensitive, and Visible, which, with a cut point of 2.9, resulted in a specificity of .96 and a sensitivity of .85. Hence, using the mean score of these items (MPQ Williams Syndrome Personality Profile), 21 of 22 participants with Williams syndrome were correctly included[1] and 17 of 20 of the participants with other developmental disabilities were correctly excluded. Two misclassified children in the mixed etiology group were different from the one misclassified according to the CBQ. These were one child with Down syndrome and one child with Pervasive Developmental Disability–Not Otherwise Specified. The participant with neurofibromatosis who showed the Williams syndrome profile using the CBQ also showed the profile using the MPQ. Findings in the literature suggest that the personality of this child is atypical because neurofibromatosis is usually associated with shyness and social withdrawal (Nilsson & Bradford, 1999; Udwin & Dennis, 1995).

DISCUSSION

Previous descriptions of children with Williams syndrome point toward a personality profile distinctively characterized by high sociability, empathy, and anxiety. In this study, we examined the effectiveness of two parental-report measures (CBQ and MPQ) at capturing this distinctive personality. Children with Williams syndrome emerged as clearly distinguishable from children with other developmental disabilities based on specific personality characteristics. Two measures of

[1]The child with Williams syndrome who was not captured by these items was not the same child as the one who was not captured by the CBQ Empathy and Shyness scales.

TABLE 10
Mean Rating and Standard Deviations for Items on MPQ Social Closeness, Social Potency, and Stress Reaction Scales[a]

Scale	*Williams Syndrome*		*Mixed Etiology*			
Item	*M*	*SD*	*M*	*SD*	*t value*	*p*
Social Closeness						
Gregarious	3.40	0.80	2.55	0.89	3.65	.002
People-Oriented	3.72	0.46	2.85	0.75	4.65	< .001
Affectionate	3.81	0.40	3.65	0.59	1.10	.36
Stress Reaction						
Tense	3.05	0.79	2.10	0.79	3.89	.001
Sensitive	3.63	0.58	2.75	0.91	3.80	.001
Even-Tempered[b]	2.72	0.98	2.20	1.06	1.67	.11
Social Potency						
Persuasive	2.27	0.97	2.05	0.94	0.75	.53
Dominance	1.59	0.59	2.30	0.98	−2.87	.01
Visible	3.54	0.59	2.65	1.04	3.46	.002

Note. MPQ = Multidimensional Personality Questionnaire.

[a]Possible scale scores range from 1 to 4, with higher ratings reflecting stronger presence of characteristic. [b]This scale is reverse-coded; high numbers reflect low Even-Temperedness.

TABLE 11
Results of ROC Analysis of MPQ Items

Item	*D*[a]	*p*	*Cut Point*[b]	*Se*	*Sp*
People-Oriented	.82	<.001	3.5	.73	.85
Gregarious	.79	.001	2.5	.91	.50
Sensitive	.78	.002	3.5	.67	.80
Tense	.78	.002	2.5	.73	.65
Visible	.75	.006	2.5	.95	.45
People-Oriented, Gregarious	.86	<.001	3.2	.82	.80
People-Oriented, Gregarious, Sensitive	.90	<.001	2.8	.91	.70
People-Oriented, Gregarious, Sensitive, Tense	.92	<.001	2.8	.91	.85
People-Oriented, Sensitive, Gregarious, Tense, Visible	.97	<.001	2.9	.96	.85

Note. ROC = receiver operating characteristic; MPQ = Multidimensional Personality Questionnaire; *Se* = sensitivity; *Sp* = specificity.

[a]*D* refers to the area under the ROC curve. [b]Ratings range from 1 to 4, with higher ratings reflecting stronger presence of characteristic.

personality yielded similarly high sensitivity and specificity for identifying the Williams syndrome personality. In particular, high mean ratings of Sociability and Empathy, as measured by the CBQ, correctly classified 21 of 22 participants with Williams syndrome and 17 of 20 participants with other developmental disabilities. Relatively high mean ratings of the items Gregarious, People-Oriented, Tense, Sensitive, and Visible together, as measured by the MPQ, also correctly classified 21 of 22 participants with Williams syndrome and 17 of 20 participants with other developmental disabilities. Hence, 8-, 9-, and 10-year-old children with Williams syndrome show a distinctive set of personality characteristics across measures. Children with Williams syndrome are much more likely to show this pattern than are children with other developmental disabilities. This finding is promising for genotype/phenotype investigations that require identification of distinctive characteristics.

The CBQ and MPQ ratings reflected very similar aspects of the Williams syndrome personality, with the MPQ perhaps more clearly capturing the undercurrent of anxiety so often reported in the literature. The distinctiveness of the Williams syndrome personality appears to lie in the focus of children with Williams syndrome on others: Children with Williams syndrome are eager to establish interactions with others, are frequently noticed by others, and show a distinctive attunement, either through empathy or sensitivity, to others' emotions. The sociability of children with Williams syndrome was reflected on the CBQ by low Shyness ratings and on the MPQ by high ratings on the items People-Oriented, Gregarious, and Visible. The anxiety of children with Williams syndrome was clearly captured by the MPQ on the items Tense and Sensitive. Although the anxiety of children with Williams syndrome is not immediately evident from examination of the CBQ findings, Derryberry and Rothbart (1997) argued that anxious adults generally tend to be more empathic than adults who are not anxious (Dias & Pickering, 1993). Thus, the undercurrent of anxiety often observed in children with Williams syndrome may be reflected in the high Empathy ratings for the Williams syndrome group on the CBQ. It appears that anxiety related to social situations is what is particularly distinctive of the children with Williams syndrome in this study.

This study included a mixed etiology group composed of children with a wide variety of diagnoses as well as children with no known etiology of developmental disorder, hence broadening the evidence for specificity of the Williams syndrome personality. The results of this study highlight the importance of comparing the personality characteristics of children with Williams syndrome with those of children with other developmental disabilities. As compared with MA or CA norms, Tomc et al. (1990) found that children with Williams syndrome were rated as significantly more approaching, significantly higher in intensity, distractibility, and negative mood, and significantly lower in persistence and threshold of excitability. The pattern of findings is quite different when comparisons are made to CA- and IQ-matched children with other forms of developmental disabilities. In particular, whereas the Williams syndrome group was found to be significantly higher in approach, there were no differences between groups for distractibility, negativity, or threshold of excitability. It is likely that the latter characteristics are a function of developmental delay rather than being syndrome-specific.

The results of this study lend support to and extend previous findings in the Williams syndrome literature. The high Social Closeness ratings indicate that children with Williams syndrome are particularly related to others, which could be seen as consistent with van Lieshout et al.'s (1998) findings of high agreeableness. The CBQ findings are consistent with those of Dykens and Rosner (1999), who found that for adolescents and adults, lack of shyness and high empathy were particularly characteristic of individuals with Williams syndrome. The results of our study indicate that these distinctive characteristics are apparent by age 8 to 10 years. The finding that children with Williams syndrome are rated by their parents as more empathic toward others than were the children in the mixed etiology group is consistent with Tager-Flusberg and Sullivan's (1999) experimental findings that children with Williams syndrome are more likely than children with Prader–Willi syndrome to behave empathically.

The interest of children with Williams syndrome in others is evident very early in their development. Mervis et al. (this issue) reported the results of two investigations of the face-watching behavior of infants or toddlers with Williams syndrome in comparison to children developing normally. Looking at faces is seen by Rothbart (1986) as reflective of sociability. In a case of an infant with Williams syndrome, the infant's tendency to look at faces intensely was particularly strong when she was interacting with a stranger. However, she also spent twice as much time looking at her mother as did MA- or CA-matched children who were developing normally. The unusually intense face-watching behavior shown by this infant when interacting with a stranger was also observed in a larger sample of infants and toddlers with Williams syndrome interacting with a physician and was distinct from the looking behavior of a large contrast group of children with other developmental disabilities. Hence, the intense looking behavior of infants and toddlers with Williams syndrome is not simply a function of their developmental delay. As discussed in Mervis et al. (this issue), very young children with Williams syndrome emerge as distinctive both in the amount of time they attend to faces and in the intensity of their gaze at faces. Hence, there is clear evidence that children with Williams syndrome have high motivation to interact with others, even from a very young age.

Implications

In this study, two different measures of personality were deliberately chosen to enable extension to younger and older individuals with Williams syndrome. Both measures successfully captured the aspects of personality central to the behavior of children with Williams syndrome, providing evidence for the construct validity of current conceptualizations of personality. The CBQ, a measure of temperament typically used with young children (age 3–8 years), and the MPQ, a measure of personality originally developed for use with adults, both succeeded in capturing the distinctiveness of the Williams syndrome personality for 8- to 10-year-olds. In future investigations, the CBQ can be used to examine the temperamental characteristics of younger children with Williams syndrome, whereas the MPQ can be used to examine the personality characteristics of older children, adolescents, and adults with Williams syndrome. This opportunity has the potential to increase our understanding of the development of temperament and personality in individuals with Williams syndrome by examining temperament and personality across the lifespan.

Relatedly, current findings provide evidence for an effective means of identifying the Williams Syndrome Personality Profile. Such an empirically derived profile is critical to genotype/phenotype investigations of personality in Williams syndrome and related genetic disorders. Williams syndrome is caused by a microdeletion of about 1.5 megabases of chromosome 7q11.23 (Morris & Mervis, 2000). Only a subset of the genes deleted in the Williams syndrome region is potentially involved in the Williams syndrome personality. Some individuals have microdeletions in the Williams syndrome region that do not span the full length of the deletion; examination of their personality may help delineate the genes relevant to personality in Williams syndrome (Frangiskakis et al., 1996). This investigation provides us with promising tools for measuring the personality phenotype of individuals with Williams syndrome or with smaller deletions within the Williams syndrome region.

In conclusion, our findings indicate that 8-, 9-, and 10-year-old children with Williams syndrome manifest a distinctive personality profile. Examination of parent ratings on the CBQ, a measure of childhood temperament, indicates that this pattern is characterized particularly by high levels of sociability and empathy. Examination of parent ratings on the MPQ, a measure of personality, similarly indicates that this pattern is characterized by an eagerness to interact with others as well as high levels of tension and sensitivity. We were able to distinguish between the Williams syndrome and mixed etiology groups with high sensitivity and specificity based on both sets of characteristics: All but one of the children with Williams syndrome fit each of the profiles; in contrast, very few of the children with other developmental disabilities showed this distinctive pattern of characteristics. These findings provide further evidence that temperamental characteristics are at least partly genetically determined (e.g., Benjamin, Ebstein, & Belmaker, 1997). The distinctiveness of the Williams syndrome personality provides the groundwork for investigations of the genetic basis of this pattern in Williams syndrome. It is important to note that we are not suggesting that only children with

Williams syndrome will show this pattern of characteristics. There are likely many pathways to a given personality. The distinctiveness of the Williams syndrome group provides a natural opportunity to investigate one such genetic pathway. Similarly, we are not suggesting that children with Williams syndrome show these fully developed characteristics even in infancy. The Williams syndrome personality phenotype is shaped both by the genetics of Williams syndrome and transactions with the environment.

ACKNOWLEDGMENTS

This research was supported by Grant No. NS35102 from the National Institute of Neurological Disorders and Stroke and by Grant No. HD29957 from the National Institute of Child Health and Human Development. We thank the participants and their families and the National Williams Syndrome Association. Mary Beth Whittle and Florence Chang assisted us with data collection. Colleen Morris, Gloria Cherney, Lauren Wakschlag, and Cathy Lord helped with participant recruitment. We are grateful to Scott Lilienfeld for providing us with the modified child parent-report version of the Multidimensional Personality Questionnaire and Mary K. Rothbart for allowing us to use the Children's Behavior Questionnaire.

REFERENCES

Benjamin, J., Ebstein, R. P., & Belmaker, R. H. (1997). Personality genetics. *Israel Journal of Psychiatry and Related Sciences, 34,* 270–280.

Block, J. H., & Block, J. (1980). The role of ego-control and ego-resiliency in the organization of behavior. In W. A. Collins (Ed.), *Development of cognition, affect, and social relations. Minnesota Symposia on Child Psychology* (Vol. 13, pp. 39–101). Hillsdale, NJ: Lawrence Erlbaum Associates, Inc.

Derryberry, D., & Rothbart, M. K. (1997). Reactive and effortful processes in the organization of temperament. *Development and Psychopathology, 9,* 633–652.

Dias, A., & Pickering, A. D. (1993). The relationship between Gray's and Eysenck's personality spaces. *Personality and Individual Differences, 15,* 297–306.

Digman, J. M. (1990). Personality structure: Emergence of the five-factor model. *Annual Review of Psychology, 41,* 417–440.

Dilts, C. V., Morris, C. A., & Leonard, C. O. (1990). Hypothesis for development of a behavioral phenotype in Williams syndrome. *American Journal of Medical Genetics Supplement, 6,* 126–131.

Dykens, E. M., & Rosner, B. A. (1999). Refining behavioral phenotypes: Personality-motivation in Williams and Prader–Willi syndromes. *American Journal on Mental Retardation, 104,* 158–169.

Frangiskakis, J. M., Ewart, A. K., Morris, C. A., Mervis, C. B., Bertrand, J., Robinson, B. F., et al. (1996). LIM-kinase1 hemizygosity implicated in impaired visuospatial constructive cognition. *Cell, 86,* 59–69.

Goldberg, L. R. (1993). The structure of phenotypic personality traits. *American Psychologist, 48,* 26–34.

Gosch, A., & Pankau, R. (1996). Psychologische aspekte beim Williams–Beuren syndrom. *Forum Kinderarzt, 9,* 8–11.

Gosch, A., & Pankau, R. (1997). Personality characteristics and behaviour problems in individuals of different ages with Williams syndrome. *Developmental Medicine and Child Neurology, 39,* 327–533.

Gray, J. A. (1987). The neuropsychology of emotion and personality. In S. M. Stahl, S. D. Iversen, & E. C. Goodman (Eds.), *Cognitive neurochemistry* (pp. 171–190). Oxford, England: Oxford University Press.

Greer, M. K., Brown, F. R., Pai, G. S., Choudry, S. H., & Klein, A. J. (1997). Cognitive, adaptive, and behavioral characteristics of Williams syndrome. *American Journal of Medical Genetics (Neuropsychiatric Genetics), 74,* 521–525.

Kaufman, A. S., & Kaufman, N. L. (1990). *Kaufman Brief Intelligence Test.* Circle Pines, MN: American Guidance Service.

Krueger, R. F., Caspi, A., Moffitt, T. E., Silva, P. A., & McGee, R. (1996). Personality traits are differentially linked to mental disorders: A multitrait-multidiagnosis study of an adolescent birth cohort. *Journal of Abnormal Psychology, 105,* 299–312.

Levine, G., & Parkinson, S. (1994). Detection, discrimination, and the theory of signal detection. In G. Levine & S. Parkinson (Eds.), *Experimental methods in psychology* (pp. 204–233). Hillsdale, NJ: Lawrence Erlbaum Associates, Inc.

Mervis, C. B., Morris, C. A., Klein-Tasman, B. P., Bertrand, J., Kwitny, S., Appelbaum, G., et al. (2003/this issue). Attentional characteristics of infants and toddlers with Williams syndrome during triadic interactions. *Developmental Neuropsychology, 23,* 245–270.

Morris, C. A., & Mervis, C. B. (2000). Williams syndrome and related disorders. *Annual Review of Genomics and Human Genetics, 1,* 461–484.

Nilsson, D. E., & Bradford, L. W. (1999). Neurofibromatosis. In S. Goldstein & C. R. Reynolds (Eds.), *Handbook of neurodevelopmental and genetic disorders in children* (pp. 350–367). New York: Guilford.

Pagon, R. A., Bennett, F. C., LaVeck, B., Stewart, K. B., & Johnson, J. (1987). Williams syndrome: Features in late childhood and adolescence. *Pediatrics, 80,* 85–91.

Reiss, S., & Havercamp, S. M. (1998). Toward a comprehensive assessment of fundamental motivation: Factor structure of the Reiss Profiles. *Psychological Assessment, 10,* 97–106.

Rothbart, M. K. (1981). Measurement of temperament in infancy. *Child Development, 52,* 569–578.

Rothbart, M. K. (1986). Longitudinal observation of infant temperament. *Developmental Psychology, 22,* 356–363.

Rothbart, M. K. (1994). Broad dimensions of temperament and personality. In P. Ekman & R. J. Davidson (Eds.), *The nature of emotion: Fundamental questions* (pp. 337–341). New York: Oxford University Press.

Rothbart, M. K., & Ahadi, S. A. (1994). Temperament and the development of personality. *Journal of Abnormal Psychology, 103,* 55–66.

Rothbart, M. K. & Derryberry, D. (1981). Development of individual differences in temperament. In M. E. Lamb & A. L. Brown (Eds.), *Advances in developmental Psychology: Vol. 1* (pp. 37–86). Hillsdale, NJ: Lawrence Erlbaum Associates, Inc.

Rothbart, M. K., Ahadi, S. A., & Hershey, K. L. (1994). Temperament and social behavior in childhood. *Merrill-Palmer Quarterly, 40,* 21–39.

Sarimski, K. (1997). Behavioural phenotypes and family stress in three mental retardation syndromes. *European Journal of Child and Adolescent Psychiatry, 6,* 26–31.

Swets, J. A. (1988). Measuring the accuracy of diagnostic systems. *Science, 240,* 1285–1293.

Tager-Flusberg, H., & Sullivan, K. (1999, April). *Are children with Williams syndrome spared in theory of mind?* Paper presented at the biennial meeting of the Society for Research in Child Development, Albuquerque, NM.

Tager-Flusberg, H., Boshart, J., & Baron-Cohen, S. (1998). Reading the windows to the soul: Evidence of domain-specific sparing in Williams syndrome. *Journal of Cognitive Neuroscience, 10,* 631–639.

Tellegen, A. (1985). Structures of mood and personality and their relevance to assessing anxiety, with an emphasis on self-report. In A. H. Tuma & J. D. Maser (Eds.), *Anxiety and the anxiety disorders* (pp. 681–716). Hillsdale, NJ: Lawrence Erlbaum Associates, Inc.

Tellegen, A., Lykken, D. T., Bouchard, T. J., Wilcox, K. J., Segal, N. L., & Rich, S. (1988). Personality similarities in twins reared apart and together. *Journal of Personality and Social Psychology, 54,* 1031–1039.

Thomas, A., & Chess, S. (1977). *Temperament and development.* New York: Bruner/Mazel.

Tomc, S. A., Williamson, N. K., & Pauli, R. M. (1990). Temperament in Williams syndrome. *American Journal of Medical Genetics, 36,* 345–352.

Udwin, O., & Dennis, J. (1995). Psychological and behavioral phenotypes in genetically determined syndromes: A review of research findings. In G. O'Brien & W. Yule (Eds.), *Behavioural phenotypes* (pp. 90–208). London: MacKeith.

Udwin, O., & Yule, W. (1991). A cognitive and behavioral phenotype in Williams syndrome. *Journal of Clinical and Experimental Neuropsychology, 13,* 232–244.

van Lieshout, C. G. M., De Meyer, R. E., Curfs, L. M. G., & Fryns, J. (1998). Family contexts, parental behaviour, and personality profiles of children and adolescents with Prader–Willi, fragile-X, or Williams syndrome. *Journal of Child Psychology and Psychiatry, 39,* 699–710.

von Arnim, G., & Engel, P. (1964). Mental retardation related to hypercalcaemia. *Developmental Medicine and Child Neurology, 6,* 366–377.

Anxiety, Fears, and Phobias in Persons With Williams Syndrome

Elisabeth M. Dykens
Division of Child and Adolescent Psychiatry
University of California, Los Angeles, Neuropsychiatric Institute

Although much research has focused on the cognitive–linguistic profile associated with Williams syndrome, studies have yet to follow up on preliminary observations suggesting increased anxiety and fears in persons with this disorder. To this aim, Study 1 compared fears in 120 participants with Williams syndrome to 70 appropriately matched persons with mental retardation of mixed etiologies. Study 2 assessed differences in parent versus child reports of fears in 36 Williams syndrome and 24 comparison group parent–child dyads. In Study 3, rates of phobia and other anxiety disorders were assessed in standardized psychiatric interviews with the parents of 51 individuals with Williams syndrome. Relative to their counterparts, persons with Williams syndrome had significantly more fears as well as a wider range of frequently occurring fears, as reported by either parents or participants themselves. Children in both groups reported more fears than their parents. Whereas generalized and anticipatory anxiety were found in 51% to 60% of the sample with Williams syndrome, specific phobia was more prevalent, with 96% showing persistent and marked fears and 84% avoiding their fears or enduring them with distress. The feasibility of cognitive–behavioral treatments for phobia is discussed, as are implications for future research.

Identified just 41 years ago, Williams syndrome has emerged as one of the field's most intriguing genetic disorders. Affecting about 1 in 20,000 people, Williams syndrome is caused by a microdeletion on one of the chromosome 7's that includes the gene for elastin (Ewart et al., 1993). Elastin insufficiency is associated with the cardiovascular disease often found in persons with this syndrome, especially supravalvar aortic stenosis (Ewart, Jin, Atkinson, Morris, & Keating, 1994). Other

---

Requests for reprints should be sent to Elisabeth M. Dykens, University of California, Los Angeles, Neuropsychiatric Institute, Division of Child and Adolescent Psychiatry, 760 Westwood Plaza, Los Angeles, CA 90024. E-mail: edykens@mednet.ucla.edu

features of Williams syndrome include musculoskeletal and renal abnormalities, distinctive facial features, and hyperacusis (Pober & Dykens, 1996).

Williams syndrome is perhaps best known for its unusual cognitive–linguistic profile, even in the face of global mental retardation. Many children and adults with Williams syndrome show significant, relative weaknesses in visual–spatial functioning, including integrating parts into a whole (Bihrle, Bellugi, Delis, & Marks, 1989). Despite these difficulties, facial recognition is well-preserved, and many persons with Williams syndrome are adept at reading and remembering faces and facial expressions (Bellugi, Wang, & Jernigan, 1994). Relative strengths in expressive language are sometimes seen, with language being characterized by well-developed vocabulary, syntax, sematics, and prosody (e.g., Reilly, Klima, & Bellugi, 1990; Udwin & Yule, 1990). Yet these linguistic strengths may not be as widespread nor as spared or pronounced as originally thought (for reviews see Dykens, Hodapp, & Finucane, 2000; Mervis, Morris, Bertrand, & Robinson, 1999).

In contrast, the maladaptive or psychiatric features of Williams syndrome have yet to be systematically studied. Such inattention to psychiatric problems may reflect diagnostic overshadowing or the tendency for clinicians and researchers to attribute psychiatric symptoms in people with mental retardation to their cognitive delay (Reiss, Levitan, & Szyszko, 1982). Yet relative to the general population, children and adults with mental retardation are actually at increased risk for maladaptive behavior and psychiatric disorders (Dykens, 1999, 2000). Many children with Williams syndrome, for example, show inattention, hyperactivity, and full-blown attention deficit hyperactivity disorder, even as compared to others with mental retardation (Einfeld, Tonge, & Florio, 1997; Preuss, 1984; Tomc, Williamson, & Pauli, 1990). Impulsivity and inattention may be associated with a "classic" Williams syndrome personality, described as overly aroused, socially disinhibited, and indiscriminately friendly (Dykens & Rosner, 1999; Gosch & Pankau, 1997).

In addition, children and adults with Williams syndrome seem to be more fearful than people with other types of mental retardation (Dykens & Rosner, 1999). Further, many individuals with Williams syndrome show high levels of generalized anxiety and worries, especially about future events and health or somatic issues (Davies, Udwin, & Howlin, 1998; Dilts, Morris, & Leonard, 1990; Einfeld et al., 1997; Udwin & Yule, 1991). These findings, however, are primarily descriptive, based on either the informal impressions of researchers or standardized global rating scales such as the Rutter Questionnaires (Rutter, 1967), the Developmental Behaviour Checklist (Einfeld & Tonge, 1994), or the Child Behavior Checklist (Achenbach, 1991). These checklists screen for a variety of behavioral or emotional problems and do not provide in-depth or diagnostic information about any one symptom such as anxiety. It thus remains unknown how anxiety is specifically manifested in people with Williams syndrome or the degree to which fears relate to full-blown phobic disorders.

A complicating factor in the assessment of fears is who is actually reporting these concerns. On the one hand, virtually all studies of fears in typically developing children rely on self-report data, often with the widely used Fear Survey Schedule for Children–Revised (FSSC–R; Ollendick, King, & Frary, 1989). On the other hand, many studies of persons with mental retardation use parents or others as informants as a means of circumventing problems with item comprehension and acquiescence bias (e.g., Heal & Selegman, 1995; Zetlin, Heriot, & Turner, 1985). In this vein, Boudlin and Pratt (1998) recently demonstrated the feasibility of administering the FSSC–R to parents of young children aged 3 to 9 years, even though parental means were somewhat lower relative to other studies using child data. In this study, then, we adopt a two-tiered approach, examining fears as reported first by parents, and then by pairs of parents and children.

In particular, three studies were conducted. Study 1 compares parental reports of fears in 120 persons with Williams syndrome to 70 participants with mental retardation of mixed etiologies. The effects of age and gender on fears were also examined. Study 2 compares child versus parent reports of fears in a subset of 36 persons with Williams syndrome and their parents and 24 persons of mixed etiologies and their parents. Study 3 assesses to what extent another subset of 51 individuals with Williams syndrome meet Diagnostic and Statistical Manual-based diagnostic criteria for specific phobia and other anxiety disorders. Taken together, these three studies provide the first in-depth look at anxiety and fears in this vulnerable population.

STUDY 1

Methods

Participants

Participants included 120 persons with Williams syndrome (59 male, 61 female) and 70 individuals with mental retardation of mixed or nonspecific etiologies (36 male, 34 female). Participants in each group ranged in age from 6 to 48 years, with participants with Williams syndrome having an average age of 16.65 years (SD = 10.79). Similarly, participants in the mixed mental retardation group had a mean age of 17.57 years (SD = 9.31). The proportion of male to female participants was also similar across groups, with male participants making up 49% (n = 59) of the Williams syndrome group and 52% (n = 37) of the group with nonspecific mental retardation.

The proportion of individuals showing mild versus moderate delay was similar across groups. Among participants with Williams syndrome, 52% showed mild levels of delay and 48% had moderate delays, based on parent reports of previously administered IQ tests. Similarly, 47% of the mixed group showed mild delay and 53% had moderate levels of delay. Level of delay was not correlated with fears in either group (*r*s = –.02 and .04, respectively).

The majority of participants with Williams syndrome (79%) were recruited through the Far West Chapter of the National Williams Syndrome Association and through referrals from university-based geneticists. Remaining persons (21%) were recruited at the July 1998 Biennial Meeting of the National Williams Syndrome Association held in Minneapolis, Minnesota. All participants had previously received clinical diagnoses of Williams syndrome, and the majority (65%) also had molecular genetic testing that confirmed these diagnoses (del 7q11.23). No differences in age, IQ level, or fears were found among participants with clinical diagnoses only versus those with clinical and molecular genetic diagnoses.

The majority of participants with mixed mental retardation (n = 45, 64%) were consecutively recruited during routine visits to an organization providing broad-based support services to persons with mental retardation. As per participants' case workers, none of these 46 individuals had Williams syndrome, 4 had autism, 2 had cerebral palsy, 3 had neurological deficits, 3 had various chromosomal rearrangements, 9 had seizure disorders, and 25 had no documented diagnoses. The remainder of persons in the mixed group (n = 25, 36%) were recruited as part of an ongoing longitudinal study on genetic disorders. Ten of these individuals had Down syndrome and 15 had Prader–Willi syndrome. Because some of these diagnostic groups were disproportionately represented, total fear scores were compared across five of the diagnostic categories (Down, Prader–Willi, seizure disorder, unknown, and all other). Because no significant differences were found (p = .97), participants were combined into a single, heterogeneous group. This type of mixed group is widely used in mental retardation behavioral research (Dykens, 1995; Hodapp & Dykens, 1994, 2001).

Procedures and Measures

Participants' parents completed questionnaires that were either mailed to them along with a stamped, return envelope or else given to them to complete during their visit to the service agency. One questionnaire asked for basic information: age of offspring, gender, IQ, and clinical diagnostic and genetic test results. Parents also completed the following survey.

Fear Survey Schedule for Children–Revised. FSSC–R (Ollendick, 1983; Ollendick et al., 1989) is a widely used inventory where 80 fears are rated on a 3-point scale: 1 (*none, no fear*), 2 (*some degree of fear*), 3 (*a lot of fear*). Because the study included both children and adults, school-related or other child-oriented items were made pertinent for adults by adding work-related concerns (e.g., "Having to stay after school or be reprimanded at work;" "Poor grades or a poor evaluation at work"). A five-factor structure has been consistently found in normative studies of the FSSC–R (e.g., King et al., 1989; Ollendick et al., 1989; Ollendick, Yule, & Ollier, 1991), and these factors are seen as well in studies of people with developmental and other disabilities (King, Josephs, Gullone, Madden, & Ollendick, 1994). Factors include fear of failure and criticism, the unknown, minor injury and small animals, danger and death, and medical issues.

Results

FSSC–R Total Scores

For the purpose of Study 1, the 190 participants were divided into three age groups. The first group had 82 children (55 Williams, 27 mixed) aged 6 to 12 years, with a mean age of 7.93 years in the Williams group ($SD = 2.81$) and 8.52 in the mixed group ($SD = 2.42$). The second group comprised 36 adolescents ages 13 to 18 years (20 Williams, 16 mixed) with a mean age of 15.65 years ($SD = 1.48$) in the Williams syndrome group and 16.10 years ($SD = 2.19$) in the group with mixed etiologies. Seventy-two adults aged 19 to 48 years (41 Williams, 31 mixed) comprised the final group, with a mean age of 28.98 years ($SD = 8.57$) in participants with Williams syndrome and 25.66 ($SD = 7.28$) in the mixed group.

A 2 × 2 × 3 (Diagnostic Group × Gender × Age Group) analysis of variance (ANOVA) was conducted using the total FSSC–R scores. The main effect for diagnostic group was significant, $F(1, 189) = 29.33$, $p < .0001$, with persons with Williams syndrome scoring significantly higher than the mixed group. Table 1 summarizes mean scores for each group. An age effect was also found, $F(2, 189) = 16.20$, $p < .0001$, but was qualified by a significant Age × Gender interaction, $F(2, 189) = 2.96$; $p < .05$. Two follow-up ANOVAs and Newman–Keuls post hocs revealed that male adults scored significantly higher than male children ($p = .039$) and that female adults scored significantly higher than female adolescents and children ($p = .0001$). Although the main effect for gender was nonsignificant, a significant interaction was found between gender and diagnostic group, $F(1, 189) = 4.47$, $p < .05$. As shown in Table 1, female participants with Williams syndrome scored significantly higher than male participants with William syndrome, whereas no gender differences were found in the mixed group. Remaining interactions terms were nonsignificant.

To further assess the relation between age and fears, correlations were conducted in each group between age and total fear scores on the FSSC–R. For the Williams syndrome group, the linear correlation was .40 ($p < .001$) and the quadratic correlation was .41 ($p < .001$). The quadratic correlation only accounted for an additional 1% of variance beyond that explained by the linear correlation. In the mixed group, the linear correlation was .47 ($p < .001$), and the quadratic

TABLE 1
Total Mean FSSC–R Scores in the Williams and Mixed Groups by Age and Gender

	Williams Syndrome Group		*Mixed Group*	
	M	*SD*	*M*	*SD*
Overall	126.24	29.31	107.00	25.63
Male	119.75	24.83	107.08	20.36
Female	132.52	32.03	106.91	30.56

	Williams Syndrome Group				*Mixed Group*			
	Male		*Female*		*Male*		*Female*	
	M	*SD*	*M*	*SD*	*M*	*SD*	*M*	*SD*
6–12 years	115.10	25.88	114.76	29.76	97.35	12.09	88.10	12.81
13–18 years	126.92	25.48	136.00	22.93	107.20	17.22	94.14	17.33
19–48 years	122.62	21.74	148.76	29.18	118.15	23.90	123.23	35.19

Note. FSSC–R = Fear Survey Schedule for Children–Revised.

correlation of .52 ($p < .001$) accounted for an additional 5% of variance. Figures 1 and 2 show the scatterplots between age and total fear scores in the Williams syndrome and mixed groups, respectively, as well as the corresponding quadratic regression lines.

FSSC–R Factors

Additional 2 × 2 × 3 ANOVAs were conducted with the five FSSC–R factors, using a Bonferroni corrected p value of .01 (.05/5 factors). As shown in Table 2, the Williams syndrome group scored significantly higher than their counterparts on all five factors. Significant age effects were found for three factors (Failure and Criticism, Injury and Small Animals, and Danger and Death), yet fears of Injury and Small Animals were qualified by significant age by gender interactions. Follow-up ANOVAs and Newman–Keuls post hocs found that adolescents and adults scored higher than children in fears of Failure and Criticism ($p < .001$) and Danger and Death ($p < .001$). In fears of Injury and Small Animals, female adolescents and adults scored higher than female children ($p < .001$).

STUDY 2

As expected, Study 1 found that relative to those with mental retardation of mixed etiologies, persons with Williams syndrome had significantly higher fear scores

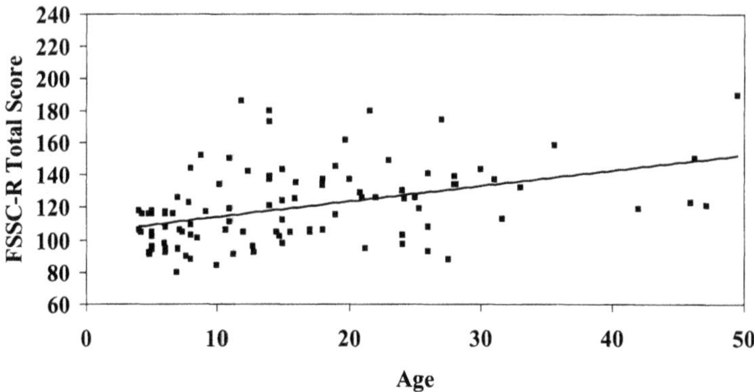

FIGURE 1 Age and total Fear Survey Schedule for Children–Revised fear scores and quadratic regression line for 120 persons with Williams syndrome; multiple $R = .41$, $R^2 = .17$.

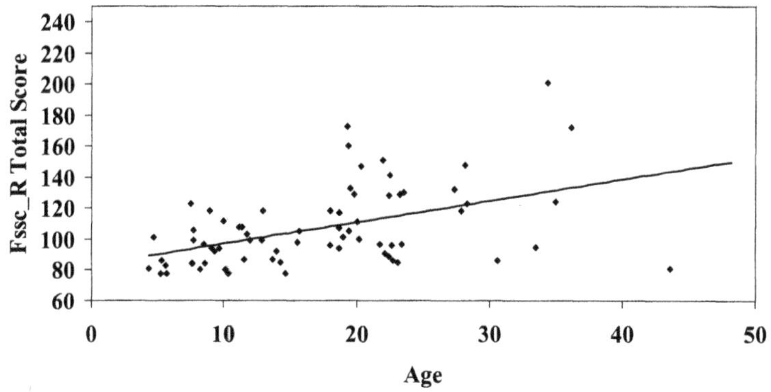

FIGURE 2 Age and total Fear Survey Schedule for Children–Revised fear scores and quadratic regression line for 70 persons with mental retardation of mixed etiologies; multiple $R = .52$; $R^2 = .27$.

on all five factors of the FSSC–R. Of concern, however, is that the mean FSSC–R scores for both the Williams and mixed groups (126.24 and 107.00, respectively) were generally lower than the means found in previous studies based on child report. Using self-report data, for example, King et al. (1994) found a total FSSC–R score of 136.58 in over 1,000 children with various types of developmental disabilities, whereas Gullone, King, and Cummins (1996) found a mean FSSC–R score of 145.37 among 187 students with mental retardation. We hypothesized that the lower means in Study 1 are likely due to our reliance on parental reports of child fears as opposed to children's self-reports of their fears. Study 2 tested this hypothesis.

TABLE 2
Mean FSSC–R Factor Scores in the Williams and Mixed Groups by Age and Gender

	Williams syndrome Group		*Mixed Group*		
	M	*SD*	*M*	*SD*	*F-Group*
Failure and Criticism	23.07	6.41	19.68	5.11	18.05**
Unknown	31.62	7.47	26.61	6.26	25.98**
Injury and Animals	36.31	9.90	31.30	9.31	19.68**
Danger and Death	21.24	7.21	17.83	5.91	21.56**
Medical	11.83	2.53	9.97	2.98	16.31**

	Males		*Females*		*Males*		*Females*			
	M	*SD*	*M*	*SD*	*M*	*SD*	*M*	*SD*	*F-Age*	*F-Age, Sex*
Failure and Criticism									16.06**	*ns*
6–12 years	20.13	5.44	20.36	6.17	18.23	3.70	16.30	1.94		
13–18 years	23.84	5.50	23.37	4.96	21.80	3.70	20.30	1.60		
19–48 years	24.75	6.41	27.72	6.53	22.35	5.24	21.29	6.60		
Unknown									*ns*	*ns*
6–12 years	30.03	5.87	30.12	7.71	24.82	2.89	22.10	2.47		
13–18 years	30.07	8.09	34.73	6.97	25.60	5.13	25.28	3.81		
19–48 years	29.56	5.93	35.76	8.28	28.28	5.73	30.23	9.08		
Injury and Animals									13.96**	4.40*
6–12 years	32.30	9.19	32.68	9.52	28.65	5.31	25.00	4.29		
13–18 years	36.15	7.51	41.36	8.77	30.40	6.65	36.71	3.90		
19–48 years	33.44	7.12	44.40	7.29	34.35	9.33	37.29	12.64		
Danger and Death									19.69**	*ns*
6–12 years	18.60	6.48	17.76	5.92	15.06	2.11	14.30	2.11		
13–18 years	23.07	7.16	23.08	6.68	17.00	2.91	14.14	1.89		
19–48 years	21.69	5.21	26.84	7.29	21.64	6.65	21.29	7.60		
Medical									*ns*	*ns*
6–12 years	12.30	2.52	11.96	2.51	9.11	2.57	9.20	3.15		
13–18 years	11.69	3.27	11.73	1.95	10.40	3.43	9.57	2.07		
19–48 years	10.95	2.14	12.84	2.65	10.28	2.61	11.06	3.65		

Note. FSSC–R = Fear Survey Schedule for Children–Revised.
*$p < .01$. **$p < .001$. *ns* = nonsignificant.

Methods

Participants

A subset of 60 families from Study 1 was enrolled in Study 2. The Williams syndrome group consisted of 36 participants (16 male, 22 female) along with their mothers. Of these, 66% were recruited during the Biennial Meeting of the National

Williams Syndrome Association and 34% were recruited through the Far West Chapter of the National Williams Syndrome Association or through local geneticists. The comparison group with mixed etiologies consisted of 24 persons (14 male, 10 female) and their mothers, who were recruited from the service agency or longitudinal study previously described. The mixed group consisted of 4 persons with unknown diagnoses, 8 with Down syndrome, and 12 with Prader–Willi syndrome. As in Study 1, we checked to ensure that fear scores were nonsignificant across these diagnoses before collapsing participants into a single, mixed comparison group ($p = .47$).

Participants in the Williams syndrome group ranged in age from 8 to 39 years, with a mean age of 20.67 years ($SD = 11.97$). Participants in the mixed group ranged in age from 8 to 30 years, with a mean of 17.87 years ($SD = 6.73$); $F(1, 59) = 1.09, p = .30$. As measured by the Kaufman Brief Intelligence Test (K–BIT; Kaufman & Kaufman, 1990), the two groups also showed comparable IQ scores; the average IQ in the Williams syndrome group was 61.25 ($SD = 13.87$) and in the mixed group it was 56.75 ($SD = 16.78$); $F(1, 59) = 1.28, p = .26$. Further, both the Matrices and Verbal Domains of the K–BIT were nonsignificant across groups. The Verbal scores averaged 64.06 and 58.79 in the Williams and mixed etiology groups, respectively; $F(1, 59) = 2.01$, $p = .16$; and the Matrices scores averaged 64.94 and 60.87, respectively; $F(1, 59) = 0.91, p = .34$.

Procedures

Participants with Williams syndrome or with mixed etiologies were individually administered the FSSC–R described in Study 1 by two trained research assistants. Individuals were first administered a neutral practice item for the FSSC–R, which included visual cues that the examiner or participants could use on an as-needed basis during the interview. Visual cues were of a neutral face ("not at all afraid") and two other faces depicting "a little afraid" and "a lot afraid." We ended the FSSC–R interview on a positive note by asking participants to describe "the things that make you feel happy."

Two tactics were taken to assess the risk of acquiescence bias, which may be a problem in collecting data directly from persons with mental retardation (Heal & Selegman, 1995). First, we obtained spontaneously generated fears from individuals in an open-ended format prior to the administration of the FSSC–R. Participants were told "I need to ask you about the kinds of things that make you feel scared or afraid. Sometimes people are afraid of different things. What things make you feel afraid or scared, what are you afraid of?" All spontaneous responses were noted, thus giving us a sense of participants' fears without the prompts and cues provided by the FSSC–R. Second, four neutral items were added to the FSSC–R (ice cream, flowers, trees, books), assessing the extent to which individuals might indiscriminately endorse items.

Participants were also individually administered the K–BIT (Kaufman & Kaufman, 1990), which assesses verbal and nonverbal reasoning in people aged 4 years through adulthood. Designed for research and screening purposes, the K–BIT has a mean of 100, a standard deviation of 15, and well-established reliability and validity. Among persons with mental retardation, the correlation is high between the K–BIT and Wechsler-based tests, and the K–BIT has been successfully used in other studies involving children and adults with mental retardation (e.g., Dykens, 1996; Dykens & Cohen, 1996; Dykens, Rosner, & Ly, 2001).

Results

Open-Ended Fears and Neutral Items

In response to the open-ended question about fears, participants with Williams syndrome spontaneously generated an average of 3.78 fears per person as opposed to 2.45 in the mixed group, $t(60) = -2.67, p < .01$. Even without the cues provided by the FSSC–R, then, individuals with Williams syndrome spontaneously generated significantly more fears than their counterparts. Spontaneous fears were not significantly related to the K–BIT Verbal IQ in either the Williams syndrome, $r = .20, p = .22$, or mixed groups, $r = .28, p = .18$.

The most frequent spontaneously mentioned fears in the Williams syndrome group were thunderstorms (47%), loud sounds (22%), death or dead people (22%), high places, including carnival rides (22%), ghosts or spooky things (19%), arguments between others (14%), and uncertainty about the future (14%). The most frequent spontaneously mentioned fears in the mixed group included ghosts or spooky things (29%), snakes (21%), high places (17%), and dark places (13%).

Very few participants endorsed fearing the neutral items that were added to the FSSC–R as another check for acquiescence bias. Two individuals with Williams syndrome endorsed having fears of "certain kinds" of books, and 1 of trees, while 1 participant in the mixed group reported a fear of flowers. In general, then, participants appeared to have discriminated among items and understood the task demands of the interview.

FSSC–R Total Scores

Given the small numbers enrolled in this study relative to Study 1, participants were not divided into age groups. Total fear scores from both parents and offspring were compared across groups in a 2 × 2 (Group × Reporter) repeated measures ANOVA. Across both groups, children reported significantly more fears than their parents, $F(1, 58) = 73.94$, $p < .001$. Mean scores for parents and children in both groups are summarized in Table 3. Among individuals with Williams syndrome, both parents and children had significantly higher FSSC–R total scores than their counterparts in the mixed group, $F(1, 58) = 21.73$, $p < .001$. The interaction term was nonsignificant.

No significant gender differences were found, although there was a trend for female participants with Williams syndrome to self-report more fears than male participants (*M*s = 168.13 and 150.13, respectively), $F(1, 37) = 3.09$, $p = .08$. K–BIT IQ was not associated with total FSSC–R scores as reported by either parents or children in either the Williams or the mixed group (*r*s = –.06, –.26, –.29, .14, respectively). Correlations were also nonsignificant between the K–BIT Verbal IQ and parent and child fears scores in both the Williams and the mixed groups (*r*s = .17, –.12, .24, and –.29, respectively).

FSSC-R Factor Scores

As shown in Table 3, repeated measures ANOVAs for the FSSC–R factors revealed a pattern of findings similar to the one found for the total FSSC–R scores. Using a Bonferroni-adjusted $p < .01$ shows that children reported significantly more fears than their parents, and parents and children in the Williams syndrome group reported significantly more fears than parents and children in the mixed group. The medical fears factor was the one exception to this pattern. No group effect was found for medical fears, and unlike the mixed group, children with Williams syndrome and their parents showed almost identical means in the medical fears factor.

Extreme Fears

Total fear scores from parents and children were also calculated using only those fears endorsed as extreme or with a rating of 3. A 2 × 2 (Group × Reporter) repeated-measures ANOVA revealed that children reported more extreme fears than their parents (see Table 3 for means and *F* and *p* values). Further, as shown in Table 3, higher total extreme fear scores were reported by both parents and children in the Williams syndrome as opposed to the mixed group.

Fear Prevalence

To obtain a better sense of the types of specific fears seen in each group, frequently occurring fears were tabulated. These were defined as items rated as a 2 or

TABLE 3
Means and Standard Deviations for Parent and Child FSSC–R Scores Across Groups

	Williams Syndrome Group				*Mixed Group*					
	Parent		*Child*		*Parent*		*Child*			
	M	*SD*	*M*	*SD*	*M*	*SD*	*M*	*SD*	*F-Group*	*F-Parent–Child*
Total FSSC–R	118.83	20.64	161.02	31.02	97.66	13.34	135.87	33.11	21.73**	73.94**
Failure and Criticism	22.00	4.99	29.30	7.28	17.66	2.94	25.08	6.77	14.38**	48.72**
Unknown	29.19	5.26	40.05	9.23	25.12	4.67	32.54	8.17	18.00**	45.82**
Injury and Animals	34.72	7.37	47.58	10.04	28.00	4.91	39.08	9.62	22.07**	64.17***
Danger and Death	19.36	5.14	30.25	6.14	15.66	2.99	24.96	7.25	17.30**	99.32**
Medical	11.58	2.60	11.77	2.73	8.79	2.69	12.08	3.83	4.30	12.68*
Extreme Fears	8.55	7.35	34.22	16.25	3.16	3.51	23.42	16.53	11.05*	110.09**

Note. FSSC–R = Fear Survey Schedule for Children–Revised.
*$p < .01$. **$p < .001$; for Medical factor, interaction term $F(1, 58) = 10.01$**.

a 3 by either parents or children and that were noted by most members (60% or more) in either the parent or the child group. As indicated in Table 4, parents of children with Williams syndrome reported 18 frequently occurring fears, whereas their children reported 50 such fears. In contrast, parents in the mixed group reported just 1 frequent fear, whereas their children reported 22 frequent fears.

Parent–Child Agreement

Correlations were nonsignificant between parent and child FSSC–R total and factor scores in both groups (e.g., *r*s = .20 and –.17 for FSSC–R total scores in the Williams and mixed groups, respectively). To obtain a clearer picture of the types of fears that parents and children agreed on, percentage agreement between the two informants was tabulated for the frequently occurring items listed in Table 4 ([agreements/[agreements + disagreements]). As shown in Table 4, adequate agreement (i.e., above 70%) was found in only four fears in the Williams syndrome group (arguments between others, bee stings, roller coaster or carnival rides, and thunderstorms) and in three items in the mixed group (roller coaster rides, war, uncertainty).

STUDY 3

Relative to others with mental retardation, Studies 1 and 2 point to elevated fears in persons with Williams syndrome, as reported by parents or children, with children reporting many more fears than their parents. It remains unclear, however, to what extent high rates of fears in Williams syndrome are associated with more conventional psychiatric diagnoses of specific phobia or other anxiety disorders. These possibilities were assessed in Study 3.

Methods

Participants

Study 3 included 51 participants (23 male, 28 female) with Williams syndrome aged 5 to 49 years, with a mean age of 15.91 years (*SD* = 10.31). These individuals were a subset of participants in Study 1. As measured by the K–BIT (Kaufman & Kaufman, 1990), the average IQ of this sample was 62.00 (*SD* = 15.44). All participants had previously received clinical diagnoses for their respective syndromes and all had molecular genetic testing (del 7q11.23) that confirmed these diagnoses. Five individuals were on medication at the time of the study; three

TABLE 4
Comparison of Parent and Child Reports of Child Fears

	Williams Syndrome Group			Mixed Mental Retardation Group		
	Child	*Parent*	*% Agreement*	*Child*	*Parent*	*% Agreement*
Frequent report by both parent and child in Williams syndrome group						
Falling from high places	92	61	64	58	25	33
Arguments between others	87	75	72	63	33	42
Mean-looking dogs	87	67	69	66	63	46
Bee stings	84	75	72	67	55	54
Thunderstorms	84	71	75	54	33	46
Parents getting sick	82	64	61	42	13	46
Being criticized	79	86	42	42	45	42
Getting cut or injured	79	67	64	65	20	46
High places	79	69	64	33	30	46
Loud noises	76	80	62	39	25	54
Shots, injections	76	83	69	70	42	38
Punished, reprimanded	76	78	64	62	42	38
Being teased	76	67	61	50	46	42
Roller coaster, carnival rides	74	86	81	54	30	75
Uncertainty, ambiguity	71	64	61	20	16	71
Going to hospital	69	67	67	37	25	63
Deep water, ocean	68	66	64	46	25	46
Making mistakes	63	70	61	20	21	67
Frequent report by child but not by parent in Williams syndrome group						
Fire, getting burned	90	58	58	71	37	50
Lost in a strange place	90	45	44	71	21	33
Being in a fight	87	50	55	62	17	30
Being hit by car, truck	84	39	44	59	38	42
Dark places	84	39	55	67	33	50
Electric shock	82	31	42	58	12	38
Drugs	81	33	42	55	8	46
Death, dead people	81	44	58	75	13	29
Bears, wolves	81	39	42	59	34	33
Nightmares	79	55	61	55	8	54
Guns	79	50	55	66	4	38
Burglar breaking in	79	39	47	75	21	37
Strangers	79	19	33	25	29	46
Germs	79	17	36	58	0	42
Being left behind	77	44	47	62	29	30

(contiinued)

TABLE 4 (*Continued*)

	Williams Syndrome Group			*Mixed Mental Retardation Group*		
	Child	*Parent*	*% Agreement*	*Child*	*Parent*	*% Agreement*
Failure experiences	76	58	55	37	4	39
Sharp objects	76	42	55	54	17	46
Spiders	75	56	66	75	46	46
Earthquakes	74	42	47	83	33	50
Bombing attacks	74	24	44	55	4	42
Being sent to principal/boss	71	50	58	62	38	50
Snakes	71	47	61	75	38	38
Ghosts, spooky things	71	45	55	67	17	33
Poor grades, work evaluation	71	39	50	50	12	46
Nuclear war	71	22	47	12	0	88
Being alone	69	39	61	68	42	58
Sight of blood	68	56	58	67	33	46
Not being able to breathe	68	33	44	33	4	62
Not fitting in with peers	66	50	61	58	21	38
Going to bed in dark	66	28	50	54	39	54
Getting sick	61	58	62	62	12	42
Cemeteries	60	3	42	32	0	66

were on stimulants and two were on selective serotonin reuptake inhibitors. No differences were found between persons on or off medication in fear scores, age, or K–BIT IQ.

Twenty-nine participants (57%) were recruited from the Far West Chapter of the National Williams Syndrome Association and from referrals through university geneticists. The remaining 22 individuals (43%) were recruited during the 1998 Biennial Meeting of the National Williams Syndrome Association. Participants derived from these two sources showed similar ages, IQs, and fear scores.

Procedures

In addition to the FSSC–R, participants' parents were individually administered the Diagnostic Interview Schedule for Children–Parent (DICA–R; Reich, Shayka, & Taibleson, 1991) by MA- or PhD-level psychologists with specialized training in working with persons with mental retardation and their families. The DICA–R is a semistructured interview administered to parents and assesses *Diagnostic and Statistical Manual of Mental Disorders* (3rd ed., rev. [*DSM–III–R*]; American Psychiatric Association, 1987) psychiatric diagnoses in children and adolescents. Consistent with our hypotheses, this study only examined the anxiety disorder domain of the DICA–R, which probes for separation anxiety disorder, avoidant disorder, overanxious disorder, specific phobia, and obsessive–compulsive disorder. DICA–R symptomatology for all diagnoses is rated on a 4-point scale—1 (*no*), 2 (*rarely*), 3 (*sometimes or somewhat*), 4 (*yes*). A rating of 3 or 4 was considered positive symptomatology.

The parent version of the DICA–R was used in light of the difficulty that many persons with mental retardation have labeling their internal states, including the time of onset, duration, and intensity of these states (e.g., Heal & Selegman, 1995). Findings from Study 2 suggest that parents may not report as many fears or other symptoms as their children. As such, data were only considered as probable or best estimates of lifetime psychiatric diagnoses (Leckman, Sholomskas, Thompson, Belanger, & Weissman, 1982).

Parents were also administered the Child Behavior Checklist (CBCL; Achenbach, 1991). The CBCL is a widely used checklist of 113 problems, which are rated 0 (*no problem*), 1 (*somewhat or sometimes true*), and 2 (*very true or often true*). The CBCL yields nine clinical domains, and three broad domains as detailed in the next section, however, in this study we used just a few items from the CBCL to supplement and clarify data analyses related to the DICA.

Results

Diagnostic Interview Schedule for Children

Table 5 summarizes the percentages of participants meeting best-estimate diagnostic criteria for the five anxiety disorders assessed by the DICA–R. Relatively few participants with Williams syndrome showed key diagnostic criteria for overanxious disorder. Whereas many participants (57%), were excessively worried about future events for at least 6 months and 51% were described as "worriers," only 16% (n = 8) showed the requisite adaptive impairment for psychiatric diagnosis. These 8 individuals ranged in age from 8 to 39 years and had a mean age of 16.24 years (SD = 8.49).

Unlike the *DSM–III–R* criteria for overanxious disorder, *Diagnostic and Statistical Manual of Mental Disorders* (4th ed. [*DSM–IV*] American Psychiatric Association, 1994) criteria for generalized anxiety disorder (which subsumes overanxious disorder) stipulates that persons must find it difficult to control their worry and that they show three or more of six symptoms (one of six for children) of sleep disturbance, restlessness, difficulty concentrating, fatigue, muscle tension, and irritability. To approximate these criteria, we identified participants who became "sick from worry" and, depending on their age, also showed one or more elevated scores of 2 on the CBCL in the five symptoms noted (muscle tension is not assessed on the CBCL). Of the 26 worriers, 17 became sick from worry, and of these, 9 showed one or more elevated symptoms of sleep disturbance, irritability,

TABLE 5
Best-Estimate Anxiety Disorder Diagnoses and Symptoms for 51 Participants with Williams Syndrome

	Percent with Diagnosis	*Percent with Symptom*[a]
Separation Anxiety Disorder	4	
Obsessive–Compulsive Disorder	2	
Avoidant Disorder	0	
Overanxious Disorder/Generalized Anxiety Disorder	16–18	
Excessively worried about future		57
A "worrier"		51
Becomes sick from worry		35
Shows an inability to relax		25
Sleep problems, fatigue, restlessness, difficulty concentrating, irritability		18
Impaired adaptive functioning		16
Specific Phobia	35	
Marked, persistent, anxiety-producing fears		96
Avoid fearful stimuli or endure with distress		84
Impaired adaptive functioning		35

[a]Percentage of those with the given diagnosis who exhibit the given symptom.

restlessness, difficulty concentrating, or fatigue on the CBCL. Thus, 18% of participants would likely meet criteria for generalized anxiety disorder, which is similar to the rate of 16% who met criteria for overanxious disorder.

In contrast, examining the key diagnostic criteria for phobia, virtually all participants, or 96%, had persistent anxiety-producing fears for 6 months or longer, and of these, 84% also avoided their feared stimuli or endured them with great distress. Thirty-five percent (n = 18) showed the fear-related adaptive impairment necessary for psychiatric diagnosis. The majority of participants, then, had what might be considered subclinical phobia, meeting all criteria for phobia except the impaired adaptive component. Six individuals (5 female, 1 male) were comorbid for phobia and overanxious disorder, and both cases of separation anxiety disorder (2 female participants) had cooccurring phobia. The 18 participants who met full criteria for phobia ranged in age from 8 to 31 years, with a mean age of 15.08 years (SD = 7.37).

Regarding subtypes of phobia, one half of the 18 participants who met full criteria for phobia had more than one subtype. The natural environment subtype was seen in 94% (72% of these had fears of thunderstorms and 55% of high places), 44% showed other types (50% of these were afraid of being alone and 35% had miscellaneous fears), and 22% showed the animal subtype.

DSM–III–R criteria for phobia are comparable to *DSM–IV*, with the exception that fears in *DSM–IV* must be "marked or excessive" as well as persistent.

Although the word "marked" was not included in the DICA–R, we checked to see if the 18 participants meeting full criteria for phobia had higher parent-reported FSSC–R total scores than their counterparts; this was indeed the case (*M*s = 123.88 and 111.82, respectively), $F(1, 49) = 3.99, p < .05$. Further, we examined the specific subtypes of phobia shown by the 18 individuals meeting full criteria and checked to ensure that the items on the FSSC–R that corresponded to these subtypes were rated a 3, or at the highest level of fear. Such correspondence was found in all 18 individuals for the natural environment and other subtypes. As 10 items relating to animals, insects, or reptiles are listed on the FSSC–R, a rating of 3 was found for at least one (but not all) of these items in the 11 participants with phobias of the animal subtype. It is likely, then, that participants had both marked and persistent fears, and would meet criteria for phobia in both versions of the *DSM*.

Although we did not administer the DICA–R to persons in the comparison group, Table 6 summarizes rates of phobia from several published studies of persons with mental retardation of mixed etiologies as well as from nonretarded children and adolescents in the general population. Relative to the 35% rate of probable phobia in our Williams syndrome sample, rates of phobia are much lower in these groups; 2.3% to 2.4% in typically developing children and adolescents, and from 0.6% to 4.3% in persons with mental retardation.

GENERAL DISCUSSION

These studies are the first to show that fears and phobias are salient manifestations of anxiety in persons with Williams syndrome. In Study 1, participants with Williams syndrome had significantly more fears than their counterparts with

TABLE 6
Rates of Phobia from This and Previously Published Studies

Study	*Sample*	*Criteria*	*Percent with Phobia*
Cooper (1997)	207 MR adults	ICD–10	4.3
Grizenko et al. (1991)	176 MR adolescents, adults	*DSM–III–R*	0.6
Moss et al. (1996)	100 MR adolescents, adults	PAS–ADD	1.0
Anderson et al. (1987)	792 children	DISC	2.4
Milne et al. (1995)	487 adolescents	K–SADS	2.3 clinical, 14.5 subclinical
This study	51 Williams syndrome	DICA–R	35 clinical, 84 subclinical

Note. MR = participant with mental retardation; *DSM–III–R* = *Diagnostic and Statistical Manual* (3rd ed., rev.); PAS–ADD = Psychiatric Assessment Schedule for Adults with Developmental Disability; DISC = Diagnostic Interview Schedule for Children; K–SADS = Schedule for Affective Disorders and Schizophrenia in School-Age Children; DICA–R = Diagnostic Interview Schedule for Children.

mixed mental retardation. Study 2 demonstrated that both parents and their children with Williams syndrome report significantly more fears than parents and their children of mixed etiologies, and that children report many more fears than parents. Consistent with these findings, Study 3 found that persons with Williams syndrome were more likely to suffer from specific phobia relative to other anxiety disorders. Collectively, findings suggest that fears are a significant, albeit newly identified, aspect of the Williams syndrome behavioral phenotype.

As depicted in Study 1, the parent-reported fears of persons with Williams syndrome showed significant age and gender effects. Whereas boys and girls aged 6 to 12 years showed the least amount of fears, fears generally increased with advancing age, often peaking in the adult years. Male adults had higher overall FSSC–R scores than male children, whereas female adults scored higher than female adolescents and children. Other studies using the FSSC–R in children with mental retardation show conflicting age results. Some samples show age-related increases in FSSC–R scores over the 7- to 18-year period, especially among female adolescents (Gullone et al., 1996), whereas others show age-related declines during this same time period (King et al., 1994).

More consistent age findings are found among typically developing children. Children generally show age-related declines in many of their fears, especially those related to immediate, tangible fears of injury, small animals, separation, the dark, and spooky things (Guarnaccia & Weiss, 1974; Gullone et al., 1996; King et al., 1994; Ramirez & Kratochwill, 1990; Vandenberg, 1993). At the same time, age-related increases are often seen in more abstract, anticipatory fears of the future and of social and performance issues, whereas medical fears may remain fairly stable (Gullone & King, 1992, 1997; King et al., 1989; Spence & McCathie, 1993).

Relative to children with or without mental retardation, participants with Williams syndrome show both similarities and differences in their fears. Similar to others, advancing age in persons with Williams syndrome was associated with more abstract fears of failure and criticism, and medical fears were relatively stable. Yet, inconsistent with previous work, participants with Williams syndrome did not show age-related declines in fears of unknown, tangible, or spooky things. Longitudinal studies are needed to clarify these cross-sectional findings, including how the type and intensity of fears change over time in male and female individuals with Williams syndrome.

Study 2 showed that fears in Williams syndrome were high regardless of the reporter; both parents and their children with Williams syndrome reported significantly higher FSSC–R scores than their counterparts in the mixed group. Yet data were striking in the magnitude of difference between child and parent reporters in either group and in the relatively poor agreement between informants. Saphare and Aman (1996) also found nonsignificant correlations between the FSSC–R scores of parents and their children with mental retardation in segregated classes, but some significant correlations between parents and children in mainstreamed classes and typically developing children in regular education classes.

Of the four items in the Williams syndrome group that had adequate agreement, two were often mentioned spontaneously by participants in the open-ended question administered prior to the FSSC–R (thunderstorms and roller coaster rides). These items may thus be more openly or frequently discussed than other fears, contributing to improved agreement. Among remaining fears with low agreement, each informant may be reporting a valid but different perspective on the problem (Achebach & Edelbrock, 1989). Parents, for example, might observe high levels of worry or anxious apprehension in their children, but underestimate specific fearful stimuli, whereas children may be less apt to report apprehension and more likely to focus on tangible fears or even physiologic discomfort. In this vein, Moss, Prosser, Ibbotson, and Goldberg (1996) found that some symptoms of anxiety (e.g., autonomic phenomena) are more frequently reported by persons with mental retardation themselves, whereas other symptoms are more frequently reported by caregivers (e.g., worrying, loss of interest). Using just one informant may thus lead to an incomplete diagnostic picture.

Acknowledging that parents may underestimate fears relative to their children, Study 3 used parental interview data to derive best-estimate diagnoses of anxiety disorders in participants with Williams syndrome. Specific phobia emerged as the most frequent anxiety disorder in the sample. Whereas 35% met all criteria for phobia, a full 84% showed subclinical phobia, meeting all criteria except impaired adaptive functioning. In contrast, and as shown by the summary of previous studies in Table 6, people with mental retardation of mixed etiologies show low rates of phobia, from 0.6% to 4.3% in various samples. Such low rates underscore the distinctiveness of fears and phobias to the Williams syndrome population.

Other symptoms of anxiety were prevalent on the DICA, primarily generalized worry (51%) and anticipatory worry about the future (57%). Only 8 participants in Study 3, or 16%, however, met criteria for overanxious disorder, whereas 18% showed symptoms indicative of generalized anxiety disorder. Six of the cases with overanxious disorder showed comorbidity with phobia, and both cases of separation anxiety also had phobia. Comorbidity was thus seen in 44% of Williams syndrome cases with DICA diagnoses, which is similar to the rate of cooccurring anxiety disorders in the general population (Kashani & Orvaschel, 1990).

Although promising, these studies have several shortcomings. One concern in Study 2 is that whereas parents in both groups underreported fears relative to their children, parental means were also low compared to the two studies to date that have examined parental responses on the FSSC–R. Sarphare and Aman (1995) found a mean parental FSSC–R total score of 124.37 in 6- to 18-year-old students in both special and regular education classrooms, and Boudlin and Pratt (1998) found an average parental FSSC–R total score of 124.04 among normal children aged 3 to 9 years. These findings raise a possible threat to validity; that is, compared to these two studies, parental means in the Williams syndrome group were not necessarily high, and parental means in the mixed group were low. The samples in these previous studies, however, were not parallel to the diagnostic groups or ages in this study, and even with a possible dampening of parental scores, group differences were still found. Further, Study 3 offsets these concerns in that, compared to those with mixed mental retardation, parents of Williams syndrome participants reported many more fears and phobias on the DICA–R.

Further, it is also possible that Williams syndrome participants inflated their fears. Indeed, whereas mean self-report fear scores in the mixed group were quite consistent with self-reported fears in previous studies, self-reported fears among participants with Williams syndrome were substantially elevated. Williams syndrome participants may have overreported their fears in part because of their social personalities and desires to please the examiner. Compared to the mixed group, however, participants with Williams syndrome had higher rates of spontaneously generated fears, and task demands or experimenter expectancies in this open-ended question were low relative to the FSSC–R interview.

Other shortcomings relate to Study 3. In particular, *DSM–III–R* criteria were used instead of *DSM–IV*, although compatibility across versions was approximated using supplemental measures and analyses. In addition, persons with Williams syndrome were not administered the DICA–R. Informant-based reporting is common in mental retardation research, yet relying solely on parents as informants may result in missed cases of phobia or other anxiety disorders in the mentally retarded population (Moss et al., 1996). Even though two of the criteria for phobia were almost at ceiling levels, parents may underestimate both specific fears and autonomic symptoms in their offspring (Moss et al., 1996). Rates of phobia may be even higher when persons with the syndrome are themselves interviewed, and studies are now underway to examine this possibility.

Another concern is that the cooccurrence of anxiety and other psychiatric disorders was not assessed. Anxiety and mood disorders, for example, often cooccur in the general population, and many adults with Williams syndrome present clinically with a mixed picture of anxiety and depressed mood (Pober & Dykens, 1996). Additional studies are needed that simultaneously assess anxiety, mood, and other disorders in persons with Williams syndrome.

A final issue is that whereas the majority of participants met key diagnostic criteria for phobia, relatively few showed impaired adaptive functioning. Persons with Williams syndrome may be similar to persons with phobia in the general population, who also typically function and adapt quite well, in part because of infrequent contact with certain fear-inducing stimuli (Craske, 1999). Alternatively, although parents were instructed to rate fear-related impairment, including possible changes from baseline states, they may have been confused about what constitutes adaptive impairment in persons who, by definition, already have adaptive delays (APA, 1994).

Even with such limitations, however, these findings have novel implications for both treatment and research. Without treatment, phobias tend to be chronic and unremitting, and many phobic individuals do not seek treatment, presumably because they function well despite their fears (Craske, 1999). As in the general population, persons with Williams syndrome may be less likely to present clinically with circumscribed fears, instead complaining of more global symptoms of anxiety, worry, rumination, maladjustment, and depression. Because phobias and other anxiety disorders may contribute over the long term to depressed mood, clinicians may want to carefully assess all these concerns in their patients with Williams syndrome.

Although treatment recommendations for persons with Williams syndrome have previously been described (Dykens & Hodapp, 1997), these should now be revised to possibly include specific cognitive–behavioral treatments for phobia and other anxiety disorders (Dykens et al., 2000). Many children and adults find relief from their phobic symptoms with cognitive restructuring, somatic exercises, and filmed or live modeling, with the treatment of choice being systematic exposure, especially *in vivo* exposure (for reviews see Craske, 1999; Ollendick & King, 1998). Studies have yet to assess the efficacy of these approaches alone or in combination with pharmacotherapy in treating phobic individuals with mental retardation (King, Ollendick, Gullone, Cummins, & Josephs, 1990). Even so, the circumscribed goals and relatively short duration of most cognitive–behavioral treatments as well as the well-developed expressive language and interpersonal strengths of many persons with Williams syndrome bode well for good therapeutic outcomes.

In addition to treatment implications, findings from this study provoke new research directions. Neurologically, for example, phobic persons show relative increases in regional blood flow in the associative visual cortex, suggesting heightened perceptual acuity related to the fight-or-flight response (Fredrickson, Wik, Annas, Ericson, & Stone-Elander, 1995). In contrast, worry is associated with activation of frontal areas and more verbal–cognitive processing effort. Studies are needed that assess these brain processes in persons with Williams syndrome, especially in light of their well-developed verbal mediation skills and of their relative sparing of the amygdala (Wang, Hesselink, Jernigan, & Doherty, 1992), which has long been implicated in the mediation of fear (Fanselow & LeDoux, 1999).

Findings on how phobias develop are also informative for Williams syndrome. As summarized by Craske (1999), phobias are thought to evolve from a generalized vulnerability involving nonspecific genetic factors (e.g., temperament), individual life experiences (e.g., early aversive or traumatic experiences, caregiver reinforcement of fear, vicarious learning), cognitive features (e.g., overestimating risk or adversity), and physiologic factors (e.g., readiness to arousal). These, in turn, interact with the severity and controllability of fearful stimuli to create phobias or anxiety disorders.

In Williams syndrome as well, high rates of fears or phobias may be associated with specific genetic or biologic vulnerabilities that interact with life experience and with certain aspects of the Williams syndrome phenotype. Fears of falling from high places or of carnival rides, for example, may relate to the joint contractures, and problems with gross motor coordination balance, and gait shown by many older children and adults with Williams syndrome (Chapman, Plessis, & Pober, 1996). Hyperacusis is seen in the vast majority of people with Williams syndrome (Van Borsel, Curfs, & Fryns, 1997) and may be directly related to elevated fears of loud sounds such as thunderstorms and sirens. Fears of arguments and of being teased, criticized, punished, or left alone may relate to the heightened social sensitivities and empathic orientation of many with Williams syndrome (Dykens & Rosner, 1999); these persons may simply bristle more than others when faced with negative social interactions.

Although further work is needed, fears and phobias in Williams syndrome may stem from interactions between biological or genetic vulnerabilities, salient physical or behavioral features of the Williams syndrome phenotype, and life experience. Indeed, because anxiety and fears are mediated by both genetic and experiential factors (Anagnostaras, Craske, & Fanselow, 1999), Williams syndrome may be a model disorder for elucidating these risk factors. Thus, although research on anxiety in Williams syndrome has just begun, this line of work may ultimately shed new light on the etiology of anxiety and fears in people with or without this complex developmental disorder.

ACKNOWLEDGMENTS

The author thanks the National Williams Syndrome Association and participating families for their enthusiastic involvement in this research. The author is also grateful to Robert M. Hodapp, Beth A. Rosner, and Deborah J. Fidler for their help with data collection and also to Dr. Hodapp for comments on an earlier draft of this article. This research was supported by NICHD Grant R0135681.

REFERENCES

Achenbach, T. M. (1991). *Manual for the Child Behavior Checklist/4-18 and 1991 Profile.* Burlington: University of Vermont, Department of Psychiatry.

Achenbach, T. M., & Edelbrock, C. (1989). Diagnostic, taxonomic, and assessment issues. In T. H. Ollendick & M. Hersen (eds.), *Handbook of child psychopathology* (pp. 53–74). New York: Plenum.

American Psychiatric Association. (1987). *Diagnostic and statistical manual of mental disorders* (3rd ed., rev.).Washington, DC: Author.

American Psychiatric Association. (1994). *Diagnostic and statistical manual of mental disorders* (4th ed.). Washington, DC: Author.

Anagnostaras, S. G., Craske, M. G., & Fanselow, M. S. (1999). Anxiety: At the intersection of genes and experience. *Nature Neuroscience, 2,* 780–782.

Anderson, J. C., Williams, S., McGee, R., & Silva, P. (1987). *DSM–III* disorders in preadolescent children. *Archives of General Psychiatry, 44,* 69–76.

Bellugi, U., Wang, P., & Jernigan, T. L. (1994). Williams syndrome: An unusual neuropsychological profile. In S. H. Browman & J. Grafram (Eds.), *Atypical cognitive deficits in developmental disorders* (pp. 23–56). Hillsdale, NJ: Lawrence Erlbaum Associates, Inc.

Bihrle, A. M., Bellugi, U., Delis, D., & Marks, S. (1989). Seeing either the forest or the trees: Dissociation in visuospatial processing. *Brain Cognition, 11,* 37–49.

Bouldin, P., & Prat, C. (1998). Utilizing parent report to investigate young children's fears: A modification of the Fear Survey Schedule for Children–II: A research note. *Journal of Child Psychology and Psychiatry, 39,* 271–277.

Chapman, C. A., Plessis, A., & Pober, B. R. (1996). Neurologic findings in children and adults with Williams syndrome. *Journal of Child Neurology, 11,* 63–65.

Cooper, S. A. (1997). Epidemiology of psychiatric disorders in elderly compared with younger adults with learning disabilities. *British Journal of Psychiatry, 170,* 375–380.

Craske, M. G. (1999). *Anxiety disorders: Psychological approaches to theory and treatment.* Boulder, CO: Westview.

Davies, M., Udwin, O., & Howlin, P. (1998). Adults with Williams syndrome. *British Journal of Psychiatry, 172,* 273–276.

Dilts, C. V., Morris, C. A., & Leonard, C. O. (1990). Hypothesis for development of a behavioral phenotype in Williams syndrome. *American Journal of Medical Genetics, 6,* 126–131.

Dykens, E. M. (1995). Measuring behavioral phenotypes: Provocations from the "new genetics." *American Journal on Mental Retardation, 99,* 522–532.

Dykens, E. M. (1996). The draw-a-person task in persons with mental retardation: What does it measure? *Research in Developmental Disabilities, 17,* 1–13.

Dykens, E. M. (1999). Direct effects of genetic mental retardation syndromes: Maladaptive behavior and psychopathology. *International Review of Research in Mental Retardation, 22,* 2–27.

Dykens, E. M. (2000). Psychopathology in children with intellectual disability. *Journal of Child Psychology and Psychiatry, 41,* 407–417.

Dykens, E. M., & Cohen, D. J. (1996). Effects of Special Olympics International on social competence in persons with mental retardation. *Journal of the American Academy of Child and Adolescent Psychiatry, 35,* 223–229.

Dykens, E. M., & Hodapp, R. M. (1997). Treatment issues in genetic mental retardation syndromes. *Professional Psychology: Research and Practice, 28,* 263–270.

Dykens, E. M., Hodapp, R. M., & Finucane, B. M. (2000). *Genetics and mental retardation syndromes: A new look at behavior and interventions.* Baltimore: Brookes.

Dykens, E. M., & Rosner, B. A. (1999). Refining behavioral phenotypes: Personality-motivation in Williams and Prader–Willi syndromes. *American Journal on Mental Retardation, 104,* 158–169.

Dykens, E. M., Rosner, B. A., & Ly, T. M. (2001). Drawings by individuals with Williams syndrome: Are people different from shapes? *American Journal on Mental Retardation, 106,* 94–107.

Einfeld, S. L., & Tonge, B. J. (1994). *Manual for the Developmental Behaviour Checklist.* Sydney/Melbourne, Australia: University of New South Wales/Monash University.

Einfeld, S. L., Tonge, B. J., & Florio, T. (1997). Behavioral and emotional disturbance in individuals with Williams syndrome. *American Journal on Mental Retardation, 102,* 45–53.

Ewart, A. K., Jin, W., Atkinson, D., Morris, C. A., & Keating, M. T. (1994). Supravalvular aortic stenosis associated with a deletion disrupting the elastin gene. *Journal of Clinical Investigation, 93,* 1071–1077.

Ewart, A. K., Norris, C. A., Atkinson, D., Jin, W., Sternes, K., Spallone, P., et al. (1993). Hemizygosity at the elastin locus in a developmental disorder, Williams syndrome. *Nature Genetics, 5,* 11–16.

Fenselow, M. S., & LeDoux, J. E. (1999). Why we think plasticity underlying Pavlovian fear conditioning occurs in the basolateral amygdala. *Neuron, 23,* 229–232.

Fredrickson, M., Wik, G., Annas, P., Ericson, K., & Stone-Elander, S. (1995). Functional neuroanatomy of visually elicited simple phobic fear: Additional data and theoretical analyses. *Psychophysiology, 32,* 43–48.

Gosch, A., & Pankau, R. (1997). Personality characteristics and behavior problems in individuals of different ages with Williams syndrome. *Developmental Medicine and Child Neurology, 39,* 527–533.

Grizenko, N., Cvejic, H., Vida, S., & Sayegh, L. (1991). Behaviour problems of the mentally retarded. *Canadian Journal of Psychiatry, 36,* 712–717.

Guarnaccia, V. J., & Weiss, R. L. (1974). Factor structure of fears in the mentally retarded. *Journal of Clinical Psychology, 30,* 540–544.

Gullone, E., & King, N. J. (1992). Psychometric evaluation of a revised fear survey schedule for children and adolescents. *Journal of Child Psychology & Psychiatry & Allied Disciplines, 33,* 987–998.

Gullone, E., & King, N. J. (1997). Three year follow-up of normal fear in children and adolescents aged 7 to 18 years. *British Journal of Developmental Psychology, 15,* 97–111.

Gullone, E., King, N. J. , & Cummins, R. A. (1996). Self-reported fears: A comparison study of youths with and without intellectual disability. *Journal of Intellectual Disability Research, 40,* 227–240.

Heal, L. W., & Selegman, C. K. (1995). Response biases in interviews of individuals with limited mental abilities. *Journal of Intellectual Disability Research, 39,* 245–250.

Hodapp, R. M., & Dykens, E. M. (1994). Mental retardation's two cultures of behavioral research. *American Journal on Mental Retardation, 98,* 675–687.

Hodapp, R. M., & Dykens, E. M. (2001). Strengthening behavioral research on genetic mental retardation syndromes. *American Journal on Mental Retardation, 106,* 4–15.

Kashani, J. H., & Orvaschel, H. (1990). A community study of anxiety in children and adolescents. *American Journal of Psychiatry, 147,* 313–318.

Kaufman, A. S., & Kaufman, N. L. (1990). *Kaufman Brief Intelligence Test Manual.* Circle Pines, MN: American Guidance Service.

King, N. J., Josephs, A., Gullone, E., Madden, C., & Ollendick, T. H. (1994). Assessing the fears of children with disability using the Revised Fear Survey Schedule for Children: A comparative study. *British Journal of Medical Psychology, 67,* 377–386.

King, N. J., Ollendick, T. H., Gullone, E., & Cummins, R. A. (1990). Fears and phobias in children and adolescents with intellectual disabilities: Assessment and intervention strategies. *Australian and New Zealand Journal of Developmental Disabilities, 16,* 97–108.

King, N. J., Ollier, K., Iacuone, R., Schuster, S., Bays, K., Gullone, E., et al. (1989). Fears of children and adolescents: A cross-sectional Australian study using the revised Fear Survey Schedule for Children. *Journal of Child Psychology and Psychiatry, 30,* 775–784.

Leckman, J. F., Sholomskas, D., Thompson, D., Belanger, A., & Weissman, M. W. (1982). Best estimate of lifetime psychiatric diagnosis. *Archives of General Psychiatry, 39,* 879–883.

Mervis, C. B., Morris, C. A., Bertrand, J., & Robinson, B. F. (1999). Williams syndrome: Findings from an integrated program of research. In H. Tager-Flusberg (Ed.), *Neurodevelopmental disorders* (pp. 65–110). Cambridge, MA: MIT Press.

Milne, J. M., Garrison, C. Z., Addy, C. L., McKeown, R. E., Jackson, K. L., Cuffe, S. P., et al. (1995). Frequency of phobic disorder in a community sample of adolescents. *American Journal of Child and Adolescent Psychiatry, 34,* 1202–1211.

Moss, S., Prosser, H., Ibbotson, B., & Goldberg, D. (1996). Respondent and informant accounts of psychiatric symptoms in a sample of patients with learning disability. *Journal of Intellectual Disability Research, 40,* 457–465.

Ollendick, T. H. (1983). Reliability and validity of the Revised Fear Survey Schedule for Children (FSSC–R). *Behaviour Research and Therapy, 21,* 685–692.

Ollendick, T. H., & King, N. J. (1998). Empirically supported treatments for children with phobic and anxiety disorders: Current status. *Journal of Clinical Child Psychology, 27,* 156-167.

Ollendick, T. H., King, N. J., & Frary, R. B. (1989). Fears in children and adolescents: Reliability and generalizability across age, gender, and nationality. *Behaviour Research and Therapy, 27,* 19–26.

Ollendick, T. H., Yule, W., & Ollier, K. (1991). Fears in British children and their relationship to manifest anxiety and depression. *Journal of Child Psychology and Psychiatry, 32,* 321–331.

Pober, B. R., & Dykens, E. M. (1996). Williams syndrome: An overview of medical, cognitive, and behavioral features. *Child and Adolescents Psychiatric Clinics of North America, 5,* 929–943.

Preus, M. (1984). The Williams syndrome: Objective definition and diagnosis. *Clinical Genetics, 25,* 422–428.

Ramirez, S. Z., & Kratochwill, T. R. (1990). Development of the fear survey for children with and without mental retardation. *Behavioral Assessment, 12,* 457–470.

Reich, W., Shayka, J. J., & Taibelson, C. (1991). *Diagnostic Interview Schedule for Children and Adolescents, parent version.* St. Louis, MO: Washington University.

Reilly, J., Klima, E. S., & Bellugi, U. (1990). Once more with feeling: Affect and language in atypical populations. *Development and Psychopathology, 2,* 367–391.

Reiss, S., Levitan, G. W., & Szyszko, J. (1982). Emotional disturbance and mental retardation: Diagnostic overshadowing. *American Journal of Mental Deficiency, 86,* 567–574.

Rutter, M. (1967). A children's behavioural questionnaire for completion by teachers. *Journal of Child Psychology and Psychiatry, 8,* 1–11.

Sarphare, G., & Aman, M. G. (1996). Parent- and self-ratings of anxiety in children with mental retardation: Agreement levels and test–retest reliability. *Research in Developmental Disabilities, 17,* 27–39.

Spence, S. H., & McCathie, H. (1993). The stability of fears in children: A two-year prospective study: A research note. *Journal of Child Psychology and Psychiatry, 34,* 579–585.

Tomc, S. A., Williamson, N. K., & Pauli, R. M. (1990). Temperament in Williams syndrome. *American Journal of Medical Genetics, 36,* 345–352.

Udwin, O., & Yule, W. (1990). Expressive language of children with Williams syndrome. *American Journal of Medical Genetics, 6,* 108–114.

Udwin, O., & Yule, W. (1991). A cognitive and behavioral phenotype on Williams syndrome. *Journal of Clinical and Experimental Neuropsychology, 13,* 232–244.

Van Borsel, J., Curfs, L. M., & Fryns, J. P. (1997). Hyperacusis in Williams syndrome: A sample survey study. *Genetic Counseling, 8,* 212–126.

Vandenberg, B. (1993). Fears of normal and retarded children. *Psychological Reports, 72,* 463–474.

Wang, P. P., Hesselink, J. R., Jernigan, T. L., & Doherty, S. (1992). Specific neurobehavioral profile of Williams syndrome is associated with neocerebellar hemispheric preservation. *Neurology, 42,* 1999–2002.

Zetlin, A. G., Heriot, M. J., & Turner, J. L. (1985). Self-concept measurement in mentally retarded adults: A micro-analysis of response styles. *Applied Research in Mental Retardation, 6,* 113–125.

For Product Safety Concerns and Information please contact our EU representative GPSR@taylorandfrancis.com
Taylor & Francis Verlag GmbH, Kaufingerstraße 24, 80331 München, Germany

www.ingramcontent.com/pod-product-compliance
Ingram Content Group UK Ltd.
Pitfield, Milton Keynes, MK11 3LW, UK
UKHW021428080625
459435UK00011B/198

* 9 7 8 0 8 0 5 8 9 6 1 2 1 *